GYNAECOLOGY BY TEN TEACHERS

Books are to be returned on or before
the last date below.

GYNAECOLOGY BY TEN TEACHERS
17th edition

Edited by

Stuart Campbell DSc (Lond), FRCP (Ed), FRCOG, FACOG (Hon)
Professor of Obstetrics & Gynaecology
St George's Hospital Medical School
London, UK

Ash Monga BMedSci, BMBS, MRCOG
Consultant Gynaecologist
Princess Anne Hospital
Southampton University Hospitals Trust
Southampton, UK

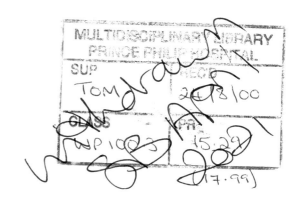

A member of the Hodder Headline Group
LONDON
Co-published in the United States of America by
Oxford University Press Inc., New York

First published in Great Britain 1919 as Diseases of Women
Eleventh edition published 1966 as *Gynaecology*

Seventeenth edition published in 2000 by
Arnold, a member of the Hodder Headline Group,
338 Euston Road, London NW1 3BH
http://www.arnoldpublishers.com

Co-published in the United States of America by
Oxford University Press Inc.,
198 Madison Avenue, New York, NY10016
Oxford is a registered trademark of Oxford University Press

Whilst the advice and information in this book are believed to be true and accurate at the date of going to press, neither the authors nor the publisher can accept any legal responsibility or liability for any errors or omissions that may be made. In particular (but without limiting the generality of the preceding disclaimer) every effort has been made to check drug dosages; however it is still possible that errors have been missed. Furthermore, dosage schedules are constantly being revised and new side effects recognized. For these reasons the reader is strongly urged to consult the drug companies' printed instructions before administering any of the drugs recommended in this book.

British Library Cataloguing in Publication Data
A catalogue record for this book is available from the British Library

Library of Congress Cataloging-in-Publication Data
A catalog record for this book is available from the Library of Congress

ISBN 0 340 71987 7 (pb)
ISBN 0 340 74081 7 (pb, International Students' Edition)

1 2 3 4 5 6 7 8 9 10

Commissioning Editor: Fiona Goodgame, Aileen Parlane
Project Editor: Catherine Barnes
Production Editor: Rada Radojicic
Production Controller: Iain McWilliams
Copy Editor & page layout: Jane Tozer
Illustrators: MTG – Sue Tyler and Kate Nardoni
Cover Design: Terry Griffiths

Typeset in 10/12 pt Minion
Printed and bound in Malta by Gutenberg Press

What do you think about this book? Or any other Arnold title?
Please send your comments to feedback.arnold@hodder.co.uk

Contents

List of contributors

Ash Monga BMedSci, BMBS, MRCOG
Consultant Gynaecologist, Dept of Obstetrics &
Gynaecology, The Princess Anne Hospital,
Southampton University Hospitals Trust,
Southampton

D Keith Edmonds MB, ChB, FRCOG, FRANZCOG
Consultant in Obstetrics & Gynaecology, Queen
Charlotte's & Chelsea Hospital, London

Simon M Kelly MB, ChB, MRANZCOG
Lecturer, Dept of Obstetrics and Gynaecology, St
George's Hospital Medical School, London

Jane E Norman MD, MRCOG
Consultant in Obstetrics & Gynaecology, Dept of
Obstetrics & Gynaecology, Glasgow Royal
Infirmary, Glasgow

P M Sean O'Brien MB, ChB, MD, FRCOG
Professor of Obstetrics & Gynaecology, North
Staffordshire Maternity Hospital, Stoke-on-Trent,
Staffordshire

Ailsa E Gebbie MB, ChB, MRCOG
Consultant in Community Gynaecology, Edinburgh
Healthcare NHS Trust, Edinburgh

Geeta Nargund MRCOG
Medical Director, The Diana Princess of Wales
Centre for Reproductive Medicine, St George's
Hospital Medical School, London

Eric Jauniaux MD, PhD
Reader in Obstetrics & Gynaecology, University
College London Medical School, London

R William Stones MD, MRCOG
Senior Lecturer, Dept of Obstetrics & Gynaecology,
The Princess Anne Hospital, Southampton

Robert W Shaw MD, FRCOG, FRCS (Edin)
Professor of Obstetrics & Gynaecology, University
of Wales College of Medicine, Cardiff

W Pat Soutter MD, MSc, FRCOG
Reader in Gynaecologic Oncology, Dept of
Obstetrics & Gynaecology, Imperial College School
of Medicine, Hammersmith Hospital, London

**Stuart Campbell DSc (Lond), FRCP (Ed), FRCOG,
FACOG (Hon)**
Professor of Obstetrics & Gynaecology, St George's
Hospital Medical School, London

Phillip E Hay MBRS, FRCP
Consultant in Genito-Urinary Medicine, The
Courtyard Clinic, St George's Healthcare NHS
Trust, St George's Hospital, London

**David W Purdie MD, FRCOG, FRCP (Edin), FSA
(Scot)**
Professor of Gynaecology, Centre for Metabolic
Bone Disease, H S Brocklehurst Building, Hull
Royal Infirmary, Hull

Fran Reader FRCOG, MFFP, BASRT Accred
Consultant in Family Planning & Reproductive
Health Care, Ipswich Hospital NHS Trust, Suffolk

**E Malcom Symonds MB BS (Adel), MD FRCOG,
FFPHM FACOG (Hon), FRANZCOG (Hon)**
Professor Emeritus, Dept of Obstetrics &
Gynaecology, University of Nottingham,
Nottingham

Preface

The word gynaecology is derived from the Greek *gynaik* meaning 'woman' and *logios* meaning 'expertise' and, therefore, it is a medical specialty devoted to disorders of the female reproductive organs and those endocrine glands that modify their function. It was originally regarded as a surgical specialty, especially for the surgical treatment of female tumours and, while this remains an important aspect, the subject has developed a wider remit covering cancer prevention, genetics, human reproduction, early pregnancy development, infertility, contraception, urinary incontinence, prolapse, the management of the menopause and the long-term problems of ageing. This book was first published under the title 'Diseases of Women by Ten Teachers' in 1919, 2 years after the publication of 'Midwifery by Ten Teachers'. It is thus the longest-standing and also the most widely read English textbook in gynaecology and it is an awesome task to ensure its continuing popularity. We have completely rewritten the text with a new team of contributors in a different format, which we hope will make the information more accessible. By doing so, we hope we have addressed the rapid changes that have occurred in this specialty.

We have tried in this book to describe the most up-to-date evidence-based gynaecological practice reflecting the extensive responsibilities that the modern gynaecologist bears for the full spectrum of a woman's reproductive health throughout her life. We have maintained the traditions of *Ten Teachers* as a comprehensive text, but we have changed the format to include summaries, key points and illustrated cases to make the information more accessible and to aid learning. We hope we have conveyed our enthusiasm for our subject and that this book will not only help you to pass examinations, but inspire some of you to take up this most diverse and interesting of specialties.

Historical Note

The history of gynaecology can be traced back to writings from the Indus civilisation in the 3rd Century B.C., but the first real scientific advances came in the 16th and 17th Centuries with the studies and publications of the great anatomists, such as **Fallopius**, who described the uterus and 'Fallopian tubes' and following the discovery of the microscope, **Regnier de Graaf**, who described the structure of the testes, ovaries and the 'Graafian' follicles, their maturation and function. The 19th Century saw the rapid progression of gynaecological surgery with a new breed of self-confident heroic, sometimes arrogant, individuals operating at great speed, because until 1850 no anaesthesia was available and there was the ever present threat of infection ready to turn a surgical triumph into disaster. Gynaecology can claim the first ever major abdominal operation, which was the removal of a 6.8 kg ovarian cyst on Christmas Day 1809 by **Ephraim McDowell** in the front room of his house in Danville, Kentucky. Subsequently McDowell carried out 13 ovariotomies with only one death which, in an age with no anaesthesia and a high risk of infection, was truly remarkable.

Perhaps the greatest of these pioneer surgeons was **James Marion Sims**, who began his surgical career in South Carolina. Over 20 years he gradually perfected the technique of repair of the vesico-vaginal fistula, a common condition which resulted from neglected obstructed labour. Sims' first patients were three Negro slaves; Lucy, Betsy and Anarchus. It took 30 operations over a period of 5 years for Sims to finally cure Anarchus by changing from silk sutures to silver wire, which resisted infection from the urine and prevented the repair from breaking down. Subsequently, the two other slaves were cured. In the course of developing these techniques, Sims developed many of the approaches and instruments used in modern vaginal surgery, such as the Sims position and the Sims speculum. Another gynaecological surgeon in the heroic mould was **Robert Lawson Tate**, a pupil of James Young Simpson (see *Obstetrics by Ten Teachers*), who was appointed to the Chair of Gynaecology in Birmingham in 1876. Tate was one of the most audacious and talented surgeons of his era and indeed, together with the great German surgeon, Bilroth, is regarded as the founder of abdominal surgery. He performed the first appendicectomy for acute appendicitis, the first salpingectomy for tubal pregnancy and was a leader in many general surgical procedures, such as cholecystectomy and partial hepatectomy. Perhaps above all, Lawson Tate was one of the first to carry out detailed and scrupulous audit of all the surgery carried out in his hospital and his staggering number of publications on all aspects of surgery gained him international acclaim. Tate was the founder and first President of the Medical Defence Union, but his reputation and fortunes fell into rapid decline following criticism of his policy of removing normal ovaries from women to treat what we would now call premenstrual syndrome. Towards the end of the 19th Century, the Viennese School of Surgery became internationally famous, especially for the radical treatment of cancer of the cervix. Foremost among these was **Ernst Wertheim**, who in 1900 described the full radical operation for this condition, which is still the standard technique used today.

The 20th Century saw the diversification of gynaecology into the multi-faceted specialty we know today. First there came techniques for screening for the pre-invasive stage of cervical cancer. **George Papanicolaou**, a Greek Pathologist working in New York, first described the cervical smear test in a landmark publication in 1941. Even before this discovery, **Hans Hinselman**, Head of the Gynaecology Department in Bonn University, had described the principles of colposcopy. Both of these techniques are still the basis for cervical cancer screening and have resulted in a substantial reduction in deaths from this condition.

Further diversification came with the development of endocrinology and an understanding of the processes of fertilisation, implantation and genetics. In parallel with this came new techniques for the clinical investigation of the pelvic organs, such as laparoscopy and ultrasound and the development of a new surgical technique called minimal access surgery (or keyhole surgery), which was pioneered by gynaecologists and later taken up by surgeons. Each of these new techniques had a vital part to play in the development of the *in vitro* fertilisation (IVF) treatment for infertility and it is in this context that these techniques will be discussed.

The first experiments in laparoscopy began in the early 1900s, but it was **Raoul Palmer**, the great French Gynaecologist, who not only developed the kind of instruments that we would recognise today, but most of their uses, not just for visualisation of the pelvis, but for surgical procedures such as tubal surgery, tubal diathermy and myomectomy. One of Palmer's pupils was **Patrick Steptoe**, who published the first English textbook on laparoscopy and who was to pioneer the use of laparoscopy for *in vitro* fertilisation. A

vital step in developing IVF was to control and stimulate the development of oocytes in the ovary. It was **Carl Gemzell**, a Swedish Gynaecologist, who was the first to use human pituitary extracts to induce ovulation and to isolate follicle stimulating hormone (FSH) and lutenising hormone (LH) from the human urine for the same purpose. Gemzell and others developed this therapy for the treatment of anovulatory infertility, but it was a necessary step for the super-ovulation treatment, where several follicles (each containing an oocyte) are stimulated in each ovary, so that several embryos can be created. The process of IVF required advances in our understanding of embryology, so that the fertilisation process can be carried out 'in vitro'. Fertilisation *in vitro* was achieved in the rabbit in 1934 by Gregory Pincus, an American Physiologist, who subsequently became the pioneer of the 'pill'. He, however, failed to achieve fertilisation of human eggs *in vitro*, because he predicted an oocyte maturation of 12 hours after the LH surge and consequently inseminated human eggs too early. It was **Robert Edwards** in Cambridge University who determined the correct maturation period of the oocyte in the human was 37 hours and he was the first to successfully fertilise a human oocyte *in vitro*. The unlikely collaboration between the high-flying scientist Robert Edwards in Cambridge and Patrick Steptoe, a Consultant Gynaecologist in the small town of Oldham in Lancashire, is the stuff of legend. Steptoe carried out the super-ovulation treatment on women with tubal infertility in Oldham and then collected the oocytes 36 hours after the LH surge at the time recommended by Robert Edwards. Edwards himself drove the 200 miles from Cambridge to Oldham each week (sometimes more than once) to attempt to fertilise the oocytes collected by Steptoe. It was 10 years of trial and error before the first IVF baby, Louise Brown, was born in 1978, thus heralding the start of modern infertility treatment and a greater understanding of early human development. The final piece of the IVF jigsaw came with developments in diagnostic ultrasound, namely the transvaginal probe. **Ian Donald**, the Professor at Glasgow University who pioneered ultrasound in Obstetrics and Gynaecology, did not himself realise the importance of the transvaginal probe, but visualised the pelvic organs with an abdominal transducer using the patient's distended bladder as a window to the pelvic organs. The transvaginal probe allowed better monitoring of ovarian follicular development and allowed the insertion of a needle directly into the ovary under ultrasound control to collect oocytes, which quickly displaced the laparoscopic technique as it avoided the need for in-patient treatment.

The modern birth control movement began with an American woman of Irish immigrant parentage, **Margaret Sanger**. This charismatic, indomitable woman opened the first Family Planning Clinic in New York in 1916, because she was horrified by the effects of unlimited reproduction among the poor and the high mortality associated with illegal abortion. Sanger met widespread opposition to her movement, but she campaigned for family planning services throughout America. When she was forbidden by the Boston civic authorities to speak on birth control, she stood on a stage with her mouth taped while a colleague read her speech. She influenced **Marie Stopes**, who set up the first Family Planning Clinic in England in 1921. It is quite staggering to realise that the timing of human ovulation in the menstrual cycle was only correctly identified by Ogino in Japan and Knaus in Austria in the 1930s which helped to formulate the 'safe period' in contraception. The major breakthrough in contraception came with the mass synthesis of oral progesterone from the Mexican yam by **Russell Marker**, an American Chemist, in the early 1940s. Subsequently, **Gregory Pincus**, the father of the 'pill' and **John Rock** produced the first report on the successful use of oral contraceptives in 1956, thus causing fundamental social changes and freeing women from the tyranny of unwanted pregnancy.

This brief selected history, can only give you a taste for the development of this most fascinating of specialties.

STUART CAMPBELL
ASH MONGA

Acknowledgements

The Editors would like to express their sincere thanks to the following people for their help with *Gynaecology by Ten Teachers* 17th edition:

Mr Kenneth Metcalfe MRCOG, FRCS, Consultant Gynaecological Oncologist and Mr Patrick Malone FRCS, Consultant Paediatric Urologist, both of Southampton University Hospitals, for contributing artwork.

Particular thanks go to Suzette Pearce at the Chalybeate Hospital, Southampton and Sue Cunningham at St George's Hospital Medical School, London for helping the Editors prepare the manuscript.

Commonly-used abbreviations

ACTH	adrenocorticotrophic hormone
AFP	alpha-fetoprotein
BEP	bleomycin and etoposide
BV	bacterial vaginosis
CIN	cervical intra-epithelial neoplasia
CMV	cytomegalovirus
COC	combined oral contraceptive pill
CRL	crown-rump length
CSF	cerebrospinal fluid
DFA	direct fluorescent antibody
DHEAS	dihydroepiandronesterone sulphate
DUB	dysfunctional uterine bleeding
EGF	epidermal growth factor
ERPC	evacuation of retained products of conception
ESR	erythrocyte sedimentation rate
ET	embryo transfer
FGF	fibroblast growth factor
FSH	follicle-stimulating hormone
FTA	fluorescent treponemal antibody
GnRH	gonadotrophin-releasing hormone
GSI	genuine stress incontinence
GUM	genitourinary medicine
hCG	human chorionic gonadotrophin
HFEA	Human Fertilization and Embryology Authority
HMG	human menopausal gonadotrophin
HOL	hairy oral leukoplakia
HPO	hypothalamus-pituitary-ovarian axis
HPV	human papilloma virus
HRT	hormone replacement therapy
HSG	hysterosalpingogram
HSV	herpes simplex virus
HWY	hundred women years
HyCoSy	hysterocontrastsonography
ICSI	intracytoplasmic sperm injection
IGFBP	insulin-like growth factor binding protein
ITP	idiopathic thrombocytopaenic purpura
IUCD	intrauterine contraceptive device
IUI	intrauterine insemination
IUS	intrauterine system
IVC	*in vitro* culture
IVF	*in vitro* fertilization
IVM	*in vitro* maturation
IVU	intravenous urogram
LAM	lactational amenorrhoea method
LCR	ligase chain reaction
LGV	*Lymphogranuloma venereum*
LH	lutinizing hormone
LLETZ	large loop excision of transformation zone
LMP	last mentrual period
LUF	lutinized unruptured follicle
MAC	*Mycobacterium avium intracellulare* complex
MCP-1	monocyte chemotactic protein 1
MMP	matrix metalloproteinase
MRI	magnetic resonance imaging
NGU	non-gonococcal urethritis
NSAIDs	non-steroidal anti-inflammatory drugs
OHSS	ovarian hyperstimulation syndrome
PAF	platelet activating factor
PCOS	polycystic ovarian syndrome
PCP	*Pneumocystis carinii* pneumonia
PCR	polymerase chain reaction
PGD	preimplantation diagnosis of genetic disease
PID	pelvic inflammatory disease
RMG	risk management group
PMS	premenstrual syndrome
POF	premature ovarian failure
RPR	rapid plasma reagin test
SARA	sexually acquired reactive arthritis
SCJ	squamocolumnar junction
SERM	selective oestrogen receptor modulators
SIL	squamous intraepithelial lesions
TA	transactional analysis
TDF	testicular determining factor
TGF	transforming growth factor
TVS	transvaginal sonography
UTI	urinary tract infection
VEGF	vascular endothelial growth factor
VCU	videocystourethrography
VTE	venous thromboembolism
VAIN	vaginal intraepithelia neoplasia
VIN	vulval intraepithelial neoplasia

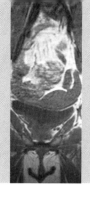

Chapter 1

The gynaecological history and examination

OVERVIEW

A careful detailed history is essential before the examination of any patient. In addition to a good general history, focusing on the history of the presenting complaint will allow you to customize the examination to elicit the appropriate signs and make an accurate diagnosis.

History

When interviewing a patient to obtain their history the consultation should ideally be held in a closed room with no one else present. Enough time should be allowed for the patient to express herself and the doctor's manner should be one of interest and understanding. It is important that a template is used for history taking as this prevents the omission of important points. A sample template is given on page 2.

Examination

It is important that the examiner smiles, introduces himself by name and, if appropriate, asks the patient's name. A handshake often helps to put the patient at ease.

Important information about the patient can be obtained on watching them walk into the examination room. Poor mobility may affect decisions regarding surgery. While obtaining a history it is possible to assess the patient's affect. A history that is taken with sensitivity will often encourage the patient to reveal more details that are relevant to future management.

Before proceeding to abdominal examination a general examination should be performed. This includes examining the hands and mucous membranes for evidence of anaemia. The supraclavicular node should always be examined, particularly on the left side where in cases of abdominal malignancy one might palpate the enlarged Virchow's node (this is also known as Troissier's sign). The thyroid gland should be palpated.

S Symptoms

History taking template

The following outline is suggested.
- Name, age, occupation.
- A brief statement of the general nature and duration of the main complaints.

History of presenting complaint

This section should focus on the presenting complaint but certain important points should always be enquired about.
- Abnormal menstrual loss.
- Pattern of bleeding – regular or irregular.
- Intermenstrual bleeding.
- Amount of blood loss – greater or less than usual.
- Number of sanitary towels or tampons used.
- Passage of clots or flooding.
- Pelvic pain – site of pain, nature and relation to periods.
- Anything that aggravates or relieves the pain.
- Vaginal discharge – amount, colour, odour, presence of blood.

Obviously if the presenting complaint is one of subfertility or is urogynaecological then the history must be appropriately tailored (see chapters 7 and 17).

Usual menstrual cycle

- Age of menarche.
- Usual duration of each period and length of cycle.
- First day of the last period.

Previous gynaecological history

This section should include any previous gynaecological treatments or surgery. The date of the last cervical smear should also be recorded.

Previous obstetric history

- Number of children with ages and birth weights.
- Any abnormalities with pregnancy, labour or the puerperium.
- Number of miscarriages and gestation at which they occurred.
- Any termination of pregnancy with record of gestation age and any complications.

Sexual and contraceptive history

- History of discomfort, pain or bleeding during intercourse.
- The use of contraception and type of contraception used.

Previous medical history

- Any serious illnesses or operations with dates.
- Family history.

Enquiry about other systems

- Appetite, weight loss, weight gain.
- Bowels.
- Micturition.
- Enquiry of other systems.

Social history

The history regarding smoking and alcohol intake should be obtained. It is important to ascertain whether the woman has a sexual partner or is married. Any family problems should be discussed and it is especially important in the case of a frail patient to enquire about home arrangements if surgery is being considered.

Summary

It is important to summarize the history in one to two sentences before proceeding to examination to alert the examiner to the salient features.

Chest and breasts should always be examined, this is particularly relevant if there is a suspected ovarian mass as there may be a breast tumour with secondaries of the ovaries known as Krukenburg tumours. In addition, a pleural effusion may be illicited as a consequence of abdominal ascites. The next step should be to proceed to abdominal and pelvic examination.

Abdominal examination

The patient should empty her bladder before the abdominal examination.

The patient should be comfortable and lying semi-recumbent with a sheet covering her from the waist down, but the area from the xiphisternum to the symphysis pubis should be left exposed. It is usual to examine the woman from her right hand side. Abdominal examination comprises inspection, palpation, percussion and, if appropriate, auscultation.

Inspection

The contour of the abdomen should be inspected and noted. There may be an obvious distension or mass (Fig. 1.1).

The presence of surgical scars, dilated veins or striae gravidarum (stretch marks) should be noted. It is important to specifically examine the umbilicus for laparoscopy scars and just above the symphysis pubis for Pfannenstiel scars (used for Caesarean Section, hysterectomy, etc.). The patient should be asked to raise her head or cough and any hernias or divarication of the rectus muscles will be evident.

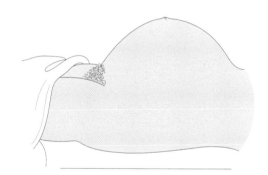

Figure 1.1 Abdominal distension.

Palpation

Firstly, if the patient has any abdominal pain she should be asked to point to the site. This area should not be examined until the end of palpation. It is usual to get the patient to cough as she may show signs of peritonism. Palpation using the right hand is performed examining the left lower quadrant and proceeding in a total of four steps to the right lower quadrant of the abdomen. Palpation should include examination for masses, liver, spleen and kidneys. If a mass is present but one can palpate below it then it is more likely to be an abdominal mass rather than a pelvic mass. It is important to remember that one of the characteristics of a pelvic mass is that one cannot palpate below it.

If the patient has pain her abdomen should be palpated gently and the examiner should look for signs of peritonism, i.e. guarding and rebound tenderness. The patient should also be examined for inguinal herniae and lymph nodes.

Percussion

Percussion is particularly useful if free fluid is suspected. In the recumbent position ascitic fluid will settle down into a horseshoe shape and dullness in the flanks can be demonstrated.

As the patient moves over to her side the dullness will move to her lower most side, this is known as 'shifting dullness'. A fluid thrill can also be elicited.

An enlarged bladder due to urinary retention will also be dull to percussion and this should be demonstrated to the examiner (many pelvic masses have disappeared after catheterization).

Auscultation

This method is not specifically useful for the gynaecological examination. However, a patient will sometimes present with an acute abdomen with bowel obstruction or a postoperative patient with ileus and therefore listening for bowel sounds may be appropriate.

Pelvic examination

Before proceeding to a vaginal examination the patient's verbal consent should be obtained and a female chaperone should be present for any intimate examination.

The external genitalia are first inspected under a good light with the patient in the dorsal position, the hips flexed and abducted and knees flexed. The left lateral position is used for examination of prolapse or to inspect the vaginal wall with a Sim's speculum (Fig. 1.2). The patient is asked to strain down to enable detection of any prolapse and also to cough, as this will show the sign of stress incontinence. After this a bivalve (Cusco's, Fig. 1.3) speculum is inserted to visualize the cervix. It is usual to warm the speculum to make the examination more comfortable for the patient. If taking a smear test this is performed at the same time.

Bimanual digital examination is then performed (Fig. 1.4). This technique requires practice. It is customary to use the fingers of the right hand in the vagina and to place the left hand on the abdomen. In a virgin or a child only a rectal examination should be performed. The left hand is used to separate the labia minora to expose the vestibule and the examining fingers of the right hand are inserted. The cervix is palpated and any hardness or irregularity noted. The abdominal hand is located just below the umbilicus and the fingers of both hands are then used to palpate the uterus. The size, shape, position, mobility and tenderness of the uterus are noted. The tips of the vaginal fingers are then placed into each lateral fornix and the adnexae are examined on each side. Except in a very thin woman the ovaries and fallopian tubes are not palpable. The uterosacral ligaments can be palpated in the posterior fornix and may be scarred or shortened in women with endometriosis.

Rectal examination

A rectal examination may be used as an alternative to vaginal examination in a virgin or a child. In addition it may be useful to differentiate between enterocele and rectocele and can be used to assess the size of a rectocele.

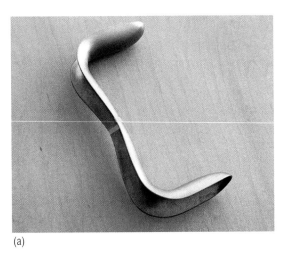
(a)

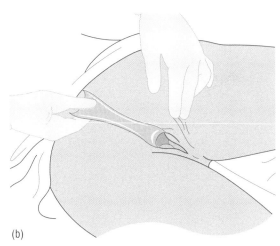
(b)

Figure 1.2 (a) Sims' speculum. (b) Sims' speculum exposing anterior vaginal wall.

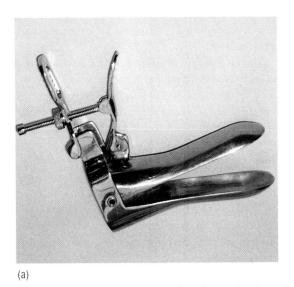
(a)

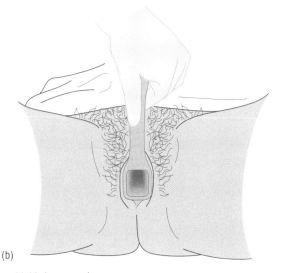
(b)

Figure 1.3 (a) Cusco's speculum. (b) Cusco's speculum in position with blades opened exposing cervix.

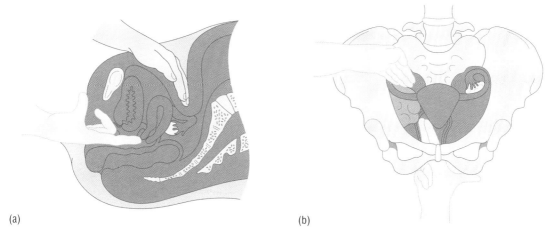

(a)

(b)

Figure 1.4 (a) Bimanual examination of the pelvis, assessing uterine size. (b) Examining the lateral fornix.

Investigations

The appropriate investigation should be performed, e.g. swabs for discharge or cervical smear.

Other investigations are discussed in chapter 15, imaging in gynaecology, chapter 12 on cervix cancer and in the appendix.

Key Points

- The consultation should be performed in a private environment in a sensitive fashion
- The examiner should introduce himself to the patient and be courteous
- The examiner should be familiar with a template and use it regularly to avoid omissions
- A chaperone should always be present for an intimate examination
- The examination should begin with inspection of the patient's hands
- The patient should be comfortable and at the end of examination the examiner should cover the exposed section and help the patient to sit up
- When presenting the history to the examiner it should be succinct and should be summarized before presenting the examination
- Remember the examiners will usually ask for a differential diagnosis

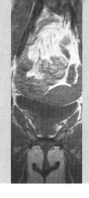

Embryology, anatomy and physiology

OVERVIEW

An understanding of the development and anatomy of the female genital tract is important in the practice of gynaecology. Both the urinary and genital systems develop from a common mesodermal ridge running along the posterior abdominal wall. Although the development of the kidneys and bladder is outside of the realm of this chapter, it is of importance to remember that congenital anomalies of the genital tract may also be associated with congenital anomalies of the urinary tract. This chapter serves as a reminder and is not a comprehensive guide to the embryology and anatomy.

EMBRYOLOGY

Development of the genital organs

During the fifth week of embryonic life the nephrogenic cord develops from the mesoderm and forms the urogenital ridge and mesonephric duct (later to form the Wolffian duct) (Fig. 2.1). The mesonephros consists of a comparatively large ovoid organ on each side of the midline with the developing gonad on the medial side of its lower portion. The paramesonephric duct later forms the Müllerian system. The fate of the mesonephric and paramesonephric ducts is dependent on gonadal secretion. Assuming female development, the two paramesonephric ducts extend caudally to project into the posterior wall of the urogenital

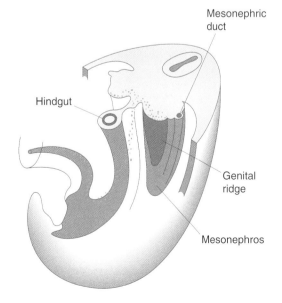

Figure 2.1 Cross sectional diagram of the posterior abdominal wall showing genital ridge.

sinus as the Müllerian tubercle. The Wolffian system degenerates.

Development of the uterus and fallopian tubes

The lower end of the Müllerian ducts come together in the midline, fuse and develop into the uterus and cervix (Fig. 2.2). At first there is a septum separating the lumina of the two ducts but later this disappears and a single cavity is formed, i.e. the uterus.

The upper parts of both ducts retain their identity and form the fallopian tubes.

The lower end of the fused Müllerian ducts beyond the uterine lumin remains solid, proliferates and forms a cord.

Development of the vagina

During the ninth week of embryonic life the cord does not open out into the sinus but makes contact with the sinovaginal bulbs which are solid out-growths

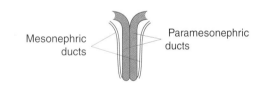

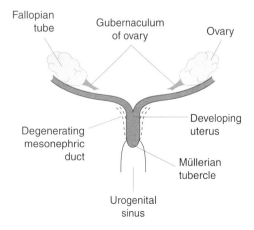

Figure 2.2 Caudal growth of paramesonephric ducts (top). Fusion to form uterus and fallopian tubes (below).

from the sinus. As the pelvic region of the fetus elongates, the sinus and Müllerian tubercle become increasingly distanced from the tubular portions, the ducts. The solid epithelial cord provides the length of the future vagina. The current view is that most of the upper vagina is of Müllerian origin. The solid sinovaginal bulbs also have to canalize to form a lower vagina and this occurs above the level of the eventual hymen so that the epithelia of both surfaces of the hymen are of urogenital sinus origin. Complete canalization of the vagina is a comparatively late event occurring in the sixth and seventh months.

Development of the external genitalia

There is overlap in timing of the formation of the external genitalia and the internal duct system.

There is a common indifferent stage consisting of two genital folds, two genital swellings and a midline anterior genital tubercle. The female development is a simple progression from these structures.

- Genital tubercle → clitoris
- Genital folds → labia minora
- Genital swellings → labia majora

A male phenotype is dependent on the production of fetal testosterone. Agents or inborn errors that prevent the synthesis or action of androgens inhibit formation of male external genitalia and the female phenotype will develop.

Development of the ovary

The primitive gonad is first evident in embryos at five weeks. It forms as a bulb on the medial aspect of the mesonephric ridge and is of triple origin from the coelomic epithelium of genital ridge, the underlying mesoderm and the primitive germ cells. There is proliferation of cells in and beneath the coelomic epithelium of the genital ridge. By five to six weeks these cells are seen spreading as ill-defined cords (sex cords) into the ridge, breaking up the mesenchyme into loose strands. The primitive germ cells are seen at first lying between the cords and then within them (Fig. 2.3).

Morphological development of the ovary occurs about two weeks later than the testes and proceeds more slowly. The sex cords develop extensively and

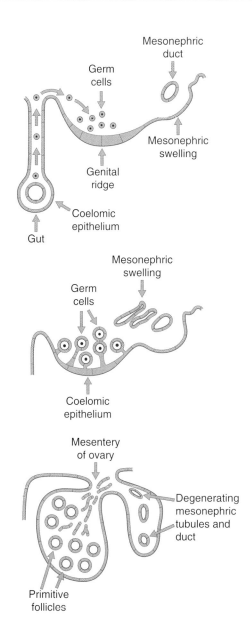

Figure 2.3 Development of the ovary.

declines. Approximately seven million germ cells are present at five months but at birth this has fallen to two million, half of which are atretic.

At the same time the ovary descends extra peritoneally in the abdominal cavity. Two ligaments develop and these appear to help control its descent, guiding it to its final position and preventing its complete descent through the inguinal ring in contrast to the testes.

ANATOMY

Anatomy is covered in some depth in the preclinical years. This is intended as a brief review.

External genitalia

The vulva

The female external genitalia, commonly referred to as the vulva, include the mons pubis, the labia majora and minora, the vestibule, the clitoris and the greater vestibular glands (Fig. 2.4). The mons pubis is composed of fibrofatty tissue, which covers the body of the pubic bones. Inferiorly it divides to become continuous with the labia majus on each

epithelial cells in this area are known as pregranulosa cells. The germ cells decrease in size by fourteen to sixteen weeks. The active growth phase causes enlargement of the gonad. The next stage involves the primitive germ cells (now known as oocytes) becoming surrounded by a ring of pregranulosa cells: stromal cells develop from the ovarian mesenchyme. Mitotic division, by which the germ cells have been increasing in numbers, then ceases and they enter the first stage of meiosis and prophase arrest. The number of oocytes is greatest before birth and thereafter

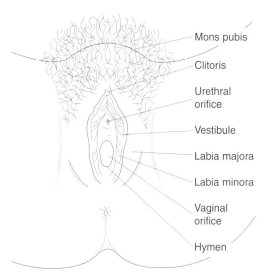

Figure 2.4 The vulva of a virgin.

side of the vulva. In the adult, the skin that covers the mons pubis bears pubic hair, the upper limit of which is usually horizontal.

The labia majora are two folds of skin with underlying adipose tissue bounding either side of the vaginal opening. They contain sebaceous and sweat glands and a few specialized apocrine glands. In the deepest part of each labium is a core of fatty tissue continuous with that of the inguinal canal and the fibres of the round ligament terminate here.

The labia minora are two thin folds of skin that lie between the labia majora. Anteriorly they divide into two to form the prepuce and frenulum of the clitoris. Posteriorly they fuse to form a fold of skin called the fourchette. They contain sebaceous glands but have no adipose tissue. They are not well developed before puberty and atrophy after the menopause. Their vascularity allows them to become turgid during sexual excitement.

The clitoris is a small erectile structure. The body of the clitoris contains two crura, the corpora cavernosa, which are attached to the inferior border of the pubic rami. The clitoris is covered by the ischiocavernosus muscle whilst bulbospongiosus muscle inserts into its root. The clitoris is about 1 cm long but has a highly developed nerve supply and is very sensitive during sexual arousal.

The vestibule is the cleft between the labia minora. The urethra, the ducts of the Bartholin's glands and the vagina open in the vestibule. The vestibular bulbs are two oblong masses of erectile tissue that lie on either side of the vaginal entrance. They contain a rich plexus of veins within the bulbospongiosus muscle. Bartholin's glands, each about the size of a small pea, lie at the base of each bulb and open via a 2 cm duct into the vestibule between the hymen and the labia minora. These are mucus-secreting, producing copious amounts during intercourse to act as a lubricant.

The hymen is a thin fold of mucous membrane across the entrance to the vagina. There are usually openings in it to allow menses to escape. The hymen is partially ruptured during first coitus and is further disrupted during childbirth. Any tags remaining after rupture are known as carunculae myrtiformes.

Age Changes

In infancy the vulva is devoid of hair and there is considerable adipose tissue in the labia majora and pubis that is lost during childhood but reappears during puberty at which time hair grows. After menopause the skin atrophies and becomes thinner. The labia minora shrink, subcutaneous fat is lost and the vaginal orifice becomes smaller.

The internal reproductive organs

Figure 2.5 shows a sagital section of the human female pelvis.

The vagina

The vagina is a fibromuscular canal lined with stratified squamous epithelium that leads from the uterus to the vulva. It is longer in the posterior wall (around 9 cm) than anteriorly (approximately 7.0 cm). The vaginal walls are normally in apposition except at the vault where they are separated by the cervix. The vault of the vagina is divided into four fornices, posterior, anterior and two lateral (Fig. 2.6).

The midvagina is a transverse slit and the lower portion is an H shape in transverse section. The vaginal walls are rugose with transverse folds. The vagina is kept moist by secretions from the uterine and cervical glands and by some transudation from its epithelial lining. It has no glands. The epithelium is thick and rich in glycogen, which increases in the postovulatory phase of the cycle. However before puberty and after the menopause the vagina is devoid of glycogen because of oestrogen deficiency.

Doderlein's bacillus is a normal commensal of the vagina breaking down the glycogen to form lactic acid and producing a pH of around 4.5. This has a protective role for the vagina in decreasing the growth of pathogenic organisms.

The upper posterior vaginal wall forms the anterior peritoneal reflection of the pouch of Douglas. The middle third is separated from the rectum by pelvic fascia and the lower third abuts the perineal body. Anteriorly the lip of the vagina is in direct contact with the base of the bladder whilst the urethra runs down the lower half in the midline to open to the vestibule. Its muscles fuse with the anterior vaginal wall. Laterally, at the fornices, the vagina is related to the attachment at the cardinal ligaments. Below this are the levator ani muscles and the ischiorectal fossae. The cardinal ligaments and the uterosacral ligaments, which form posteriorly from the parametrium, support the upper part of the vagina.

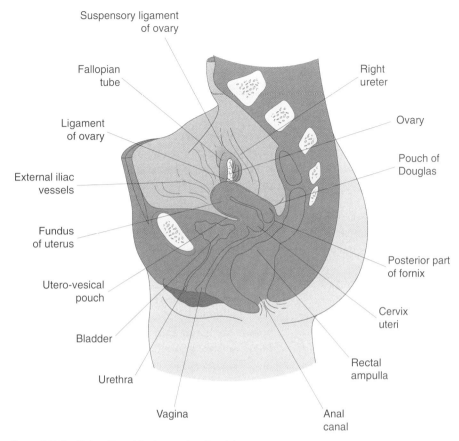

Figure 2.5 Sagittal section of the human female pelvis.

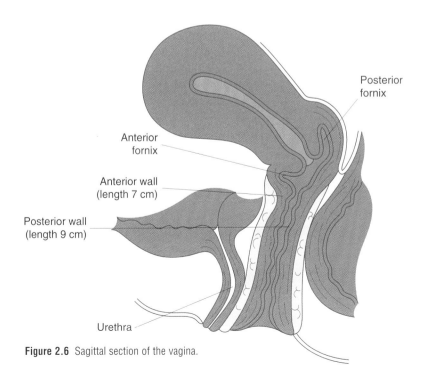

Figure 2.6 Sagittal section of the vagina.

Age changes

At birth, the vagina is under the influence of maternal oestrogens so the epithelium is well developed. After a couple of weeks the effects of the oestrogens disappear and the pH rises to 7 and the epithelium atrophies. At puberty the reverse occurs and finally at the menopause the vagina tends to shrink and the epithelium atrophies.

The uterus

The uterus is shaped like an inverted pear tapering inferiorly to the cervix and in the non-pregnant state is situated entirely within the pelvis. It is hollow and has thick muscular walls. Its maximum external dimensions are approximately 7.5 cm long, 5 cm wide and 3 cm thick (Fig. 2.7).

An adult uterus weighs about 70 g. In the upper part the uterus is termed the body or corpus. The area of insertion of each fallopian tube is termed the cornu and that part of the body above the cornu, the fundus. The uterus tapers to a small central constricted area, the isthmus, and below this is the cervix which projects obliquely into the vagina and can be divided into vaginal and supravaginal portions (Fig. 2.8).

The cavity of the uterus is the shape of an inverted triangle and when sectioned coronally the fallopian tubes open at the lateral angles. The constriction at the isthmus where the corpus joins the cervix is the anatomical internal os. Seen microscopically, the site of the histological internal os is where the mucous membrane of the isthmus becomes that of the cervix.

The uterus consists of three layers – the outer serous layer (peritoneum), the middle muscular layer (myometrium), and the inner mucous layer (endometrium).

The peritoneum covers the body of the uterus and posteriorly, the supravaginal portion of the cervix. The serous coat is intimately attached to a subserous fibrous layer except laterally where it spreads out to form the leaves of the broad ligament.

The muscular myometrium forms the main bulk of the uterus and comprises interlacing smooth muscle fibres intermingling with areolar tissue, blood vessels, nerves and lymphatics. Externally these are mostly longitudinal but the larger intermediate layer has interlacing longitudinal, oblique and transverse fibres. Internally they are mainly longitudinal and circular.

The inner endometrial layer has tubular glands that dip into the myometrium. The endometrial layer is covered by a single layer of columnar epithelium. Ciliated prior to puberty, this epithelium is mostly lost due to the effects of pregnancy and menstruation. The endometrium undergoes cyclical changes during menstruation and varies in thickness between 1 and 5 mm.

The cervix

The cervix is narrower than the body of the uterus and is approximately 2.5 cm in length. Due to antiflexion or retroflexion the long axis of the cervix is rarely the same as the long axis of the body of the uterus. Anterior and lateral to the supravaginal portion is cellular connective tissue, the parametrium. The posterior aspect is covered by peritoneum of the pouch of Douglas. The ureter runs about 1 cm laterally to the supravaginal cervix. The vaginal portion projects into the vagina to form the fornices.

The upper part of the cervix mostly consists of involuntary muscle, whereas the lower part is mainly fibrous connective tissue. The mucous membrane of the endocervix has anterior and posterior columns from which folds radiate out, known as the arbor vitae. It has numerous deep glandular follicles that secrete a clear, alkaline mucus, the main component of physiological vaginal discharge. The epithelium of the endocervix is cylindrical and also ciliated in its upper two-thirds and changes to stratified squamous epithelium around the region of the external os. This

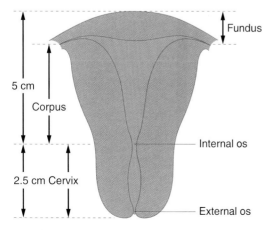

Figure 2.7 Uterine dimensions.

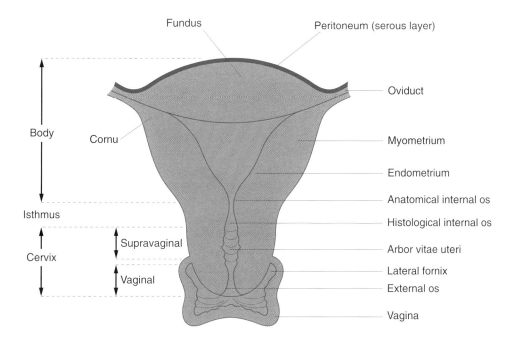

Figure 2.8 Coronal section of uterine cavity.

squamocolumnar junction is also known as the transformation zone and is an area of rapid cell division and approximately 90 per cent of cervical carcinoma arises in this area.

Position of uterus
The longitudinal axis of the uterus is, approximately, at right angles to the vagina and normally tilts forwards. This is termed anteversion. The uterus is usually also flexed forwards on itself at the isthmus – antiflexion. In around 20 per cent of women this tilt is not forwards but backwards – retroversion and retroflexion. This does not have a pathological significance.

Age changes
The disappearance of maternal oestrogens after birth causes the uterus to decrease in length by around one-third and in weight by about one-half. The cervix is then twice the length of the uterus.

At puberty, however, the corpus grows much faster and the size ratio reverses. After the menopause the uterus atrophies, the mucosa becomes very thin, the glands almost disappear and the wall becomes relatively less muscular. These changes affect the cervix more than the corpus, cervical loops disappear and the external os becomes more or less flush with the vault.

The fallopian tubes

Each fallopian tube extends outwards from the uterine cornu to end near the ovary. At the abdominal ostium the tube opens into the peritoneal cavity, which is therefore in communication with the exterior of the body via the uterus and the vagina. The tubes or oviducts convey the ovum from the ovary towards the uterus, which provides oxygenation and nutrition for sperm, ovum and zygote should fertilization occur.

The fallopian tube (Fig. 2.9) runs in the upper margin of the broad ligament, part of which, known as the mesosalpinx, encloses it so that the tube is completely covered with peritoneum except for a narrow strip along this inferior aspect. Each tube is about 10 cm long and is described in four parts:
1. the interstitial portion;
2. the isthmus;
3. the ampulla;
4. the infundibulum, or fimbrial portion.

The interstitial portion lies within the wall of the uterus, while the isthmus is the narrow portion adjoining the uterus. This passes into the widest and longest portion, the ampulla. This in turn terminates

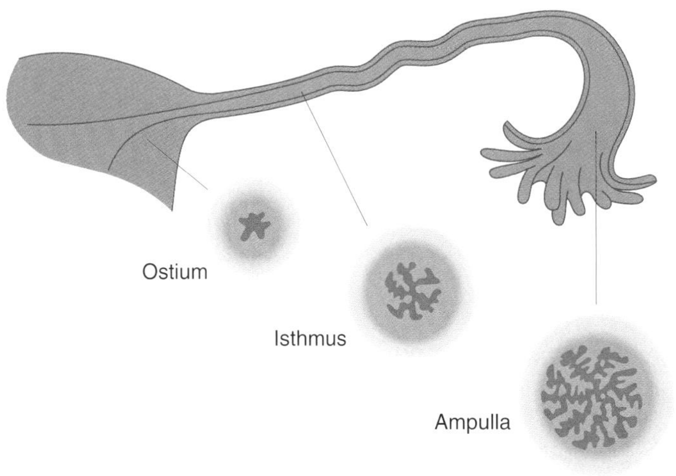

Figure 2.9 The fallopian tube.

Ostium

Isthmus

Ampulla

in the extremity known as the infundibulum where the funnel-shaped opening of the tube into the peritoneal cavity is surrounded by finger-like processes, called fimbriae, into which the muscle coat does not extend. The inner surfaces of the fimbriae are covered by ciliated epithelium, which is similar to the lining of the fallopian tube itself. One of these fimbriae is longer than the others and extends to, and partly embraces, the ovary. The muscle fibres of the wall of the tube are arranged in an inner circular and an outer longitudinal layer.

The tubal epithelium forms a number of branched folds, or plicae, which run longitudinally; the lumen of the ampulla is almost filled with these folds. The folds have a cellular stroma, but at their bases the epithelium is only separated from the muscle by a very scanty amount of stroma. There is no submucosa and there are no glands. The epithelium of the fallopian tubes contains two functioning cell types: the ciliated cells, which act to produce a constant current fluid in the direction of the uterus; and the secretary cells, which contribute to the volume of tubal fluid. Changes occur under the influence of the menstrual cycle but there is no cell shedding during menstruation.

The ovaries

The size and appearance of the ovaries depends on both age and the stage of the menstrual cycle. In the young adult they are almond-shaped, solid, a greyish-pink and approximately 3 cm long, 1.5 cm wide and 1 cm thick.

In the child the ovaries are small structures approximately 1.5 cm long. They have a smooth surface and at birth they contain between one and two million primordial follicles, some of which will ripen into mature follicles in the reproductive years. The ovaries increase to adult size in the months preceding puberty. This considerable increase is brought about by proliferation of the stromal cells and by the commencing maturation of the ovarian follicles. After the menopause no active follicles are present and the ovary becomes a small shrunken structure with a wrinkled surface.

The ovary is the only intra-abdominal structure not to be covered by peritoneum. Each ovary is attached to the cornu of the uterus by the ovarian ligament, and at the hilum to the broad ligament by the mesovarium, which contains its supply of vessels and nerves. Laterally each ovary is attached to the suspensary ligament of the ovary with folds of peritoneum, which become continuous with that overlying the psoas major.

Anterior to the ovary lie the fallopian tubes, the superior portion of the bladder and the uterovesical pouch. It is bound behind by the ureter where it runs downwards and forwards in front of the internal iliac artery.

Structure

The ovary (Fig. 2.10) has a central vascular medulla consisting of loose connective tissue containing many elastin fibres and non-striated muscle cells. It has an outer thicker cortex, denser than the medulla, consisting of networks of reticular fibres and fusiform cells, although there is no clear-cut

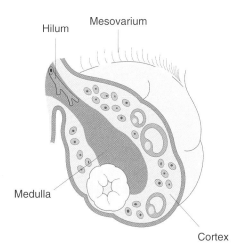

Figure 2.10 The ovary.

demarcation between the two. The surface of the ovaries is covered by a single layer of cuboidal cells, the germinal epithelium. Beneath this is an ill-defined layer of condensed connective tissue, the tunica albuginea, which increases in density with age. At birth, numerous primordial follicles are found mostly in the cortex but some are found in the medulla. With puberty some form each month into graafian follicles which at later stages of their development form corpora lutea and ultimately atretic follicles, the corpora albicans.

Vestigial structures
Vestigial remains of the mesonephric duct and tubules are always present in young children, but are variable structures in adults. The epoophoron, a series of parallel blind tubules, lies in the broad ligament between the mesovarium and the fallopian tube. The tubules run to the rudimentary duct of the epoophoron, which runs parallel to the lateral fallopian tube. Situated in the broad ligament, between the

epoophoron and the uterus are occasionally seen a few rudimentary tubules, the paroophoron. In a few individuals, the cordal part of the mesonephric duct is well developed, running alongside the uterus to the internal os. This is the duct of Gartner.

The bladder, urethra and ureter

The bladder

The average capacity of the bladder is 400 mL. The bladder is lined with transitional epithelium. The involuntary muscle of its wall is arranged in an inner longitudinal layer, a middle circular layer and an outer longitudinal layer.

The ureters open into the base of the bladder after running medially for about 1 cm through the vesical wall. The urethra leaves the bladder in front of the ureteric orifices; the triangular area lying between the ureteric orifices and the internal meatus is known as the trigone. At the internal meatus the middle layer of vesical muscle forms anterior and posterior loops round the neck of the bladder, some fibres of the loops being continuous with the circular muscle of the urethra.

The base of the bladder is related to the cervix, with only a thin layer of connective tissue intervening. It is separated from the anterior vaginal wall below by the pubocervical fascia, which stretches from the pubis to the cervix.

The urethra

The female urethra is about 3.5 cm long, and has a slight posterior angulation at the junction of its lower

Figure 2.11 The bladder and urethra.

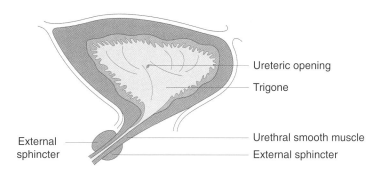

External sphincter

Ureteric opening

Trigone

Urethral smooth muscle

External sphincter

and middle thirds. It is lined with transitional epithelium. The smooth muscle of its wall is arranged in outer longitudinal and inner circular layers. As the urethra passes through the two layers of the urogenital diaphragm (triangular ligament) it is embraced by the striated fibres of the deep transverse perineal muscle (compressor urethrae), and some of the striated fibres of this muscle form a loop on the urethra. Between the muscular coat and the epithelium is a plexus of veins. There are a number of tubular mucous glands and, in the lower part, a number of crypts, which occasionally become infected. In its upper two-thirds the urethra is separated from the symphysis by loose connective tissue, but in its lower third it is attached to the pubic ramus on each side by strong bands of fibrous tissue called the pubourethral ligaments. Posteriorly it is related to the anterior vaginal wall, to which it is firmly attached in its lower two-thirds. The upper part of the urethra is mobile, but the lower part is relatively fixed. Figure 2.11 depicts the bladder and urethra.

Medial fibres of the pubococcygeus of the levator ani muscles are inserted into the urethra and vaginal wall. When they contract they pull the anterior vaginal wall and the upper part of the urethra forwards, forming an angle of about 100° between the posterior wall of the urethra and the bladder base. On voluntary voiding of urine the base of the bladder and the upper part of the urethra descend and this posterior angle disappears, so that the base of the bladder and the posterior wall of the urethra come to lie in a straight line. It was formerly claimed that absence of this posterior angle was the cause of stress incontinence but this is probably only one of a number of mechanisms responsible.

The ureter

As the ureter crosses the brim of the pelvis it lies in front of the bifurcation of the common iliac artery. It runs downwards and forwards on the lateral wall of the pelvis to reach the pelvic floor, and then passes inwards and forwards, attached to the peritoneum of the back of the broad ligament, to pass beneath the uterine artery. It next passes forwards through a fibrous tunnel, the ureteric canal, in the upper part of the cardinal ligament. Finally it runs close to the lateral vaginal fornix to enter the trigone of the bladder.

Its blood supply is derived from small branches of the ovarian artery, from a small vessel arising near the iliac bifurcation, from a branch of the uterine artery where it crosses beneath it, and from small branches of the vesical arteries.

Because of its close relationship to the cervix, the vault of the vagina and the uterine artery, the ureter may be damaged during hysterectomy (Fig. 2.12). Apart from being cut or tied, in radical procedures the ureter may undergo necrosis because of interference with its blood supply. It may be displaced upwards by fibromyomata or cysts which are growing between the layers of the broad ligament and may suffer injury if its position is not noticed at operation.

The rectum

The rectum extends from the level of the third sacral vertebra to a point about 2.5 cm in front of the coccyx, where it passes through the pelvic floor to become continuous with the anal canal. Its direction follows the curve of the sacrum and it is about 11 cm in length.

The front and sides of the upper third are covered by the peritoneum of the rectovaginal pouch; in the middle third only the front is covered by the peritoneum. In the lower third there is no peritoneal covering and the rectum is separated from the posterior wall of the vagina by the rectovaginal fascial septum. Lateral to the rectum are the two uterosacral ligaments, beside which run some of the lymphatics draining the cervix and vagina.

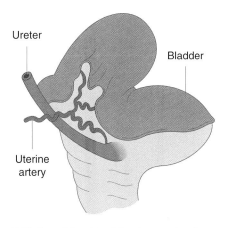

Figure 2.12 The relationship of the uterus and ureter.

The pelvic muscles, ligaments and fasciae

The pelvic diaphragm

The pelvic diaphragm is formed by the levator ani muscles (Fig. 2.13).

Levator ani muscles

Each is a broad, flat muscle, the fibres of which pass downwards and inwards. The two muscles, one on either side, constitute the pelvic diaphragm. The muscle arises by a linear origin from:

- the lower part of the body of the os pubis;
- the internal surface of the parietal pelvic fascia along the white line;
- the pelvic surface of the ischial spine.

The levator ani muscles are inserted into:

- the pre-anal raphé and the central point of the perineum where one muscle meets the other on the opposite side;
- the wall of the anal canal, where the fibres blend with the deep external sphincter muscle;
- the postanal or anococcygeal raphé, where again one muscle meets the other on the opposite side;
- the lower part of the coccyx.

The muscle is described in two parts; the pubococcygeus arises from the pubic bone and the anterior part of the tendinous arch of the pelvic fascia (white line), and the iliococcygeus, which arises from the posterior part of the tendinous arch and the ischial spine.

The medial borders of the pubococcygeus muscles pass on either side from the pubic bone to the pre-anal raphé. They thus embrace the vagina, and on contraction have some sphincteric action. The nerve supply is from the third and fourth sacral nerves.

The pubococcygeus muscles support the pelvic and abdominal viscera, including the bladder. The medial edge passes beneath the bladder and runs laterally to the urethra, into which some of its fibres are inserted. Together with fibres from the opposite muscle they form a loop which maintains the angle between the posterior aspect of the urethra and the bladder base. During micturition this loop relaxes to allow the bladder neck and upper urethra to open and descend.

Urogenital diaphragm

The urogenital diaphragm (triangular ligament) lies below the levator ani muscles and consists of two layers of pelvic fascia, which fill the gap between the descending pubic rami. The deep transverse perineal muscle (compressor urethrae) lies between the two layers, and the diaphragm is pierced by the urethra and the vagina.

The perineal body

This is the perineal mass of muscular tissue that lies between the anal canal and the lower third of the vagina. Its apex is at the lower end of the rectovaginal septum, at the point where the rectum and posterior vaginal walls come into contact. Its base is covered with skin and extends from the fourchette to the anus. It is the point of insertion of the superficial perineal muscles and is bounded above by the levator ani muscles where they come into contact in the midline between the posterior vaginal wall and the rectum.

The pelvic peritoneum

The peritoneum is reflected from the lateral borders of the uterus to form, on either side, a double fold of peritoneum – the broad ligament. This is not a

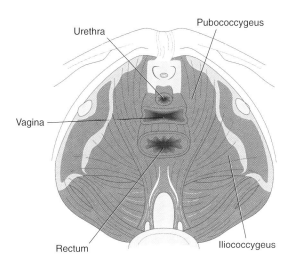

Figure 2.13 Diagrammatic representation of the superior aspect of the pelvic floor.

ligament but a peritoneal fold, and it does not support the uterus. The fallopian tube runs in the upper free edge of the broad ligament as far as the point at which the tube opens into the peritoneal cavity. The part of the broad ligament that is lateral to the opening is called the infundibulopelvic fold, and in it the ovarian vessels and nerves pass from the side wall of the pelvis to lie between the two layers of the broad ligament. The mesosalpinx, the portion of the broad ligament which lies above the ovary, is layered; between its layers are to be seen any Wolffian remnants which may be present. Below the ovary the base of the broad ligament widens out and contains a considerable amount of loose connective tissue, called the parametrium. The ureter is attached to the posterior leaf of the broad ligament at this point.

The ovary is attached to the posterior layer of the broad ligament by a short mesentery (the mesovarium) through which the ovarian vessels and nerves enter the hilum.

The rectovaginal pouch has already been described. It will be noted that while the vagina does not have any peritoneal covering in front, behind it is in contact with the rectovaginal pouch for about 2 cm where the vagina is separated from the abdominal cavity only by the peritoneum and thin fascia. The peritoneal cavity can be opened by posterior colpotomy at this point.

The ovarian ligament and round ligament

The ovarian ligament lies beneath the posterior layer of the broad ligament and passes from the medial pole of the ovary to the uterus just below the point of entry of the fallopian tube.

The round ligament is the continuation of the same structure and runs forwards under the anterior leaf of peritoneum to enter the inguinal canal, ending in the subcutaneous tissue of the labium majus. Together, the ovarian and round ligaments are homologous with the testis of the male.

The pelvic fascia and pelvic cellular tissue

Connective tissue fills the irregular spaces between the various pelvic organs. Much of it is loose cellular tissue, but in some places it is condensed to form strong ligaments which contain some smooth muscle fibres and which form the fascial sheaths which enclose the various viscera. The pelvic arteries, veins, lymphatics, nerves and ureters run through it.

The cellular tissue is continuous above with the extraperitoneal tissue of the abdominal wall, but below it is cut off from the ischiorectal fossa by the pelvic fascia and the levator ani muscles. There is a considerable collection of cellular tissue in the wide base of the broad ligament and at the side of the cervix and vagina, spoken of as the parametrium. The pelvic fascia may be regarded as a specialized part of this connective tissue. Anatomists describe parietal and visceral components.

The parietal pelvic fascia lines the wall of the pelvic cavity, covering the obturator internus and pyramidalis muscles. There is a thickened tendinous arch (or white line) on the side wall of the pelvis. It is here that the levator ani muscle arises and the cardinal ligament gains its lateral attachment. Where the parietal pelvic fascia encounters bone, as in the pubic region, it blends with the periosteum. It also forms the upper layer of the urogenital diaphragm (triangular ligament).

Each viscus has a fascial sheath, which is dense in the case of the vagina and cervix and at the base of the bladder, but is tenuous or absent over the body of the uterus and the dome of the bladder. Various processes of the visceral pelvic fascia pass inwards from the peripheral layer of the parietal pelvic fascia. From the point of view of the gynaecologist, certain parts of the visceral fascia are of particular importance, as follows.

The cardinal ligaments (transverse cervical ligaments) provide the essential support of the uterus and vaginal vault. These are two strong fan-shaped fibromuscular expansions which pass from the cervix and vaginal vault to the side wall of the pelvis on either side.

The uterosacral ligaments run from the cervix and vaginal vault to the sacrum. In the erect position they are almost vertical in direction and support the cervix.

The bladder is supported laterally by condensations of the vesical pelvic fascia one each side, there is also a sheet of pubocervical fascia which lies beneath it anteriorly.

Arteries supplying the pelvic organs

The ovarian artery

Because the ovary develops on the posterior abdominal wall and later migrates down into the pelvis it derives its blood supply directly from the abdominal aorta. The ovarian artery arises from the aorta just below the renal artery and runs downwards on the anterior surface of the psoas muscle to the pelvic brim, where it crosses in front of the ureter and then passes into the infundibulopelvic fold of the broad ligament. The artery divides into branches that supply the ovary and tube and then run on to reach the uterus, where they anastomose with the terminal branches of the uterine artery.

The internal iliac (hypogastric) artery

This vessel is about 4 cm in length and begins at the bifurcation of the common iliac artery in front of the sacroiliac joint. It soon divides into anterior and posterior divisions; the branches that supply the pelvic viscera are all from the anterior division.

The uterine artery provides the main blood supply to the uterus. The artery first runs downwards on the lateral wall of the pelvis, in the same direction as the ureter. It then turns inwards and forwards, lying in the base of the broad ligament. By this change of direction the artery crosses above the ureter, at a distance of about 2 cm from the uterus, at the level of the internal os. On reaching the wall of the uterus the artery turns upwards to run tortuously to the upper part of the uterus where it anastomoses with the ovarian artery. In this part of its course it sends many branches into the substance of the uterus.

The artery supplies a branch to the ureter as it crosses it, and shortly afterwards another branch is given off to supply the cervix and upper vagina.

The vaginal artery is another branch of the internal iliac artery that runs at a lower level to supply the vagina.

The vesical arteries are variable in numbers. They supply the bladder and terminal ureter. One usually runs in the roof of the ureteric canal.

The middle rectal artery often arises in common with the lowest vesical artery.

The pudendal artery is another branch of the internal iliac artery. It leaves the pelvic cavity through the sciatic foramen and, after winding round the ischial spine, enters the ischiorectal fossa where it gives off the inferior rectal artery. It terminates in branches that supply the perineal and vulval structures, including the erectile tissue of the vestibular bulbs and clitoris.

The superior rectal artery

This artery is the continuation of the inferior mesenteric artery and descends in the base of the pelvic mesocolon. It divides into two branches, which run on either side of the rectum and supply numerous branches to it.

The pelvic veins

The veins around the bladder, uterus, vagina and rectum form plexuses which intercommunicate freely.

Venous drainage from the uterine, vaginal and vesical plexuses is chiefly into the internal iliac veins.

Venous drainage from the rectal plexus is via the superior rectal veins to the inferior mesenteric veins, and the middle and inferior rectal veins to the internal pudendal veins and so to the iliac veins.

The ovarian veins on each side begin in the pampiniform plexus that lies between the layers of the broad ligament. At first there are two veins on each side accompanying the corresponding ovarian artery.

Higher up the vein becomes single; that on the right ends in the inferior vena cava and that on the left in the left renal vein.

The pelvic lymphatics

Lymph draining from the lower extremities and the vulval and perineal regions is all filtered through the inguinal and superficial femoral nodes before continuing along the deep pathways on the side wall of the pelvis. One deep chain passes upwards lateral to the major blood vessels, forming in turn the external iliac, common iliac and para-aortic groups of nodes.

Medially another chain of vessels passes from the deep femoral nodes through the femoral canal to the obturator and internal iliac groups of nodes. These last nodes are interspersed among the origins of the branches of the internal iliac artery, receiving lymph directly from the organs supplied by this artery, including the upper vagina, cervix and body of the uterus.

From the internal iliac and common iliac nodes afferent vessels pass up the para-aortic chains, and finally all the lymphatic drainage from the legs and pelvis flows into the lumbar lymphatic trunks and the cisterna chyli at the level of the second lumbar vertebra. From here all the lymph is carried by the thoracic duct through the thorax, with no intervening nodes, to empty into the junction of the left subclavian and internal jugular veins.

Tumour cells that penetrate or bypass the pelvic and para-aortic nodes are rapidly disseminated via the great veins at the root of the neck.

Lymphatic drainage from the genital tract

The lymphatic vessels from individual parts of the genital tract drain into this system of pelvic lymph nodes in the following manner (Fig. 2.14)

The vulva and the perineum medial to the labiocrural skin folds contain superficial lymphatics which pass upwards towards the mons pubis and then curve laterally to the superficial inguinal and femoral nodes. Drainage from these is through the fossa ovalis into the deep femoral nodes. The largest of these, lying in the upper part of the femoral canal, is known as the node of Cloquet.

The vagina: the lymphatics of the lower third follow the vulval drainage to the superficial inguinal nodes, whereas those from the upper two-thirds pass upwards to join the lymphatic vessels of the cervix.

The cervix: the lymphatics pass either laterally in the base of the broad ligament or posteriorly along the uterosacral ligaments to reach the side wall of the pelvis. Most of the vessels drain to the internal iliac, obturator and external iliac nodes, but vessels also pass directly to the common iliac and lower para-aortic nodes, so that radical surgery for carcinoma of the cervix should include removal of all these node groups on both sides of the pelvis.

The corpus uteri: nearly all the lymphatic vessels join those leaving the cervix and therefore reach similar groups of nodes.

A few vessels at the fundus follow the ovarian channels, and there is an inconsistent pathway along the round ligament to the inguinal nodes.

The ovary and fallopian tube have a plexus of vessels which drain along the infundibulopelvic fold to the para-aortic nodes on both sides of the midline. On the left these are found around the left renal pedicle, whilst on the right there may be only one node intervening before the lymph flows into the thoracic duct, thus accounting for the rapid early spread of metastatic carcinoma to distant sites such as the lungs.

The bladder and urethra: the drainage is to the iliac nodes, whilst the lymphatics of the lower part of the urethra follow those of the vulva.

The rectum: the lymphatics from the lower anal canal drain to the superficial inguinal nodes, and the remainder of the rectal drainage follows pararectal channels accompanying the blood vessels to both the internal iliac nodes (middle rectal artery) and the para-aortic nodes at the origin of the inferior mesenteric artery.

Nerves of the pelvis

Nerve supply of the vulva and perineum

The pudendal nerve arises from the second, third and fourth sacral nerves.

As it passes along the outer wall of the ischiorectal fossa it gives off an inferior rectal branch and divides into the perineal nerve and the dorsal nerve of the clitoris. The perineal nerve gives the sensory supply to the vulva; it also innervates the anterior part of the external anal sphincter and levator ani, and the superficial perineal muscles. The dorsal nerve of the clitoris is sensory.

Sensory fibres from the mons and labia also pass, in the ilioinguinal and genitofemoral nerves, to the first lumbar root. The posterior femoral cutaneous nerve carries sensation from the perineum to the small sciatic nerve, and thus to the first, second and third sacral nerves.

The main nerve supply of the levator ani muscles comes from the third and fourth sacral nerves.

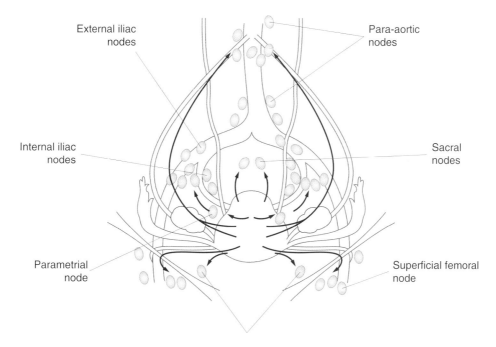

External iliac
nodes

Para-aortic
nodes

Internal iliac
nodes

Sacral
nodes

Parametrial
node

Superficial femoral
node

Figure 2.14 The lymphatic drainage of the female genital organs.

Nerve supply of the pelvic viscera

To describe what can be seen on dissection of the extensive autonomic nerve supply of the pelvic organs is one thing – to determine the physiological functions of the various parts of the system is another.

Nerve fibres of the preaortic plexus of the sympathetic nervous system are continuous with those of the superior hypogastric plexus, which lies in front of the last lumbar vertebra and is wrongly called the presacral nerve. Below, the superior hypogastric plexus divides, and on each side its fibres are continuous with fibres passing beside the rectum to join the uterovaginal plexus (inferior hypogastric plexus, or plexus of Frankenhäuser). This plexus lies in the loose cellular tissue posterolateral to the cervix below the uterosacral folds of peritoneum.

Parasympathetic fibres from the second, third and fourth sacral nerves join the uterovaginal plexus. Fibres from (or to) the bladder, uterus, vagina and rectum join the plexus. The uterovaginal plexus contains a few ganglion cells, so it is likely that a few motor nerves have their relay stations there and then pass onwards with the blood vessels to the viscera.

The ovary is not innervated by the nerves already described but from the ovarian plexus, which surrounds the ovarian vessels and joins the preaortic plexus high up.

This description has avoided any conjecture as to the particular function of the sympathetic and parasympathetic nerves, and no opinion has been expressed as to whether the various nerves carry sensory or motor impulses. Clinical facts are few. It is evident that afferent sensory impulses are often carried in the superior hypogastric plexus. If this is divided during presacral neurectomy, pain from the bladder and uterus can often be blocked. Apart from a transient pelvic hyperaemia there is no change in the motor function of either bladder or uterus. At an ordinary hysterectomy the uterovaginal plexus is not disturbed, but after a more extensive Wertheim operation there may be painless atony and distension of the bladder, which is attributed to loss of bladder sensation because the sacral connections of the uterovaginal plexus have been divided.

The motor effects are even less certain than the sensory. Stimulation of the cut lower end of the hypogastric plexus seems to have no effect on the bladder or the uterus. Although it has been stated that the parasympathetic nerves are excitatory to the musculature of the body of the uterus and inhibitory to that of the cervix, and that the sympathetic has the opposite effect, there is not general agreement about this.

The myometrium contains both α- and β- adrenergic receptors and also cholinergic receptors. In the non-pregnant uterus the balance of their action is uncertain, but during pregnancy strong stimulation of β-receptors with β-mimetic drugs such as isoxsuprine will inhibit myometrial activity.

Key Points

- The nephrogenic cord develops from the mesoderm and forms the urogenital ridge and the mesonephric duct. The para-mesonephric duct which later forms the müllerian system is the precursor of female genital development
- The lower end of the müllerian ducts come together in the midline, fuse and develop into uterus and cervix
- Most of the upper vagina is of müllerian origin. The lower vagina forms from the sinovaginal bulbs
- The primitive gonad is first evident at 5 weeks of embryonic life and forms on the medial aspect of the mesonephric ridge.
- The size and ratio of the cervix to uterus changes with age and parity
- Vaginal ph is normally acidic and has a protective role for decreasing the growth of pathogenic organisms
- An adult uterus weighs about 70 grams and consists of three layers; the peritoneum, the myometrium and the endometrium
- The cervix is narrower than the body of the uterus and is approximately 2.5 cm in length, the ureter runs about 1 cm lateral to the supravaginal cervix
- The epithelium of the cervix in its lower third is stratified squamous variety and the junction between this and the columnar epithelium is where most cervical carcinoma arises
- The ovary is the only intraperitoneal structure not covered by peritoneum
- The main supports to the pelvic floor are the connective tissue and levator ani muscles. The main supports of the uterus are the uterosacral ligaments which are condensations of connective tissue.
- The ovarian arteries rise from the aorta whilst the right ovarian vein drains into the venacava, the left ovarian vein usually drains into the left renal vein
- The major nerve supply of the pelvis comes from the pudendal nerves which arise from the second, third and fourth sacral nerves

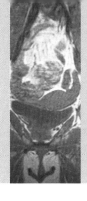

Chapter 3

Normal and abnormal sexual development and puberty

OVERVIEW

Sexual differentiation and normal subsequent development are fundamental to the continuation of the human species. In recent years our understanding of the control of this process has greatly increased. Following fertilization the human embryo will differentiate into a male or female fetus, and subsequent development is genetically controlled. This chapter describes the processes involved and discusses the subsequent evolution to full maturation.

Sexual differentiation

The means by which the embryo differentiates is controlled by the sex chromosomes. This is known as genetic sex. The normal chromosome complement is 46 chromosomes, including 22 autosomes derived from each parent. An embryo that contains 46 chromosomes and has the sex chromosomes XY will develop as a male. If the sex chromosomes are XX the embryo will differentiate into a female. The resulting development of the gonad will create either a testis or an ovary. This is known as gonadal sex. Subsequent development of the internal and external genitalia give phenotypic sex or the sex of appearance, and finally cerebral differentiation to a male or female orientation is known as brain sex.

Genetic sex

In the developing embryo with a genetic complement of 46 XY it is the presence of the Y chromosome which determines that the undifferentiated gonad will become a testis (Fig. 3. 1). Absence of the Y chromosome will result in development of an ovary. On the short arm of the Y chromosome is a region known as the SRY gene, which is responsible for the determination of testicular development as it produces a protein known as testicular determining factor (TDF). TDF directly influences the undifferentiated gonad to become a testis. When this process occurs the testis also produces Müllerian inhibitor.

The undifferentiated embryo contains both Wolffian and Müllerian ducts. The Wolffian ducts have

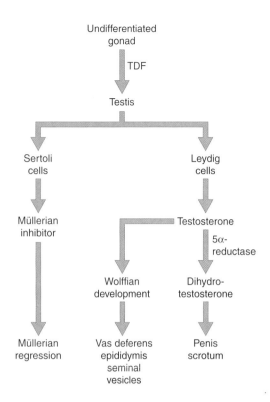

Figure 3.1 Male differentiation.

the potential to develop into the internal organs of the male, and the Müllerian ducts into the internal organs of the female. If the testis produces Müllerian inhibitor the Müllerian ducts regress.

The testis differentiates into two cell types, Leydig cells and Sertoli cells. The Sertoli cells are responsible for the production of Müllerian inhibitor, which leads to Müllerian regression. The Leydig cells produce testosterone which promotes the development of the Wolffian duct leading to the development of vas deferens, the epididymis and the seminal vesicles. Testosterone by itself does not have a different effect on the cloaca; in order to exert its androgenic effects it needs to be converted by the cloacal cells through the enzyme 5α-reductase to dihydrotestosterone. These androgenic effects lead to the development of the penis and the scrotum. The absence of a Y chromosome and the presence of two X chromosomes means that Müllerian inhibitor is not created, and the Müllerian ducts persist in the female (Fig. 3.2). The absence of testosterone means that the Wolffian ducts regress, and the failure of androgen to affect the cloaca leads to an external female phenotype.

Abnormal development

Any aberration in development that results in an unexpected developmental sequence of events may be mediated in a number of ways.

Chromosome abnormalities

In an embryo which loses one of its sex chromosomes the total complement of chromosomes will be reduced to 45, leaving a fetus viable only where this is 45 XO (Turner's syndrome). Here the absence of the second X chromosome or Y chromosome means there is no testicular development and therefore the phenotype is female (Fig. 3.3). The gonad, however, is unable to complete its development and, although it initially differentiates to be an ovary, the oogonia are unable to complete their development and at birth only the stroma of the ovary is present (streak ovaries). Thus, in Turner's syndrome the absence of a functional ovary means that there is no oestrogen production at puberty and secondary sexual characteristics cannot develop. As the genes involved in achieving final height are shared by the sex chromosomes, the absence of one sex chromosome will also lead to short stature.

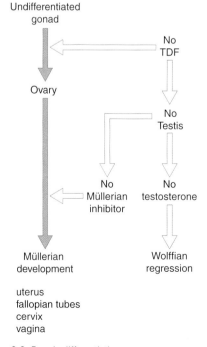

Figure 3.2 Female differentiation.

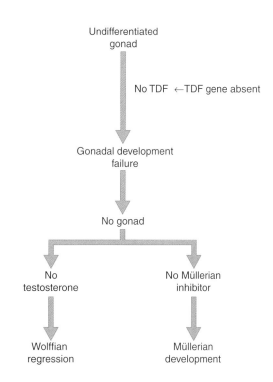

Figure 3.3 Turner's syndrome.

Figure 3.4 XY gonadal agenesis.

In females who have an XY karyotype, a mutation at the site on the short arm of the Y chromosome resulting in failure of production of TDF will mean there is no testicular development (XY gonadal agenesis). The default phenotypic state is female (Fig. 3.4). In these circumstances the absence of a testis means that the internal genitalia will persist as a result of the development of Müllerian structures and the Wolffian ducts will regress. The external genitalia will be female.

Gonadal abnormalities

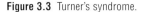

In males, a number of gonadal abnormalities may exist. The first is known as the vanishing testis syndrome; an XY fetus develops testes that then undergo atrophy. The reason for this remains speculative, although torsion, thrombosis and viral infections have been suggested. However, the failure of the development of the testes leads to a female default state, as above (similar to Fig. 3. 4).

In Leydig cell hypoplasia the Leydig cells responsible for the production of testosterone either completely fail to produce this or produce it in only small quantities. A range of abnormalities may result, dependent on the level of androgen produced and therefore the phenotype may range from female through to the hypospadiac male.

In XY gonadal dysgenesis a genetic abnormality leads to an abnormal testicular development. The testis fails to secrete androgen or Müllerian inhibitor, resulting in an XY female. If the genetic abnormality leads to an enzyme deficiency in the biosynthetic pathway to androgen, testosterone will fail to be secreted by the testis. However, some androgen may be produced depending on which enzyme is absent in the pathway. Therefore some effect on the external genitalia may be possible and a varying degree of virilism will occur. If the biosynthetic production of Müllerian inhibitor is deficient then, of course, its absence will mean the persistence of the Müllerian duct. This is an extremely rare syndrome.

In the female, gonadal dysgenesis may occur, and in this situation (similar to Turner's syndrome), the gonad is present only as a streak. These individuals have been found to have small fragments of a Y chromosome and, as a result of this, the gonad may undergo mitotic change which leads to the development of a gonadal tumour, e.g. a gonadoblastoma.

The Müllerian structures remain and the Wolffian structures regress, because of the absence of testes. At puberty the failure of development of the ovary will mean that there is no possibility for the production of oestradiol, and a failure of secondary sexual characteristic growth will occur.

In the rare condition known as mixed gonadal dysgenesis, there is a testis and a streak gonad in the same individual. The chromosome complement is typically 46 XX or a mosaic with a Y component. Here strangely, the Wolffian structures develop only on the side of the testis, but all Müllerian structures regress. The external genitalia in this rare condition may be ambiguous, depending on the functional capacity of the testis.

In true hermaphrodites the gonad may develop into either a testis or an ovary, or a combination of the two known as an ovotestis. Here a number of permutations may occur with either a testis and an ovary, or an ovotestis with a testis, an ovary or another ovotestis (Fig. 3.5). This usually results from a mosaic XX:XY karyotype and the predominance of either ovarian or testicular tissue in the gonad depends on the percentage of cell lines in the mosaic. As can be seen from Figure 3.5, the combination of gonads will determine the degree of virilization. The greater the testicular component the more virilized the resulting development, and the greater the testicular component the more likely the presence of Müllerian inhibitor will be. Thus in the true hermaphrodite it is possible to get co-existent Müllerian and Wolffian structures in terms of

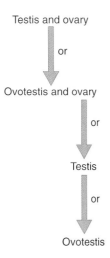

Figure 3.5 True hermaphrodite.

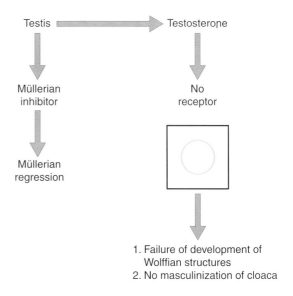

1. Failure of development of Wolffian structures
2. No masculinization of cloaca

Figure 3.6 XY female – androgen insensitivity.

internal development and varying degrees of masculinization of the external genitalia depending on the combination of gonads.

Internal genitalia abnormalities

In males there are three fundamental changes which may lead to abnormalities of the internal genitalia. The first of these is androgen insensitivity (Fig. 3.6). In this condition the fetus fails to develop androgen receptors due to mutations in the androgen receptor gene. Failure to possess the receptor means that, although the testis will be producing testosterone, the androgenic effect cannot be translated into the end organ as it is not recognized by the cell wall. The result here is that the fetus develops in the default female state, as it is unable to recognize the androgenic impact. This is the commonest type of XY female and the Wolffian ducts regress as they also have no androgen receptor. However, the Müllerian ducts also regress because the testis is normal and produces Müllerian inhibitor. These girls present with primary amenorrhoea at puberty.

A further aberration in XY females also exists with a condition known as 5α-reductase deficiency (Fig. 3.7). As outlined above, this enzyme is responsible for the conversion of testosterone to dihydrotestosterone resulting in virilization of the cloaca. If this enzyme is

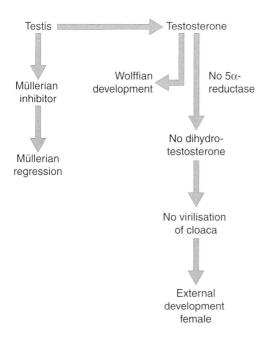

Figure 3.7 XY female – 5α reductase deficiency.

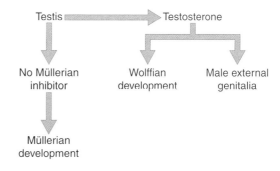

Figure 3.8 XY female – absent Müllerian inhibitor.

absent then the external genitalia will be female but the internal genitalia will be male. The Müllerian ducts will regress. Here again, this female will present with primary amenorrhoea. Finally, a rare condition known as Müllerian inhibitory deficiency may mean that an XY male may have persistent Müllerian structures due to the absence of Müllerian inhibitory factor, and co-existent male and female internal structures (Fig. 3.8).

In 46 XX females a genetic defect which results in failure of development of the uterus, cervix and vagina is known as the Rokitansky syndrome. This is the second most common cause of primary amenorrhoea in women, the first being Turner's syndrome. Here the ovaries are normal, and the external genitalia are normally female. The internal genitalia are either absent or rudimentary. Variations on this may lead to development of the vagina without development of the uterus, or development of the uterus without subsequent development of the cervix or vagina and a functional uterus may result. The aetiology of this developmental abnormality remains to be clarified. It is, however, very likely a genetic defect in the genes responsible for the development of the internal female genitalia. These genes, known as the homeobox genes, are likely to possess either deletions, which may be partial or complete, or point mutations, and as a consequence of these variations the resulting structures of the internal genitalia will vary in their development. However, the overall effect of this developmental abnormality is a failure of uterine and vaginal development, leading to infertility. These patients will present at puberty with either primary amenorrhoea or in circumstances when a small portion of uterus may be functional, with cyclical abdominal pain due to retained menstrual blood.

Two other developmental abnormalities may occur. The first of these is maldevelopment of the uterus, and here fusion defects occur from the extreme of a double uterus with a double cervix through to the normally fused uniform uterus. These abnormalities have been classified and result from the failure of fusion of the paramesonephric ducts at their lower border. A maldeveloped uterus may be associated with some degree of reproductive failure.

The development of the vagina involves a down growth of the vaginal plate and subsequent union of this with the cloaca and thereafter cannulization. This process can also fail leading to transverse vaginal septae, where the passage of the vagina is interrupted and therefore at puberty menstrual blood is trapped in an upper vagina which does not connect to the lower vagina. In the unusual condition of a double uterus, a double vagina can also exist and failure to develop the full double vaginal system may result in a blind hemivagina, again leading to a collection of menstrual blood at puberty.

External genitalia abnormalities

In males the external genitalia may fail to develop from a number of the above reasons, and the phallus may be underdeveloped leading to hypospadias. In hypospadias the urethra often fails to reach the end of the phallus or penis, and urine exits from the base of the penis.

In females the external genitalia may be virilized giving a masculine appearance. This is most commonly seen in a condition known as congenital adrenal hyperplasia. In this condition an enzyme defect in the adrenal gland, usually 21-hydroxylase deficiency, prevents the fetal adrenal from producing cortisol (Fig. 3.9). Failure of production of cortisol means that the feedback mechanism on the hypothalamus leads to an elevation of adrenocorticotrophic hormone (ACTH). This in turn stimulates the adrenal gland to undergo a form of hyperplasia and the excessive production of steroid precursors (17-hydroxyprogesterone) means the adrenal gland produces excessive amounts of androgen. This androgen enters the fetal circulation and impacts on the developing cloaca thereby leading to virilization. The female child is then born with a degree of phallic enlargement and the lower part of the vagina may be obliterated by the development of a male-type perineum and hence a vaginal orifice is not apparent. Virilization of the cloaca can also occur if the fetus is exposed to androgen from the mother ingesting an androgenic drug or, in many cases, the virilization is idiopathic. The end result in both of these circumstances is known as the intersex state. At birth, investigation of the chromosomes, the endocrine status of the infant and ultrasound of the internal organs will lead to a rapid diagnosis revealing whether the child is a female with a virilization state, which is most likely to be congenital adrenal hyperplasia, or a male that has been under masculinized.

Brain sex

The sex of orientation of a human is influenced by many factors. Theories exist that this is genetically predetermined and it is most likely that our sexual orientation is in fact determined by our sexual make up. However, this may be influenced by androgen exposure *in utero* or by other genetic and environmental factors, which impact on this function. Enormous care has to be taken in those individuals who are uncertain as to their sexual orientation before a final decision is taken on the sex of rearing.

Puberty

The hypothalamo-pituitary–ovarian axis is functionally complete during the latter half of fetal life. Follicle-stimulating hormone (FSH) levels are suppressed from 20 weeks' gestation by the production of oestrogen by the placenta and by the fetus itself. At birth the fetus is separated from its placenta and therefore the major source of oestrogen is removed. The FSH level then rises in response to the hypo-oestrogenic state of the fetus and remains elevated for some 6 to 18 months after birth. During this time it is suppressed due to the central inhibition of the production of gonadotrophin-releasing hormone (GnRH), which controls the pituitary production of FSH. The mechanism by which this is achieved remains speculative, but almost certainly is controlled by a gene in the GnRH cell nucleus in the hypothalamus. It is possible that there is a relationship between the production of leptin, a peptide produced by fat cells, and the subsequent control of this gene.

During childhood FSH pulses are almost undetectable, and at around the age of 8 or 9 years a change gradually occurs in the function of the GnRH cell. It begins with the production of single nocturnal spikes of GnRH and subsequently FSH. These spikes of FSH increase in frequency during the night-time hours over 1–2 years. Eventually, the frequency of pulses increases such that FSH pulses are detectable in the daylight hours, and thereafter after 4–5 years a fully functional production of GnRH with normal adult frequency and pulse amplitude leads to the establishment of the ovulatory menstrual cycle. Puberty therefore occurs over a total of 5 to 10 years, and involves five types of development (see box below).

The physiology of puberty

The sequence of events that occurs in the physical change resulting in the adult fertile female is usually the growth spurt followed by breast development, followed by pubic hair growth, followed by menarche, followed finally by axillary hair growth. Although this is the sequence of events in 70 per cent of girls, variations on this often occur. The description of pubertal development is credited to Tanner. He has classified the stages of development into five stages for breast growth and pubic hair growth.

The breast bud responds to the production of oestradiol by the ovary, which is itself reliant on GnRH production as outlined above. The breast grows in phases; initially the body of the breast grows, this is then superseded by areolar development which leads to a pronounced areola in comparison with the rest of the breast, and at this stage the breast has reached Tanner stage 4. Finally the breast tissue grows to become confluent with the areola and the breast has then completed its development.

Pubic hair growth begins on the labia and extends gradually up onto the mons and then into the inguinal regions. It is perfectly normal for pubic hair to extend along the midline up towards the umbilicus, and this is often misconstrued by women as being abnormal.

The growth spurt begins around age 11 years in girls, and the rate at which growth occurs increases from around 6–10 cm per year for around two years. Finally the effect of oestrogen on the end plate of the femur causes fusion and growth ceases, and by age 15 most girls have achieved their final height.

Menarche, the first menstrual period, occurs at any age between nine and 17 years. As one would imagine, the hypothalamo-pituitary–ovarian axis is not fully mature at the time of menarche and subsequent menstrual cycles are commonly irregular. Menstrual loss may also vary enormously, as a result of the immaturity of the axis. It takes between five and eight years from the time of menarche for women to develop ovulatory cycles 100% of the time. In understanding the menstrual difficulties that might arise during adolescent life, this piece of physiology is important to bear in mind.

Five stages of puberty

- Growth spurt
- Breast development
- Pubic hair growth
- Menstruation
- Axillary hair growth

Common clinical presentations and problems

Turner's syndrome

Patients with this condition may present at two ages in their life, either soon after birth or, more rarely, at a time of delayed puberty. The manner of presentation in infancy is variable. In the first few months of life there may be unexplained oedema of the hands and feet, loose folds of skin at the neck and occasionally unusual facies. In older children the oedema usually disappears, although it can persist, but the main feature of the growing child is the shortness of stature. It is this that suggests to the clinician the possibility of a sex chromosome anomaly. As the child grows a wide carrying angle of the arms may become apparent, the neck may become webbed in its appearance and the chest becomes broad with widely spaced nipples. Individuals occasionally have associated features such as colour blindness, co-arctation of the aorta and short metatarsals (Fig. 3.10). As these girls approach puberty they have streak ovaries and are, therefore, incapable of producing oestradiol. The hypothalamus and pituitary function normally and therefore FSH levels and leutinizing hormone (LH) levels are elevated due to ovarian failure. As mentioned previously, their internal genitalia are otherwise normal and investigation will reveal a karyotype which is typically 45 XO and measurement of gonadotrophins will show markedly elevated FSH and LH.

Treatment of this condition falls into two phases. Firstly the induction of puberty, which involves the administration of hormone replacement therapy. In order to ensure that secondary sexual characteristics appear normally, oestrogen is administered orally beginning at an extremely low dose and gradually increasing over a number of years. As puberty itself takes five years to complete, the same time frame should be anticipated when puberty is induced by exogenous oestrogen. The introduction of progesterone to the regime usually occurs after 18 months to two years when withdrawal bleeds from the patient's functioning uterus will occur.

The second phase of treatment is at a time when the patient desires a pregnancy. As she is deficient of oocytes, pregnancy can only be achieved with the aid of a donor egg and a sperm from the patient's partner used to create an embryo which is then transferred to

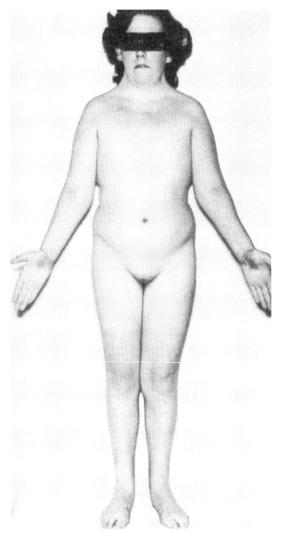

Figure 3.10 Turner's syndrome.

the recipient's uterus. Pregnancy progresses thereafter normally, although childbirth may be difficult because of the short stature.

If the investigations reveal a diagnosis of 46 XX gonadal dysgenesis, then the gonads have a 30 per cent risk of developing a gonadoblastoma, a malignant tumour of the ovary, and therefore patients should be advised that their gonads be removed. Again these women require induction of puberty in the same way as a Turner's syndrome patient.

XY females

These patients present at puberty with primary amenorrhoea. In the case of patients with androgen insensitivity, they are phenotypically normal females with breast development because their testes have produced androgen at puberty, which is converted peripherally to oestrogen by aromatase activity in fat cells. This oestrogen then enters the circulation and induces breast growth. It is common for breast growth to be complete at the time of presentation.

However, the absence of an androgen receptor means that pubic hair and axillary hair is either very scanty or absent. Their vagina is short and, of course, the uterus and tubes are absent. The testes may be found in the lower abdomen, groins or, rarely, in the labia majora. These girls may well have presented in childhood with inguinal herniae which have been operated on and the gonads will have been discovered at that stage and removed. If this has not been the case and the testes are still present, then advice that they should be removed because of the risk of malignancy should be given. The clinical appearance of these patients makes the diagnosis straightforward, and only confirmation by karyotype is necessary.

Oestrogen will need to be administered to these women in order to maintain their female body habitus, but the failure of the development of the Müllerian structures means pregnancy is impossible, except in those cases of XY gonadal agenesis or the XY female with absent Müllerian inhibitor only.

Intersex

Ambiguous genitalia are usually diagnosed at birth when the infant is clearly neither male nor female. In these circumstances gender assignment should be withheld until the infant can be fully evaluated. A very sensitive approach to the clinical situation must be taken. The parents will obviously be anxious to learn as swiftly as possible whether their child is male or female. Initially the most important investigation is a karyotype, and such facilities now exist that the karyotype can be determined within 24 hours on white blood cells taken from the infant.

The most common cause of ambiguous genitalia is congenital adrenal hyperplasia. Therefore, as we know that these are females with a masculinized vulva, ultrasound of the pelvis will reveal a normal uterus and ovaries. This, in conjunction with a karyotype of 46 XX, will almost always clinch the diagnosis. These children fail to produce cortisol and have high levels of circulating 17-hydroxyprogesterone, another investigative test that should be performed. The infants require cortisol supplementation in order to avoid an adrenal crisis. Further investigation may be required if the karyotype is 46 XY, and these possibilities are outlined earlier in the chapter.

Vaginal atresia

The presentation of an adolescent with primary amenorrhoea and normal secondary sexual characteristics should raise the possibility of congenital absence of the vagina as the primary concern until proven otherwise. Here the clinical story is a simple one, with the absence of establishment of menses. Clinical examination of the vulva will reveal a normal external appearance. However, parting the labia will reveal an absent vagina. An ultrasound examination of the pelvis will then confirm the absence of the development of the internal genitalia, but the presence of normal ovaries. The management of these patients is extremely sensitive, as their diagnosis will cause them great distress. Teenage girls are emotionally labile during puberty and adolescent development and the news that they have no vagina and no uterus is very distressing to them and to their parents.

It is impossible currently to offer any help for the absence of the uterus. However, it is possible to create a vagina so that sexual intercourse may occur normally. This may be created in one of two ways, either non-surgically or surgically. The non-surgical technique involves the use of graduated glass dilators, which will stretch the small vagina that they have into a fully functional vagina. This may be achieved over six to eight weeks of gradual dilatation, which is performed by the patient herself. In order for this technique to be successful, which it will be in some 85 per cent of girls, the motivation must be appropriate and will usually only be successful if they are in an established relationship leading towards the desire for sexual intercourse. In those patients in whom this cannot be successfully achieved, a surgical approach may be necessary to create a vagina. Various techniques have been described in order to achieve this using a number of materials, either skin grafts, amnion or bowel. Again subsequent to the surgery, dilators are required in order to maintain the surgically-created neovagina.

Obstructive outflow tract problems

Two varieties of outflow tract problems exist in the developmental abnormalities observed by gynaecologists in their female patients. The first of these is known as transverse vaginal septae. The simplest and most common is the imperforate hymen, where menstrual blood is trapped behind a thin hymenal membrane. This situation is easily resolved by a cruciate incision which releases the menstrual blood, subsequent sexual activity is normal and there are no sequelae at all.

In cases where a transverse vaginal septum results from failure of cannulization of the vagina, septae may occur at three levels. Either at the lower third of the vagina, the middle third or in the upper third. They all present with cyclical abdominal pain, and the development of a pelvic mass as menstrual blood accumulates in the vagina, thereby distending it. In some cases the vagina may distend to give a mass which may extend to the umbilicus. Investigation of these circumstances demands an ultrasound that will demonstrate the presence of a haematocolpos (blood in the vagina) (Fig. 3.11). Having established the anatomical defect, surgery is required to correct the absent portion by its excision and reconstruction of the vagina thereby creating a normal result, normal menstrual drainage and the ability of the vagina to function normally both for sexual intercourse and for subsequent conception.

In the situation of a vertical septal defect, here a midline septum persists between two hemivaginas, one of which has successfully developed and the other has failed to reach the perineum. In these circumstances the hemiuterus on the blind side bleeds into the blind hemivagina creating a hemihaemato-

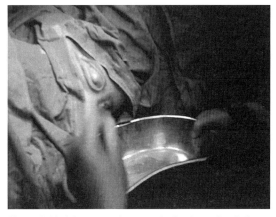

Figure 3.11 A haematocolpos seen in the theatre just before incision.

Common clinical presentations and problems

Conditions	Signs and symptoms	Investigations
Turner's syndrome	oedema of hands and feet short stature webbed neck wide carrying angle broad chest	FSH and LH karyotype 45 XO
XY females	primary amenorrhoea usually normal breast development scanty/absent pubic and axillary hair absent uterus and tubes undescended/maldescended testes	karyotype 46 XY
Intersex	ambiguous genitalia at birth	karyotype 46XX
Vaginal atresia	primary amenorrhoea normal secondary sexual characteristics absent vagina and uterus normal ovaries	

colpos. Here cyclical abdominal pain occurs with increasing severity, but this time the patient does have periods because the other hemiuterus and vagina function normally. Excision of the midline septum results in proper drainage of the menstrual flow, thereby resolving the problem.

Menorrhagia in adolescence

Menstrual problems in adolescence are very common, and may manifest themselves in a number of ways. The periods may be irregular and very heavy and occasionally result in marked anaemia, or they may be very scant and infrequent and cause equal concern. As outlined above, the important understanding of the physiology of the onset of the menstrual cycle and its subsequent development to normal is imperative for the clinician to manage these patients correctly.

In the former group of heavy menstrual loss, if the patient is not anaemic it is unnecessary to offer any treatment other than reassurance. If the patient does become anaemic then some control of menstrual loss must be undertaken. This is best achieved either by progestogens or by the oral contraceptive pill. Here control of the cycle will result until such times as the hypothalamo-pituitary–ovarian axis has matured.

In the group of patients who have very infrequent periods a further investigation may be required, and this is best carried out by assessing levels of gonadotrophins and by ultrasound of the ovary. In some circumstances a diagnosis of polycystic ovary syndrome may be made and these patients may require menstrual cycle control also in the form of the oral contraceptive pill. They also may develop oligomenorrhoea later in life, which may contribute towards an infertility problem that may require some attention. However, it is important to remember that the vast majority of these teenage girls will eventually establish a normal menstrual cycle and be fertile. The clinician is well advised to be cautious in giving advice about fertility potential as anxiety may be falsely invoked with incorrect advice.

Precocious puberty

Occasionally pubertal changes may occur earlier than the normal age range, and have been known to occur as early as three or four years of age. Most cases of precocious puberty are idiopathic, but result from activation of the gene in the GnRH cell prematurely. The sequence of events that occur subsequently mimics normal puberty, and therefore ovulatory cycles may result in very young children if they are not treated. In fact pregnancy has been known to occur in five and six year olds in whom sexual maturity has been reached. Precocious puberty, however, may also result from abnormal situations, e.g. a granulosa cell tumour which produces oestradiol, and subsequently this will lead to pubertal development, or from pituitary or hypothalamic tumours, which lead to FSH production, e.g. craniopharyngioma.

In investigating these children the exclusion of a serious tumour is of primary importance and imaging techniques can be used to achieve this. As the majority is idiopathic then treatment is targeted at down regulation of the pituitary using GnRH analogues.

New developments

Laparoscopic techniques have been developed to help form a neovagina in cases of vaginal atresia. Although more invasive than using dilators, they allow faster formation of a functional vagina.

Key Points

- Genetic sex is determined by the presence of the sex chromosomes X or Y
- The presence of a Y chromosome determines male development, the absence of a Y chromosome leads to a female phenotype
- In Turner's syndrome the absence of a second X chromosome leads to streak ovaries
- If the testis fails to develop or cannot function the default state is female
- True hermaphrodites have the presence of both ovarian and testicular tissue. The effect is determined by the dominant cell line
- Congenital absence of the uterus and vagina is the second most common cause of primary amenorrhoea
- Uterine maldevelopment does not usually result in reproductive failure
- External genitalia in girls may be virilized by excessive androgen exposure *in utero*
- Puberty is genetically determined and controlled from the hypothalamus

References for further reading

Edmonds DK, *Paediatric and Adolescent Gynaecology.* Oxford: Butterworths, 1989.

Edmonds DK, *Normal and Abnormal Development of the Genital Tract in Obstetrics and Gynaecology for Postgraduates.* Oxford: Blackwell, 1998.

Edmonds DK, *Gynaecological Disorders of Childhood and Adolescence in Obstetrics and Gynaecology for Postgraduates.* Oxford: Blackwell, 1998.

Moore K, Persaud M (eds). *The Developing Human* edited by London: Saunders, 1995.

Paediatric and Adolescent Gynaecology Sanfilippo. London: Saunders, 1998.

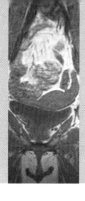

The normal menstrual cycle

OVERVIEW

Women in the western world each have around 400 menstrual cycles during the course of their lifetimes. In the UK, disorders of menstruation are one of the commonest reasons why women present to their general practitioner. An understanding of the physiology of the normal menstrual cycle is also required in order to tackle subjects such as infertility and the prevention of unwanted pregnancy. This chapter aims to describe the mechanisms that take place during the normal menstrual cycle. At each stage, the clinical relevance of menstrual cycle physiology will be emphasized.

Introduction

The most obvious manifestation of the normal menstrual cycle is the presence of regular menstrual periods. These occur as the endometrium is shed following failure of implantation or fertilization of the oocyte. Menstruation is initiated in response to changes in steroids produced by the ovaries, which themselves are controlled by the pituitary and hypothalamus.

The ovary

Within the ovary, the menstrual cycle can be divided into three phases:
- the follicular phase;
- ovulation;
- the luteal phase.

Follicular phase

The development of the oocyte is the key event in the follicular phase of the menstrual cycle. The ovary contains thousands of primordial follicles that are in a continuous state of development from birth, through periods of anovulation, such as pregnancy, to the menopause. These initial stages of follicular development are independent of hormonal stimulation. In the absence of the correct hormonal stimulus however, follicular development fails at the preantral stage, with ensuing follicular atresia. Development beyond the preantral stage is stimulated by the pituitary hormones, (luteinizing hormone [LH] and follicle-stimulating hormone [FSH]), which can be considered as key regulators of oocyte development.

At the start of the menstrual cycle, FSH levels begin to rise as the pituitary is released from the negative feedback effects of progesterone, oestrogen and inhibin. Rising FSH levels rescue a cohort of follicles from atresia, and initiate steroidogenesis. Figure 4.1 shows hormonal changes throughout the ovarian and menstrual cycles.

Steroidogenesis

The basis of hormonal activity in preantral to pre-ovulatory follicles is described as the 'two cell, two gonadotrophin' hypothesis. Steroidogenesis is compartmentalized in the two cell types within the follicle: the theca and granulosa cells. The two cell, two gonadotrophin hypothesis states that these cells are responsive to the gonadotrophins, LH and FSH respectively.

Within the theca cells, LH stimulates the production of androgens from cholesterol. Within granulosa cells, FSH stimulates the conversion of thecally-derived androgens to oestrogens (aromatization) (Fig. 4.3). In addition to its effects on aromatization, FSH is also responsible for proliferation of granulosa cells. Although other mediators are now known to be important in follicular development, this hypothesis is still the cornerstone to understanding events in the ovarian follicle. The respective roles of FSH and LH in follicular development are evidenced by studies on women undergoing ovulation induction in whom endogenous gonadotrophin production has been suppressed. If pure FSH alone is used for ovulation induction, an ovulatory follicle can be produced but oestrogen production is markedly reduced. Both FSH and LH are required to generate a normal cycle with adequate amounts of oestrogen.

Androgen production within the follicle may also regulate development of the preantral follicle. Low levels of androgens enhance aromatization and therefore increase oestrogen production. In contrast, high androgen levels inhibit aromatization and produce follicular atresia. A delicate balance of FSH and LH is required for early follicular development. The ideal situation for the initial stages of follicular devel-

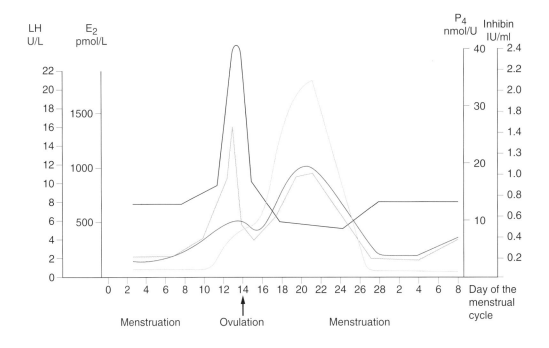

Figure 4.1 Pituitary and ovarian hormones during the menstrual cycle. (LH, luteinizing hormone; inhibin; E2, oestradiol; P4, progesterone.)

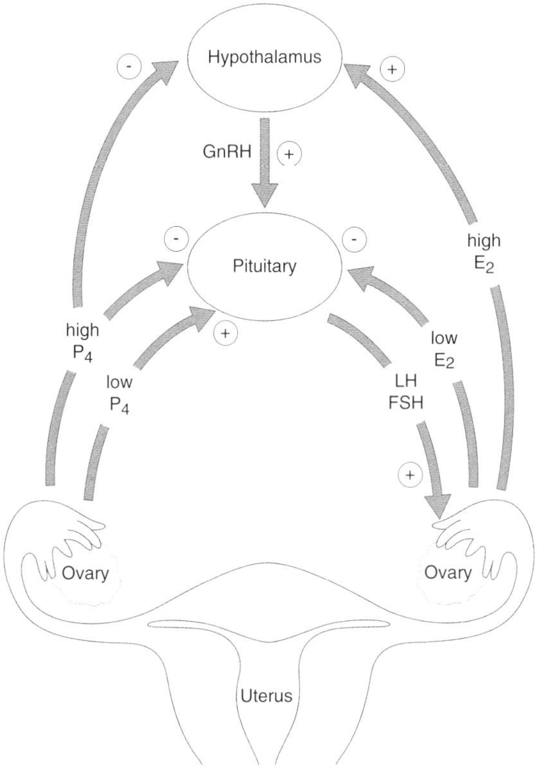

Figure 4.2 Hypothalamo-pituitary–ovarian axis showing positive and negative feedback of hormones. It should be noted that the mechanism by which low oestrogen induces negative feedback of LH and FSH production is uncertain. (P_4 = Progesterone; E_2 = Oestrogen.)

opment is low LH levels and high FSH levels, as seen in the early menstrual cycle. If LH levels are too high, theca cells produce large amounts of androgens causing follicular atresia.

Selection of the dominant follicle

The developing follicle grows and produces steroid hormones under the influence of the gonadotrophins LH and FSH. These gonadotrophins rescue a cohort of preantral follicles from atresia. However, normally only one of these follicles is destined to grow to a pre-ovulatory follicle and be released at ovulation – the dominant follicle.

The selection of the dominant follicle is the result of complex signalling between the ovary and the pituitary. In simplistic terms, the dominant follicle is the largest and most developed follicle in the ovary at the mid-follicular phase. Such a follicle has the most efficient aromatase activity and the highest concentration of FSH-induced LH receptors. The dominant

follicle therefore produces the greatest amount of oestradiol and inhibin. Inhibin further amplifies LH-induced androgen synthesis, which is used as a substrate for oestradiol synthesis. These features mean that the largest follicle therefore requires the lowest levels of FSH (and LH) for continued development. At the time of follicular selection, FSH levels are declining in response to the negative feedback effects of oestrogen. The dominant follicle is therefore the only follicle that is capable of continued development in the face of falling FSH levels.

Ovarian–pituitary interaction is crucial to the selection of the dominant follicle, and the forced atresia of the remaining follicles. Figure 4.2 depicts the positive and negative feedback mechanisms of the hypothalamo-pituitary–ovarian axis. When this interaction is bypassed, as in ovulation induction with the administration of exogenous gonadotrophins, many follicles continue to develop and are released at ovulation with an ensuing multiple gestation rate of around 30 per cent. During *in vitro* fertilization (IVF) the production of many ovulatory follicles is desired since the oocytes are harvested, and fertilized *in vitro*, and the number of embryos replaced can be carefully controlled. However, if such multiple follicular development occurred unchecked in the normal cycle, it would lead to the production of multiple gestations of high-order numbers, with their associated problems.

Inhibin and activin

Although folliculogenesis, ovulation and the production of progesterone from the corpus luteum can be explained largely in terms of the interaction between pituitary gonadotrophins and sex steroids, it is becoming clear that other autocrine or paracrine mediators also play a role. One of the most important of these is inhibin.

Inhibin was originally described as a testicular product that inhibited pituitary FSH production, hence its name. However, inhibin is also produced by a variety of other cell types, including granulosa cells within the ovary. Granulosa cell inhibin production is stimulated by FSH but in women, as in men, inhibin attenuates FSH production. Within the ovary, inhibin enhances LH-induced androgen synthesis. The production of inhibin is a further mechanism by which FSH levels are reduced below a threshold at which only the dominant follicle can respond, ensuring atresia of the remaining follicles.

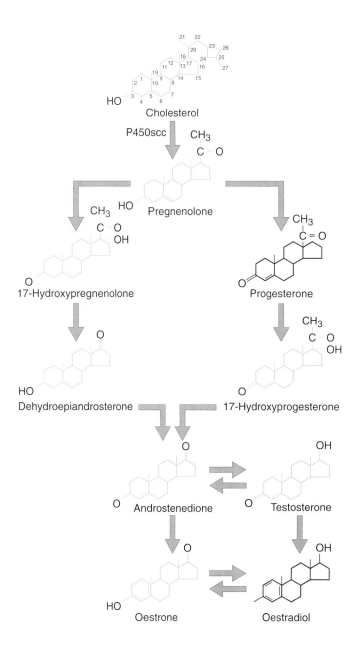

Figure 4.3 Ovarian steroidogenesis. The ovary has the capacity to synthesize oestradiol from cholesterol. The major products of the ovary are oestradiol and progesterone although small amounts of testosterone and androstenedione are also produced.

Activin is a peptide that is structurally related to inhibin. It is produced both by the granulosa cells of antral follicles, and also by the pituitary gland. The action of activin is almost directly opposite to that of inhibin in that it augments pituitary FSH secretion, and increases FSH binding to granulosa cells. Granulosa cell activin production therefore appears to amplify the effects of FSH within the ovarian follicle.

Insulin-like growth factors
Insulin-like growth factors (IGF-I and IGF-II) act as paracrine regulators. Circulating levels do not change during the menstrual cycle, but follicular fluid levels increase towards ovulation, with the highest level found in the dominant follicle. The actions of IGF-I and -II are modified by their binding proteins: insulin-like growth factor binding proteins (IGFBPs).

In the follicular phase, IGF-I is produced by theca cells under the action of LH. IGF-I receptors are present on both theca and granulosa cells. Within the theca, IGF-I augments LH-induced steroidogenesis. In granulosa cells, IGF-I augments the stimulatory effects of FSH on mitosis, aromatase activity and inhibin production. In the preovulatory follicle, IGF-I enhances LH-induced progesterone production from granulosa cells. Following ovulation, IGF-II is produced from luteinized granulosa cells, and acts in an autocrine manner to augment LH-induced proliferation of granulosa cells.

Ovulation

Late in the follicular phase, FSH induces LH receptors on granulosa cells. Oestrogen is an obligatory co-factor in this effect. As the dominant follicle develops further, follicular oestrogen production increases. The production of oestrogen is eventually sufficient that the threshold required for oestrogen to exert a positive feedback effect on pituitary LH secretion is achieved. Once this occurs, LH levels increase, at first quite slowly (day 8 to day 12 of the menstrual cycle) and then more rapidly (day 12 onwards). During this time, LH induces luteinization of granulosa cells in the dominant follicle, so that progesterone is produced. Progesterone further amplifies the positive feedback effect of oestrogen on pituitary LH secretion, leading to a surge of LH. Ovulation occurs 36 hours after the onset of the LH surge. The LH surge is one of the best methods by which the time of ovulation can be determined, and is the event detected by most over-the-counter 'ovulation predictor' kits.

The periovulatory FSH surge is probably induced by the positive feedback effects of progesterone. In addition to the rise in LH, FSH and oestrogen that occur around ovulation, a rise in serum androgen levels also occurs. These androgens are derived from the stimulatory effect of LH on theca cells, particularly those of the non-dominant follicle. This rise in androgens may have an important physiological effect in the stimulation of libido, ensuring that sexual activity is likely to occur at the time of ovulation when the woman is at her most fertile.

Prior to the release of the oocyte at the time of ovulation, the LH surge stimulates the resumption of meiosis, a process which is completed after the sperm enters the egg. In order for the ovary to release the oocyte at ovulation, breakdown of the follicular wall is required. This event is coordinated by LH, FSH and progesterone which stimulate the activity of proteolytic enzymes such as plasminogen activators (which produce plasmin, which stimulates collagenase activity) and prostaglandins. Prostaglandins not only stimulate the activity of proteolytic enzymes, but also promote an inflammatory-type response within the follicle wall, and by stimulation of smooth muscle activity may help extrusion of the oocyte.

The crucial importance of prostaglandins and other eicosanoids in the process of ovulation is demonstrated by studies showing that inhibition of prostaglandin production may result in failure of release of the oocyte from the ovary, despite apparently normal steroidogenesis (the luteinized unruptured follicle syndrome, LUF). Although LUF appears to be an uncommon cause of infertility, women wishing to become pregnant should be advised to avoid taking prostaglandin synthetase inhibitors such as aspirin and ibuprofen which may inhibit oocyte release.

Luteal phase

The luteal phase is characterized by the production of progesterone from the corpus luteum within the ovary. The corpus luteum is derived both from the granulosa cells that remain after ovulation, and from some of the theca cells which differentiate to become theca lutein cells. The granulosa cells of the corpus luteum have a vacuolated appearance associated with the accumulation of a yellow pigment, lutein, from where the corpus luteum derives its name. Extensive vascularization within the corpus luteum ensures that the granulosa cells have a rich blood supply providing the precursors for steroidogenesis.

The production of progesterone from the corpus luteum is dependent on continued pituitary LH secretion. However, serum levels of progesterone are such that LH and FSH production is relatively suppressed. This effect is amplified by moderate levels of oestradiol and inhibin that are also produced by the corpus luteum. The low levels of gonadotrophins mean that the initiation of new follicular growth is inhibited for the duration of the luteal phase.

Luteolysis
The duration of the luteal phase is fairly constant, being around 14 days in most women. In the absence of pregnancy and the production of human chorionic gonadotrophin (hCG) from the implanting

embryo, the corpus luteum regresses at the end of the luteal phase, a process known as luteolysis. The control of luteolysis in women remains obscure. As the corpus luteum dies, oestrogen, progesterone and inhibin levels decline. The pituitary is released from the negative feedback effects of these hormones and gonadotrophins, particularly FSH, start to rise. A cohort of follicles which happen to be at the pre-antral phase are rescued from atresia and a further menstrual cycle is initiated.

Summary of ovarian events

Follicular phase
- LH stimulates theca cells to produce androgens
- FSH stimulates granulosa cells to produce oestrogens
- The most advanced follicle at mid-follicular phase becomes the dominant follicle
- Rising oestrogen and inhibin produced by the dominant follicle inhibit pituitary FSH production
- Declining FSH levels cause atresia of all but the dominant follicle

Ovulation
- FSH induces LH receptors
- LH surge
- Proteolytic enzymes within the follicle cause follicular wall breakdown and release of the oocyte

The luteal phase
- The corpus luteum is formed from granulosa and theca cells retained after ovulation
- Progesterone produced by the corpus luteum is the dominant hormone of the luteal phase
- In the absence of pregnancy, luteolysis occurs 14 days after ovulation

Pituitary gland

The process of follicular development, ovulation and the maintenance of the corpus luteum has been described in terms of ovarian physiology. In reality however, the ovary, pituitary and hypothalamus act in concert (the hypothalamo-pituitary–ovarian axis) to ensure the growth and development of (ideally) one ovarian follicle, and to maintain hormonal support of the endometrium to allow implantation.

The pituitary hormones LH and FSH are, as we have seen, key regulators of folliculogenesis. The output of LH and FSH from the pituitary gland is stimulated by pulses of gonadotrophin-releasing hormone (GnRH) produced by the hypothalamus and transported to the pituitary in the portal circulation. The response of the pituitary is not constant but is modulated by ovarian hormones, particularly oestrogen and progesterone. Thus low levels of oestrogen have an inhibitory effect on LH (negative feedback) whereas high levels of oestrogen actually stimulate pituitary LH production (positive feedback). In the late follicular phase, serum levels of oestrogen are sufficiently high so that a positive feedback effect is triggered thus generating the periovulatory LH surge. In contrast, the combined contraceptive pill produces serum levels of oestrogen in the negative feedback range, so that measured levels of gonadotrophins are low.

The mechanism of action of the positive feedback effect of oestrogen involves an increase in GnRH receptor concentrations and an increase in GnRH production, whilst the mechanism of the negative feedback effect of oestrogen is uncertain.

In contrast to the effects of oestrogen, low levels of progesterone have a positive feedback effect on pituitary LH and FSH secretion. Such levels are generated immediately prior to ovulation, and contribute to the FSH surge. High levels of progesterone such as those seen in the luteal phase inhibit pituitary gonadotrophin production. Negative feedback effects of progesterone are generated both via decreased GnRH production, and via decreased sensitivity to GnRH at the pituitary level. Positive feedback effects of progesterone operate at the pituitary level only and involve increased sensitivity to GnRH. Importantly, progesterone can only have these effects if there has been prior priming by oestrogen.

As we have seen, oestrogen and progesterone are not the only hormones to have an effect on pituitary gonadotrophin secretion. The peptide hormones inhibin and activin have opposing effects on gonadotrophin production: inhibin attenuates pituitary FSH secretion whereas activin stimulates it.

The hypothalamus

The hypothalamus, via the pulsatile secretion of GnRH, stimulates pituitary LH and FSH secretion. Production of GnRH not only has a permissive effect on gonadotrophin production, but alterations in amplitude and frequency of GnRH pulsation throughout the cycle are also responsible for some fine tuning of gonadotrophin production (see section on pituitary gland above).

The importance of GnRH secretion is seen in disorders such as anorexia nervosa, and the amenorrhoea associated with excessive exercise. In these disorders, GnRH production is suppressed leading to anovulation and amenorrhoea. Ovulation can be restored in these women by the administration of GnRH in a pulsatile manner (although this should be approached carefully since pregnancy is relatively contraindicated in women whose body weight is significantly below average).

It is important to remember that GnRH is produced in a pulsatile manner to exert its physiological effect. Drugs that are GnRH agonists (e.g. buserelin and goserilin) are widely used in gynaecology for the treatment of endometriosis and other disorders. Although these drugs act as GnRH agonists, they cause a decrease in pituitary LH and FSH secretion. The reason for this is that these agonists are long-acting and the continued exposure of the pituitary to moderately high levels of GnRH causes down-regulation and desensitization of the pituitary. LH and FSH production is therefore markedly decreased. Ovarian steroidogenesis is suppressed so that serum oestrogen and progesterone fall to postmenopausal levels. Most women become amenorrhoeic whilst taking GnRH agonists. A potential disadvantage of the currently available GnRH agonists is that such down-regulation and desensitization of the pituitary takes up to three weeks to exert its effects. The initial effect of GnRH administration is to stimulate pituitary LH and FSH production, leading to increased ovarian steroidogenesis. When a patient commences GnRH therapy, this temporary increase in ovarian steroidogenesis leads to a vaginal bleed within the first month of administration and it is important to warn the patient of this.

The endometrium

We have already described the changes in the hypothalamo-pituitary–ovarian axis during the menstrual cycle. These changes occur whether or not the uterus is still present. Menstruation, which occurs in the presence of the uterus, is the most obvious external manifestation that regular menstrual cycles are occurring. The changes in the endometrium that occur during the menstrual cycle are described below.

Menstruation

As the corpus luteum dies at the end of the luteal phase, circulating levels of oestrogen and progesterone fall precipitously (see Figure 4.1). In an ovulatory cycle, where the endometrium is exposed to oestrogen and then progesterone in an orderly manner, the endometrium becomes 'decidualized' during the second half of the cycle to allow implantation of the embryo. Decidualization is an irreversible process, and if implantation does not occur, programmed cell death (apoptosis) ensues. Menstruation is the shedding of the 'dead' endometrium and ceases as the endometrium regenerates.

Menstruation is initiated by the withdrawal of oestrogen and progesterone. Such an effect can be produced experimentally and women receiving oestrogens and progestogens in the form of the combined contraceptive pill or hormone replacement therapy will experience a 'withdrawal bleed' on completion of a pack. Immediately prior to menstruation, the endometrium regresses. Endometrial venous drainage is inhibited and vasodilation ensues. Thereafter, a sequence of intense spiral artery vasoconstriction followed by relaxation is generated. These events lead to ischaemia and tissue damage, shedding of the functional endometrium (the stratum compactum and stratum spongiosum) and bleeding from fragments of arterioles remaining in the basal endometrium.

Menstruation ceases as the damaged spiral arteries vasoconstrict and the endometrium regenerates. Thus, haemostasis in the endometrial vessels differs from haemostasis elsewhere in a number of important aspects. Normally, bleeding from a damaged vessel is stemmed by platelet accumulation, fibrin deposition and platelet degranulation. Such events may however lead to scarring. In the endometrium, scarring would significantly inhibit function (as seen in Ashermann's syndrome) and an alternative system of haemostasis is therefore required. Vasoconstriction is the mechanism by which haemostasis is initially secured in the endometrium. Scarring is minimized by enhanced fibrinolysis, which breaks down blood clots. Later, repair of the endometrium and new blood vessel formation (angiogenesis) lead to complete cessation of bleeding within 5–7 days from the start of the menstrual cycle.

The involvement of oestrogen and progesterone withdrawal in the process of menstruation is certain, but the paracrine mediators involved in each part of the process are less clear. The vasoconstrictors prostaglandin $F_{2\alpha}$, endothelin-1 and platelet activating factor (PAF) are known to be produced within the endometrium and seem likely candidates for vessel constriction, both initiating and controlling menstruation. These mediators may be balanced by the effect of vasodilator agents such as prostaglandin E_2, prostacyclin (PGI), and nitric oxide (NO) which are also produced by the endometrium.

Endometrial repair involves both glandular and stromal regeneration and angiogenesis. Both vascular endothelial growth factor (VEGF) and fibroblast growth factor (FGF) are found within the endometrium, and both are powerful angiogenic agents. Increasing evidence suggests that oestrogen-induced glandular and stromal regeneration is mediated by epidermal growth factor (EGF). Other growth factors such as transforming growth factors (TGFs) and IGFs, and the interleukins, particularly interleukin-1 (IL-1), may also be important.

Increased understanding of the agents involved in menstruation may improve attempts to control pathologically excessive menstruation. Prostaglandin synthetase inhibitors such as mefenamic acid (Ponstan) are widely used in the UK as a first line treatment for menorrhagia. They are thought to increase the ratio of the vasoconstrictor prostaglandin PGF_{2a} to the vasodilator prostaglandin PGE_2. Although mefenamic acid does reduce menstrual loss, the mean reduction is only in the order of 20–25 per cent in women with true menorrhagia and the search for more effective agents has therefore continued.

The proliferative phase/follicular phase

Once endometrial repair is completed, usually at around day 5–6 of the cycle, menstruation ceases. Within the endometrium, the remainder of the follicular phase is characterized by glandular and stromal growth, hence the name 'the proliferative phase'. During this time, the epithelium lining the endometrial glands changes from a single layer of low columnar cells to pseudostratified epithelium with frequent mitoses. The stromal component of the endometrium re-expands, and is infiltrated by bone marrow-derived cells. The massive development taking place in the endometrium is reflected in the increase in endometrial thickness, from 0.5 mm at menstruation to 3.5–5 mm at the end of the proliferative phase.

Secretory phase/luteal phase

The postovulatory or luteal phase of the menstrual cycle is characterized by endometrial glandular secretory activity – hence the name the secretory phase. Under the action of progesterone, oestrogen-induced cellular proliferation is inhibited, and the depth of the endometrium remains fixed. Despite this, some elements continue to grow, leading to increased tortuosity of both the glands and spiral arteries in order to fit into the endometrial layer.

Shortly after ovulation, subnuclear intracytoplasmic granules appear in glandular cells. These vacuoles progress to the apex of the glandular cells and their contents are released into the endometrial cavity. Peak secretory activity occurs at the time of implantation, seven days after the gonadotrophin surge. Progesterone is essential for the induction of endometrial secretory changes and these changes are only seen after ovulation in the absence of exogenous steroid therapy. In former years, histological examination of luteal phase endometrium was commonly performed to confirm that ovulation had occurred (Fig. 4.4).

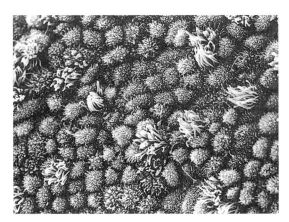

Figure 4.4 Scanning electron micrograph of the normal endometrium at the secretory phase of the menstrual cycle. (Illustration kindly provided by Dr Gill Irvine.)

However, access to inexpensive, accurate steroid hormonal assays has rendered this invasive test obsolete, so that ovulation is now confirmed by serum progesterone measurements in the luteal phase.

Within the stroma, oedema is induced in the secretory phase under the influence of oestrogen and progesterone. The predominant bone marrow-derived cell within the endometrium is the large granulated lymphocyte which has properties similar to the natural killer cell, and is thought to be important in regulating trophoblast invasion during implantation. In the late secretory phase, progesterone induces irreversible decidualization of the stroma. Histologically, decidualization is initiated around blood vessels. The surrounding stromal cells display increased mitotic activity, nuclear enlargement and a basement membrane is generated (Fig. 4.5a and b).

Immediately prior to menstruation, three distinct zones of the endometrium can be seen. The basalis is the basal 25 per cent of the endometrium, which is retained during menstruation and shows few changes during the menstrual cycle. The mid-portion is the stratum spongiosum with oedematous stroma and exhausted glands. The superficial portion (the uppermost 25 per cent) is the stratum compactum with prominent decidualized stromal cells. The withdrawal of oestrogen and progesterone leads to col-

> ## Summary of endometrial events
>
> ### Menstruation
> - Menstruation is initiated largely by arteriolar vasoconstriction
> - The functional layer (upper 75 per cent) is shed
> - Menstruation ceases due to vasoconstriction and endometrial repair
> - Fibrinolysis inhibits scar tissue formation
>
> ### Proliferative phase
> - Characterized by oestrogen-induced growth of glands and stroma
>
> ### Luteal phase
> - Characterized by progesterone-induced glandular secretory activity
> - Decidualization induced in late secretory phase
> - Decidualization is an irreversible process and leads to endometrial apoptosis and menstruation unless pregnancy occurs

lapse of the decidualized endometrium, repeated vasoconstriction and relaxation of the spiral arterioles, and consequent shedding of the endometrium. The onset of menstruation heralds the end of one menstrual cycle and the beginning of the next.

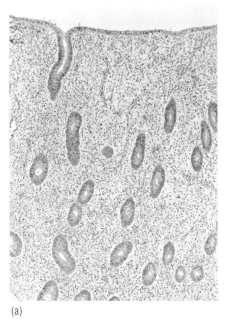

(a)

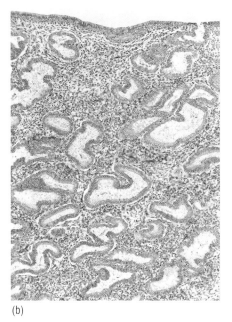

(b)

Figure 4.5 Tissue sections of normal endometrium stained with haematoxylin and eosin during the proliferative (a) and secretory (b) phase of the menstrual cycle. (Illustration kindly provided by Dr Colin Stewart.)

Clinical features of the normal menstrual cycle

Medical students are taught that the normal menstrual cycle is 28 days long (from the start of one cycle to the start of the next) and that the usual duration of menstrual flow is 4–6 days. In fact, only 15 per cent of women have a perfect 28-day cycle, and any cycle of between 21 and 35 days long can be regarded as normal. Menstrual cycles are longest immediately after puberty and in the five years leading up to the menopause, corresponding to the peak incidence of anovulatory cycles. The length of the menstrual cycle is determined by the length of the follicular phase. Once ovulation occurs, luteal phase length is fairly fixed at 14 days in almost all women.

The duration of menstrual flow also varies between women from 2–8 days. The amount of menstrual flow peaks on the first or second day of menstruation. The normal volume of menstrual loss is 30 mL per month. A menstrual loss of greater than 80 mL is considered to be excessive – this level is rather arbitrary and corresponds to the threshold at which iron deficiency anaemia may ensue unless treated.

Clinical points

Hormone assays
- Pituitary and ovarian hormones change constantly throughout the menstrual cycle
- A single blood test at a random point in the menstrual cycle is of little value
- Hormonal assays should be carefully timed to give the maximum information
1. To determine whether a patient is ovulating:
- Measurement of serum progesterone is the most helpful test
- Progesterone of $\geq$ 10 nmol/L indicates that ovulation has occurred
- Blood should be withdrawn in the mid-luteal phase (normally day 21 of the cycle)
- The results can only be interpreted if a menstrual period occurs around seven days after sampling
2. To determine whether a patient is menopausal:
- Measurement of serum gonadotrophins is the most helpful test
- Elevated gonoadotrophins indicate that the stock of ovarian follicles is exhausted
- Blood should be withdrawn within five days after menstruation to avoid the mid-cycle surge
- Abnormal results should be confirmed by repeat sampling

Ovarian cysts
- The preovulatory follicle reaches a diameter of 20 mm
- These follicles contain fluid and can be seen on ultrasound examination
- A 'cyst' of up to 20 mm in diameter in a premenopausal women at mid-cycle is likely to be a preovulatory follicle
- In practice, single unilocular ovarian cysts of up to 50 mm in diameter are likely to be functional cysts
- The appropriate initial management of a functional cyst is observation by serial ultrasound

New developments

Oocyte growth *in vitro*
During *in vitro* fertilization, exogenous gonadotrophins are administered to stimulate follicular growth within the ovary. The administered dose of gonadotrophins has to be controlled carefully to achieve adequate follicular growth with minimal side effects. Ideally, many ovulatory follicles should be generated and harvested prior to ovulation. However, such a process requires intensive monitoring which is time-consuming for both the patient and physician.

At present, follicular growth can only be achieved *in vivo*. In future, it may be possible to culture primordial follicles *in vitro* from frozen ovarian biopsies. If ovulatory follicles could be generated, this would be a major advance – the adverse effects of gonadotrophin therapy could be avoided, and there would be no need for frequent hospital attendances for scans and hormone assays during ovulation induction. Moreover, ovarian biopsies could be taken (before pelvic radiotherapy, for example) and stored until required.

GnRH antagonists
We have seen that the use of GnRH agonists is associated with an initial increase in ovarian steroidogenesis until down regulation of the pituitary is achieved. GnRH antagonists have now been developed and are currently undergoing phase III clinical trials. GnRH antagonists will inhibit the action of GnRH at the pituitary and therefore reduce LH and FSH secretion. The use of GnRH antagonists will avoid the initial stimulatory effect of GnRH agonists at the pituitary gland, hence a therapeutic effect will be achieved more rapidly, and some of the side effects of the GnRH agonists will be prevented.

🔑 Key Points

- An intact hypothalamo-pituitary–ovarian axis is required for normal menstruation
- The ovary should ideally produce only one ovulatory follicle each cycle
- Pituitary–ovarian dialogue ensures selection of the dominant follicle and atresia of the remaining follicles
- Ovulation occurs 36 hours after the start of the mid-cycle LH surge
- Progesterone produced by the corpus luteum induces decidualization of the endometrium
- The embryo can only implant in the decidualized endometrium
- In the absence of pregnancy, the life span of the corpus luteum is 14 days
- Following luteolysis, steroid hormone levels fall, the endometrium dies, and menstruation occurs

References for further reading

Cameron IT, Irvine G, Norman JE. Menstruation. In: Hillier SG, Kitchener HC, Neilson JP (eds). *Scientific Essentials of Reproductive Medicine.* London: WB Saunders, 1996. 208–18.

Ferrin MJ. The menstrual cycle: an integrative view. In: Adashi EY, Rock JA, Rosenwaks Z (eds). *Reproductive Endocrinology, Surgery and Technology*, Philadelphia, USA: Lippincott–Raven, 103–22.

Speroff L, Glass RH, Kase NG. Regulation of the menstrual cycle. In: *Clinical gynecologic endocrinology and infertility.* 5th Edn. Baltimore, USA: Williams and Wilkins, 1994, 183–230.

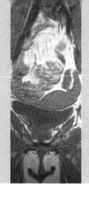

Disorders of the menstrual cycle

OVERVIEW

Menstrual disorders are very common. Over the last century a reduction in family size and the introduction and widespread acceptance of contraception and sterilisation have resulted in a significant increase in the number of menstrual periods that an individual woman will experience within her reproductive life. They are the single leading cause of referral to hospital gynaecology clinics. They can lead to major social and occupational disruption and often affect an individual's psychological wellbeing. It is essential that clinicians involved in treating women with menstrual problems do so with a compassionate and empathetic manner. They must also have a clear objective understanding of the various disorders that commonly present.

Introduction

In order to understand the various abnormalities of the menstrual cycle it is important firstly to grasp the basic concepts of normal menstrual physiology. This topic has been covered in Chapter 4.

To summarize briefly, normal menses is essentially a 'breakdown, remodelling and repair' process. The actual events that lead to endometrial breakdown are predominantly local events. These events are precipitated by a fall in steroid hormones at the end of the menstrual cycle. Local factors implicated in breakdown include lysosomes (tissue breakdown enzymes), metalloproteinases and endothelins (vasoconstrictive agents). The production of these local substances is associated with a recognizable premenstrual increase in inflammatory cells such as lymphocytes and macrophages within the endometrial stroma.

The bleeding associated with normal menses is, in fact, derived primarily from the spiral arterioles. A number of substances may have an influence on bleeding from these vessels. Oestrogen has a direct vasodilatory effect whilst progesterone has an opposing effect. Both of these sex steroids also regulate local production of prostaglandins, which are powerful vasoactive agents. (An imbalance of the ratio between these prostaglandins may be associated with heavy menstrual bleeding). Finally, fibrinolysis does occur in the endometrium and a disturbance in this process may prevent clot formation and lead to excessive bleeding.

The process of remodelling and repair of the epithelium and vascular endothelium is essential to stop menstrual flow. For this process growth factors such as vascular endothelial growth factor (VEGF) and fibroblast growth factor appear to have a major role. The levels of circulating sex steroids also influence these factors.

ABNORMAL UTERINE BLEEDING

Abnormal uterine bleeding is a descriptive term applied to any alteration in the normal pattern of menstrual flow. Table 5.1 outlines the classical terminology applied to abnormal uterine bleeding. However, from a practical point of view abnormalities in menstrual flow may take the form of:

- excessive flow;
- prolonged flow;
- intermenstrual bleeding.

Menorrhagia is one of the commonest gynaecological complaints seen in practice and accounts for approximately 12 per cent of all referrals to a general gynaecology clinic. Among women aged 16 to 45 years it has an incidence of around 30 per cent and remains the commonest indication for hysterectomy.

The average menses lasts for 3–7 days with a mean blood loss of 35 mL. Menorrhagia is generally defined as a blood loss of greater than 80 mL as women who lose this amount or more will consistently have a lower haemoglobin and haematocrit value.

However, accurate measurements of menstrual blood loss are used only as a research tool. Therefore in the clinical setting the assessment of blood loss is highly subjective. In fact it has been shown that 30 per cent of women who consider their periods to be normal actually lose more than 80 mL and 15 per cent of women consider their periods to be heavy when losing 20 mL or less.

Aetiology

Abnormal uterine bleeding can be classified as organic or non-organic. At least 50 per cent of women with menorrhagia have no identifiable pathology (i.e. non-organic). This pattern is called dysfunctional uterine bleeding (DUB).

Non-organic causes

Most cases of DUB (at least 85 per cent) are due to a failure of ovulation as a result of an alteration in neuro-endocrinological function. Therefore DUB can be further classified as anovulatory or ovulatory.

Table 5.1 – Classical nomenclature of abnormal uterine bleeding

Menorrhagia	prolonged and increased menstrual flow
Metrorrhagia	regular intermenstrual bleeding
Polymenorrhoea	menses occurring at <21 day interval
Hypermenorrhoea	excessive regular menstrual bleeding
Menometrorrhagia	prolonged menses and intermenstrual bleeding
Amenorrhoea	absence of menstruation for more than 6 months
Oligomenorrhoea	Menses at intervals of >35 days

Anovulatory

This tends to occur in women at the extremes of reproductive age and is typified by an irregular cycle. It is more common in obese women.

Ovulatory

This pattern is more common in women aged 35 to 45 years and is typified by regular heavy and often painful menstrual periods. It may be due to an inadequate production of progesterone by the corpus luteum.

Organic causes

The major organic causes of abnormal uterine bleeding include the following conditions.

Local disorders

Myomata or fibroids may cause excessive bleeding particularly when they are located below the endometrium (submucous).

Adenomyosis, which is the presence of endometrial tissue embedded within the myometrium, is a well-recognized cause of painful periods. It may also be associated with heavy menstrual bleeding.

Endocervical polyps/endometrial polyps or hyperplasia classically cause intermenstrual bleeding due to erratic and irregular shedding of the endometrium.

Intrauterine contraceptive devices (IUCD) are known to be associated with an alteration in menstrual flow in many women. Periods may become heavier and longer in duration. It is thought that IUCD insertion elevates circulating levels of plasminogen activator leading to an increase in fibrinolytic activity. Newer generation progesterone- releasing IUCDs actually reduce blood loss and may be used as a form of therapy.

Pelvic inflammatory disease (PID) may cause heavy or erratic menstrual bleeding due, predominantly, to a local endometrial inflammatory response. Severe pelvic infection may affect ovarian function and, secondarily, lead to abnormal menstrual bleeding.

Malignancy of the cervix or uterus may present with abnormal bleeding. The presence of postcoital bleeding should lead to the possibility of a cervical lesion in particular. Postmenopausal bleeding should be treated seriously as it may herald an underlying endometrial malignancy.

Hormone-producing tumours such as granulosa-theca cells of the ovary are known to be strongly associated with abnormal uterine bleeding due to their production of significant amounts of oestrogen hormone. Rarely, lesions such as lipoid-cell tumours or arrhenoblastomas elaborate amounts of oestrogens or androgens to influence menstrual flow.

Trauma to the lower genital tract should also be considered as a cause for an acute presentation of abnormal bleeding. Postcoital lacerations to the vagina can occur and in many situations a history may not be readily forthcoming. Bleeding from other sites, such as the gastrointestinal and urinary tract should also be considered.

Rarities such as arteriovenous malformations in the uterus have also been reported.

Systemic disorders

Endocrine disorders may manifest themselves as an abnormality of menstruation. The following conditions may be associated with menstrual dysfunction.
- Hyper- or hypothyroidism.
- Diabetes mellitus.
- Adrenal disease.
- Prolactin disorders.

These disorders most likely interfere with the normal feedback mechanisms that regulate the secretion of gonadotrophin-releasing hormone (GnRH) from the hypothalamus, gonadotrophins from the pituitary and sex steroids from the ovary.

Disorders of haemostasis are a significant cause of abnormal menstrual bleeding, particularly in teenagers presenting with heavy bleeding. Approximately 20 per cent of teenagers who present with this problem will have an underlying coagulopathy. Of those who require hospitilization for blood transfusion, at least 50 per cent will have a coagulopathy. Specifically, disorders such as von Willebrand's disease, idiopathic thrombocytopaenic purpura (ITP) and deficiencies of factors II, V, VII and XI are the most commonly diagnosed disorders.

Liver disorders may interfere with the metabolism of oestrogen. In addition there may be a reduced production of hepatically-derived coagulation factors.

Renal disease may alter the excretion of oestrogen and progesterone.

Medications such as steroid hormones, neuroleptics, anticoagulants and cytotoxic agents frequently lead to abnormal uterine bleeding.

Pregnancy

In women of reproductive age, the possibility of pregnancy-related bleeding must always be considered in any patient presenting with abnormal uterine bleeding. Conditions such as miscarriage, ectopic pregnancy, gestational trophoblastic disease and postpartum haemorrhage may present as a complaint related to abnormal menstruation.

Management

Diagnosis

It is important to have an efficient and systematic approach to determining the cause of abnormal uterine bleeding. The essential elements of this approach involve the following.

History

Initially this should be directed at providing a description of the pattern of abnormal menstrual bleeding as this will help to guide further evaluation. It is important to get some gauge of the severity of the bleeding pattern. Actual blood loss is highly subjective but a general impression may be gained by ascertaining how many pads or tampons a patient is using and at what frequency these are changed. The use of menstrual pictograms as illustrated in Figure

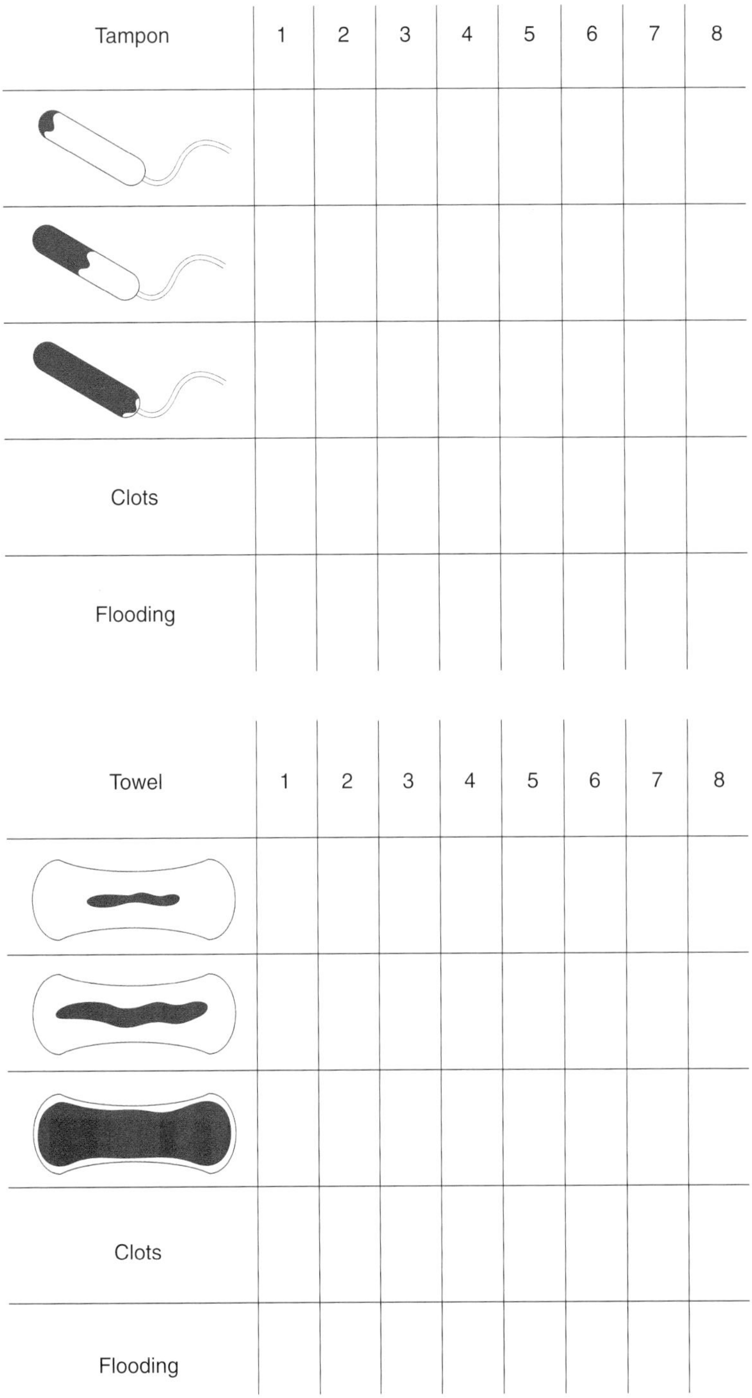

Figure 5.1 Menstrual pictogram.

5.1 may be useful in order to help quantify or compare menstrual losses. The duration of the abnormal pattern of bleeding should be determined. It is important to note the presence of other cyclical symptoms such as dysmenorrhoea, abdominal bloating, breast tenderness or any psychological disturbance. It is also useful to ask specifically for the presence of postcoital or intermenstrual bleeding, as these are potentially important markers for serious underlying pathology.

A detailed account of the patient's reproductive history covering issues such as past obstetric and gynaecological history, current and past contraceptive use, cervical smear history and sexual history are all crucial to a thorough assessment.

Clinical examination

Patients' vital signs, height and weight should be documented.

A general examination looking for stigmata of underlying systemic disease is important. It is essential to specifically look for signs of endocrine disorders: hirsutism, striae, thyroid enlargement or nodularity, skin pigment changes. An assessment of normal secondary sexual characteristics should be performed. Look for ecchymoses or petechiae, which may suggest an underlying coagulopathy. Palpation of the abdomen for liver enlargement and the presence of pelvic masses as well as palpation of regional lymph nodes should also be done routinely.

The vulval region should be examined for any external evidence of bleeding or signs of local infection. Speculum examination of vagina and cervix should routinely be performed and vaginal/cervical swabs and a cervical smear taken if clinically indicated. Bimanual palpation to assess for uterine or adnexal enlargement or tenderness is also mandatory. A rectal examination may also be necessary if bleeding from the bowel is suspected.

Laboratory investigations

There are a number of laboratory investigations that may be relevant. The patient's history and examination will guide the selection of various tests.

A full blood count is an essential investigation in a patient with abnormal bleeding.

Serum βhCG should be requested if any possibility of pregnancy exists.

Thyroid function tests.

A mid-luteal progesterone level test is performed when a patient has a regular cycle only. A level greater than 30 nmol/L is indicative of ovulation.

Serum androgens may be elevated in patients with polycystic ovarian syndrome or rarely due to adrenal conditions or androgen-producing tumours. If signs of hyperandrogenism are present then the following tests should be considered:

- testosterone;
- dihydroepiandrosterone sulphate (DHEAS);
- sex-hormone-binding globulin;
- androstendione.

Prolactin. Hyperprolactinaemia may result in anovulation, which can cause abnormal uterine bleeding. The presence of galactorrhoea should also be a warning to the possibility of an elevated prolactin level.

Coagulation screen/bleeding time is important to request if a bleeding disorder is suspected.

Renal/liver function tests should be requested if a systemic condition or malignancy is suspected.

Imaging techniques

Transvaginal ultrasound

This is an excellent tool for evaluating pelvic structures and pathology. It is useful for determining both the size and shape of the uterus and adnexal structures. For example, it will demonstrate the size and site of uterine myomata. It may be useful at identifying areas of adenomyosis and remains the gold standard method of diagnosing polycystic ovaries. Transabdominal ultrasound may be used in particular cases, especially in women who have not been sexually active.

New developments with Doppler ultrasound will provide information on pelvic vascularity while 3-D ultrasound will aid the diagnosis of congenital uterine abnormalities.

Computerized tomography/magnetic resonance imaging

These techniques are more invasive but in certain conditions will afford a greater level of detail and delineation of pelvic structures and abnormalities.

Endometrial sampling

An endometrial biospy is an integral component of evaluating abnormal uterine bleeding, particularly in women of more than 35 years of age or younger women if there has been a history of chronic anovulation. It provides a direct histological evaluation of the endometrium.

Hysteroscopically directed biopsy

This is the gold standard procedure as it provides visualization of the entire uterine cavity and allows specifically directed biopsy. Traditionally, dilatation and curettage has been performed. However, when this is combined with hysteroscopy the accuracy of the diagnostic process is improved. Hysteroscopy is ideally performed during the proliferative phase of the menstrual cycle when the endometrium is at its thinnest.

Aspiration techniques

There are a variety of out-patient aspiration techniques that can be used for endometrial sampling. The main principal being that these provide a rapid screening test. It is important to note their limitations in that the sample obtained may not be representative of the endometrium as a whole. It is reasonable to have a low threshold for proceeding to hysteroscopy with persistent abnormal bleeding in light of a 'normal' aspiration endometrial sample.

Treatment

In the acute situation the main priorities of treatment involve:
- resuscitation;
- correction of anaemia;
- arresting ongoing bleeding.

As previously noted, the majority of women with abnormal bleeding have no identifiable pathology, i.e. DUB. However, this should be a diagnosis of exclusion and a full evaluation of the patient for pathologic causes should be performed prior to longer-term treatment being instituted.

In most circumstances patients will present with mild to moderate levels of bleeding in an out-patient setting. Treatment options available include both medical and surgical modalities. A full discussion of treatment options should be entered into with each patient. In general, particularly with DUB, medical options should be considered first before surgery is contemplated.

Medical therapies

Hormonal treatments

Progestagens are mainly indicated in patients with anovulatory bleeding, to reverse the effects of oestrogen-mediated endometrial proliferation and induce endometrial maturation. They can be used in an acute situation to halt heavy menstrual bleeding (usually oral medroxyprogesterone, 10 mg given daily for ten days). When used cyclically for 21 days per cycle they have been shown to reduce mean blood loss by 15–30 per cent. They appear to have a minimal role in ovulatory bleeding.

Combined oral contraceptives are often prescribed, particularly for younger patients who also require contraception. Despite widespread use there is very little data available demonstrating an effective role in reducing menstrual blood flow.

Danazol is a derivative of testosterone that acts on the hypothalamus–pituitary–ovarian axis and on the endometrium itself. It is a competitive inhibitor of the sex steroids to their individual receptors. It is an effective treatment for heavy menstrual bleeding and may reduce blood loss by up to 60 per cent. Androgenic side effects, such as weight gain, hirsutism, acne and voice changes, may make it unacceptable to many patients.

GnRH analogues such as buserelin, naferelin or goserelin may be used in selected cases. They effectively induce a medical menopause by suppressing gonadotrophin output from the pituitary. They should not be prescribed for longer than six months (even with oestrogen 'add-back' therapy) because of the risk of osteoporosis.

Hormone replacement therapy (HRT) may be useful in controlling heavy menstrual bleeding in women who are perimenopausal.

Levenorgestral-releasing IUCDs are very effective at controlling heavy menstrual bleeding. Blood volume reductions of up to 80 per cent have been reported with this device. Progestagen released directly from the coil appears to act locally on the endometrium. Current devices are active for up to seven years.

Antifibrinolytics

Tranexamic acid acts on the premise that fibrinolytic activity is significantly increased in women with heavy menstrual periods. As much as an 80 per cent reduction in menstrual flow may be achieved in some patients. It is prescribed during menstruation only and is often effective in the acute situation. It is contraindicated in patients who have a history of thromboembolism and those who have reduced levels of antithrombin III.

Ethamsylate is not widely used but is thought to reduce blood loss by increasing capillary wall strength as well as exhibiting an antifibrinolytic effect. It is also taken only during menstruation.

Antiprostaglandins (non-steroidal anti-inflammatory drugs, NSAIDs)

Mefenamic acid is the most widely used antiprostaglandin for women with heavy or painful periods. Antiprostaglandins act by inhibiting the enzyme cyclo-oxygenase thereby reducing local prostaglandin levels. There is ample evidence demonstrating that women with excessive menstrual bleeding have higher levels of prostaglandin E2 and prostaglandin F2α. The exact mechanism by which these elevated levels of prostaglandins cause excessive bleeding remains unclear. Antiprostaglandins may reduce menstrual flow by as much as 30 per cent. They are also beneficial in reducing dysmenorrhoea a common accompaniment to heavy menstrual bleeding. They are taken only during menstruation and are contraindicated in patients with a history of peptic or gastric ulceration.

Surgical therapies

Surgical treatment is usually reserved for patients in whom medical treatments have failed. Occasionally surgical treatment is indicated in the acute situation. Dilatation and curettage in an acute situation can reduce haemorrhage in 75–80 per cent of cases.

Below is a list of surgical treatment options available. Approximately 20–40 per cent of patients with abnormal uterine bleeding will ultimately require some form of surgical intervention.

Endometrial resection and ablation

This procedure involves the resection or ablation of the endometrium so that a layer of fibrous tissue replaces it. It has been used for women with refractory dysfunctional bleeding and in patients with submucous fibroids. Techniques used include diathermy, laser, radiofrequency-induced ablation and thermal balloon ablation. The primary advantages of these procedures are:

- it may be performed as a day case procedure;
- there is a shorter operating time (30–45 minutes average duration);
- there are fewer postoperative complications compared to hysterectomy.

Approximately 20–40 per cent of patients who undergo this procedure will continue to experience some menstrual bleeding, albeit reduced. In around 20–30 per cent of patients there is no improvement in their bleeding pattern.

Optimal treatment results are achieved when the following criteria are met.

- Patients older than 35 years – there appears to be higher recurrence rates for bleeding (approximately 10 per cent recurrence rate per year) than when the procedure is performed in younger women.
- DUB – although it can be used to resect small submucous fibroids.
- Uterus less than 10 weeks in size – poor results achieved when fibroids are present or uterine cavity is greater than 10 cm.
- Best performed during proliferative phase of cycle or after pretreatment with danazol or a progestagen. Pretreatment is usually instituted six weeks prior to surgery.
- No endometriosis or adenomyosis are present.

In addition, it is also a recommendation that endometrial histology is evaluated prior to surgery in order to exclude the possibility of atypical endometrial hyperplasia or, indeed, carcinoma. Seeding of endometrial carcinoma following resection has been reported.

Myomectomy

This procedure involves the surgical removal of fibroids from the uterus. It is generally indicated in patients who have symptomatic uterine fibroids who wish to retain their fertility. There is approximately a 15 per cent risk of hysterectomy during the procedure due to intractable bleeding.

Hysterectomy

This is generally reserved as a final treatment option for patients who have not responded to medical therapy or to more conservative surgical options. Within the UK the lifetime risk for a woman undergoing hysterectomy is approximately 20 per cent. In situations where significant pathology is present then hysterectomy may be considered as an earlier treatment option. In all situations fully informed consent from the patient must be gained before proceeding to hysterectomy. In general however studies would indicate that satisfaction rates for the judicious use of hysterectomy are very high.

There are a variety of hysterectomy techniques available including:

- total abdominal hysterectomy;
- subtotal hysterectomy (involves preservation of the cervix);

- vaginal hysterectomy;
- laparoscopic-assisted vaginal hysterectomy.

Patients also need to be counselled about possible oophorectomy during hysterectomy. This is no longer routinely advocated but should be considered in the following situations.
- There is co-existant ovarian pathology.
- There exists a family history of ovarian, breast or bowel cancer.
- The patient is over 45 years of age and is close to the menopause or there are associated menopausal symptoms.
- There is a history of severe pelvic pain.
- The patient has severe premenstrual syndrome.

If oophorectomy is performed then postoperative HRT should also be discussed with the patient.

Recent developments

There have been some recent developments in surgical treatment modalities. Predominantly these relate to less invasive methods of treating symptomatic uterine fibroids. Both laparoscopic myolysis and embolization techniques have been reported to be successful modes of treatment.

Post menopausal bleeding

Although not strictly a disorder of the menstrual cycle any discussion of abnormal uterine bleeding would not be complete without including Post Menopausal Bleeding (PMB). As an entity any bleeding after the menopause should be viewed as abnormal essentially until proven otherwise.

In the majority of cases, atrophic vaginitis is responsible. This results from a loss of structural integrity within the vagina secondary to the hypoestrogenic state characteristic of the post menopause.

However it is important to consider the following pathological causes:
- *Endometrial Hyperplasia* – found in around 15% of cases of PMB
- *Endometrial Polyps* – occur in up to 10% of women with PMB
- *Endometrial Malignancy* – may be present in 7–10% of women with PMB
- *Cervical Malignancy* – peak incidence occurs in 5th and 6th decades. May present with post-

menopausal bleeding, often with an offensive blood stained discharge.
- *Uterine Sarcoma* – although very uncommon they may present with postmenopausal bleeding.

The common association of endometrial carcinoma with PMB deserves special consideration. There are a number of risk factors where endometrial pathology is likely to be more prevalent:
- *Age* – the association of endometrial carcinoma and PMB increases with age so that 60% of women in their 80's with PMB will have endometrial carcinoma.
- *Nulliparity* – is associated with a higher lifetime risk of endometrial carcinoma.
- *Obesity* – adipose tissue increases the amount of circulating endogenous oestrogens.
- *PCOS* – a history of chronic anovulation with prolonged endometrial exposure to oestrogens increases the risk of endometrial malignancy.
- *Unopposed oestrogen exposure* – although now uncommon, the injudicious use of oestrogen replacement therapy without progesterone can lead to endometrial hyperplasia and carcinomatous change.
- *Tamoxifen* – used as adjunctive therapy for breast cancer but can lead to endometrial hyperplasia or malignancy. Patients taking tamoxifen should have a regular gynaecological assessment.
- *Oestrogen producing tumours* – such as Granulosa cell tumours.
- *Glandular cells on cervical smear* – approximately 5% of post menopausal women with normal endometrial cells on a cervical pap smear will have underlying endometrial carcinoma.
- *Past medical history* – conditions such as diabetes, hypertension, previous cancer of the breast, colon or ovary are more likely to indicate a pathologic cause for PMB.

Management

The basic premise is that an underlying pathology needs exclusion in all cases of PMB. In most cases endometrial sampling will be required.

An initial thorough examination looking for signs of systemic disease is extremely important. Pelvic examination should include an evaluation of the oestrogenic state of the vagina and cervix. Characteristic findings include a pale and thin appearance of the vaginal mucosa often with a loss of the normal rugae. A cervical smear is a routine component of the investigation of PMB. High vaginal swabs should be taken if discharge is present.

The use of ultrasound as an initial step at investigation has some advantages. It is less invasive, sensitive, cheaper and allows visualisation of other pelvic structures. An endometrial thickness of 4 mm or more is used to identify those cases that require further investigation. It is particularly useful in older patients who are less likely to tolerate more invasive investigations.

However, those patients who have persistent bleeding or have a detectable abnormality on ultrasound require endometrial sampling.

Outpatient aspiration techniques can be used but hysteroscopically directed biopsy should be performed if bleeding continues despite a normal aspiration sample.

Treatment will be directed at the underlying aetiology. If the investigation reveals no underlying pathology then hypoestrogenic atrophic changes are the most likely cause and can be treated with systemic or local hormonal replacement. Any detected pathology requires appropriate treatment.

AMENORRHOEA

Amenorrhoea is defined as the absence of menstruation. It may be classified as either primary or secondary amenorrhoea. There are, of course, physiological situations where amenorrhoea is normal, namely pregnancy, lactation and prior to the onset of puberty.

- Primary amenorrhoea – This condition relates to females who fail to develop secondary sexual characteristics by 14 years of age or who fail to menstruate by 16 years of age.
- Secondary amenorrhoea – This is defined as the cessation of menstruation for more than six months in a normal female of reproductive age that is not due to pregnancy.

Aetiology

A useful method of classifying the various causes of amenorrhoea is to group them as follows.

- Reproductive outflow tract abnormalities.
- Ovarian disorders.
- Pituitary disorders.
- Hypothalamic disorders.
- Miscellaneous endocrine disorders.

Reproductive outflow tract abnormalities

Müllerian agenesis

This results from a congenital absence of vagina or uterus or both. It is called the Mayer-Rokitansky-Küster-Huaser syndrome and affects approximately 1 in 4000 females. Ovarian function is usually normal. Diagnosis may be suspected by the absence of vagina and uterus on perineal and rectal examination and confirmed by ultrasound examination. Associated renal abnormalities are not uncommon.

Transverse vaginal septum

This results from an embryological failure of the lower third of the vagina to canalize. In most cases the rest of the genital tract is normal. Occurrence is much less frequent compared to Müllerian agenesis. Ultrasound is usually crucial in determining this diagnosis by demonstrating a normal uterus, ovaries and the presence or absence of a septum.

Androgen insensitivity (testicular feminization)

These patients have a congenital defect of androgen receptors despite normal circulating levels of testosterone. They have an XY karyotype but because of an absent response to testosterone they develop female external genitalia. They lack a uterus and have an absent or blind vagina. The gonads in such patients need excision as they carry a 20 per cent risk of malignancy.

Imperforate hymen

This results from an absent orifice in the vaginal hymen, which remains asymptomatic until puberty. Classical presentation is of a bulging haematocolpos at the hymenal ring in conjunction with a history of cyclical symptoms.

Cervical stenosis

This is a rare condition but may be found after cervical surgery, radiation therapy or following chronic cervical infection.

Asherman's syndrome

This refers to the presence of intrauterine adhesions that can occur following overvigorous uterine curettage or infection.

Ovarian disorders

Anovulation

Chronic anovulation may result in menstrual irregularity or amenorrhoea. Polycystic ovarian syndrome is the most common cause but it may arise from a variety of other endocrine disorders including hyperprolactinaemia.

Gonadal dysgenesis

Gonadal dysgenesis usually results in bilateral rudimentary gonads leading to primary amenorrhoea, sexual infantilism and elevated gonadotrophin levels. There are a variety of chromosomal disorders that can produce this condition, e.g. Turner's syndrome (45 XO and mosaic forms). Pure gonadal dysgenesis which have a normal 46 XX karyotype but with streak gonads and no secondary sexual development. Swyers syndrome is rare and is most likely the result of a loss of germ cells early in fetal life. The gonads in these patients also have malignant potential and require excision prior to puberty.

Premature ovarian failure

This is defined by the onset of menopausal symptoms and elevated gonadotrophin levels before the age of 40 years. Generally the cause is unknown but in other circumstances may result from irradiation, chemotherapy or an autoimmune process.

Resistant ovary syndrome

This occurs when elevated gonadotrophin levels occur despite the presence of viable follicles within the ovary. It is believed to result from a defect in the LH/FSH receptor complex. In most cases it is a temporary condition.

Pituitary disorders

Pituitary adenomas

These include in particular prolactinomas, which cause hyperprolactinaemia. This may result in an impaired pulsatile secretion of gonadotrophins and, as a consequence, amenorrhoea or oligomenorrhoea. Although most are microadenomas, some are larger macroadenomas which may cause visual symptoms due to compression of the optic chiasm. Hyperprolactinaemia is the primary cause of amenorrhoea in 20 per cent of cases.

Pituitary insufficiency

This is essentially a failure of the pituitary to secrete gonadotrophins. In females the most common cause is a result of severe obstetric haemorrhage causing necrosis of the pituitary (Sheehan's syndrome).

Hypothalamic disorders

Functional hypogonadotrophic hypogonadism

Essentially a variety of conditions may lead to a reduction in gonadotrophin secretion mediated by the hypothalamus.

Exercise: Menstrual irregularities are common in competitive athletes. It is known that a minimum of 17 per cent body fat by weight is required for the initiation of menarche and around 20 per cent is required to maintain menses. In addition, the stress of performance and increased levels of circulating endorphins can reduce GnRH production from the hypothalamus.

Stress: Emotionally stressful events such as those involved with work, relationships, death or illness of a close family member, or travel may cause amenorrhoea.

Weight loss: Considerable weight loss to or below 15–20 per cent of ideal body weight are often associated with menstrual disturbance or amenorrhoea. Anorexia nervosa is an extreme form of this condition.

Pseudocyesis: Or false pregnancy is an interesting condition of unknown aetiology. It appears to be a voluntary alteration of hypothalamic function in women desirous of pregnancy. Interestingly there are often elevated levels of prolactin (often enough to cause galactorrhoea) and LH.

Drug-induced amenorrhoea: This may occur with the use of drugs such as Depo-Provera, danazol, GnRH agonists and some neuroleptic medications. Approximately 1 per cent of women discontinuing the combined oral contraceptive pill will experience a period of 'postpill amenorrhoea'.

The aetiology is unknown but is more common in women who take the pill continuously without a regular pill-free period. In most cases menses resumes within 3–6 months.

Nonfunctional hypogonadotrophic hypogonadism

Space-occupying lesions: The hypothalamus may be partially or completely destroyed by lesions such as craniopharyngiomas, tuberculosis or sarcoidosis. In addition they may be associated with focal neurologic symptoms.

Kallmann's syndrome: A congenital disorder characterized by primary amenorrhoea, infantile sexual development and anosmia.

Miscellaneous endocrine disorders

There are a number of other endocrine conditions that may present with amenorrhoea:
- Hypothyroidism: TSH is usually elevated which results in an elevated prolactin level;
- Cushing's syndrome: Increased adrenal activity leads to a hyperandrogenic state.

Management

History

A detailed history is essential to formulate a correct diagnosis in a patient with amenorrhoea. It is necessary to consider the possibility of pregnancy as a cause for amenorrhoea as this is the leading cause of secondary amenorrhoea. Obviously whether the patient presents with primary or secondary amenorrhoea will guide the history taking to a certain extent.

Particular points of note related to a diagnosis of primary amenorrhoea are:
- developmental history;
- presence or absence of cyclical symptoms;
- history of chronic illness;
- excessive weight loss/presence of an eating disorder;
- excessive exercise;
- history or family history of anosmia.

In addition historical factors that may be important for a diagnosis of secondary amenorrhoea are:

- age of onset of menarche;
- menstrual/contraceptive and reproductive history;
- past medical and surgical history;
- presence of menopausal symptoms;
- current medications;
- family history of premature menopause;
- development of any virilizing signs or galactorrhoea;
- psychological history;
- recent stressful events (past or present history of depression or an eating disorder).

Examination

In addition to a general examination particular emphasis should be placed on the following areas of clinical examination.
- Height – an abnormality in appropriate height for age may reflect an underlying chromosomal disorder (patients with Turner's syndrome are often short, whereas patients with androgen insensitivity are often tall).
- Development of secondary sexual characteristics or any evidence of abnormal virilization.
- Visual field disturbance or papilloedema may imply a pituitary lesion.
- Pelvic examination is essential as this may detect a structural outflow abnormality. An examination under anaesthesia may be required to help identify such abnormalities. Also look for evidence of atrophic effects of hypo-oestrogenism within the lower genital tract.

Investigations

Depending on the history and examination the following investigations may be indicated.
- Serum βhCG – to exclude possible pregnancy.
- Prolactin – a useful test particularly in secondary amenorrhoea as, excluding pregnancy, hyperprolactinaemia is the leading cause of amenorrhoea.
- Thyroid function tests – these should be performed in all patients with amenorrhoea.
- Gonadotrophin – elevated levels will confirm premature ovarian failure. Reduced levels indicate a pituitary (primary pituitary hypogonadism is rare) or hypothalamic disorder (functional or non-functional). GnRH stimulation tests may be

helpful in distinguishing between a pituitary and hypothalamic cause.

- Androgen profile – hyperandrogenism can cause amenorrhoea most commonly associated with polycystic ovarian syndrome. Rarely adrenal disorders or androgen-secreting tumours may be the cause.
- Karyotype – indicated in women with primary amenorrhoea and in women less than 30 years of age who present with premature ovarian failure.
- Autoimmune screen – indicated in women with premature ovarian failure. Ovarian auto-antibodies are found in a small number of women.
- Imaging – ultrasound or CT/MRI scanning may be useful in determining complex structural abnormalities of the pelvic organs or for identifying intracranial lesions.

Treatment

The treatment of a patient with amenorrhoea is specific to the diagnosis.

Medical therapy

Premature ovarian failure is managed as for the menopause. In most circumstances this will involve commencing HRT in order to prevent deleterious sequelae as a result of oestrogen withdrawal.

Anovulation may be managed by cyclic progestagens or by oral contraceptive. In patients desiring pregnancy, ovulation induction agents such as clomiphene or gonadotrophins may be used.

Hyperprolactinaemia responds well to the use of dopamine agonists such as bromocriptine.

Pituitary insufficiency can be managed by replacing target organ hormones as well as HRT as for a menopausal patient.

Hypogonadotrophic hypogonadism is also managed with cyclic HRT. Patients are generally responsive to pulsatile GnRH therapy when pregnancy is desired.

Surgical therapy

Outflow tract disorders: Patients with vaginal agenesis can undergo formation of a functional neo-vagina. A transverse vaginal septum or imperforate hymen will require excision.

Dysgenetic gonads: Patients will require these gonads to be removed because of the high incidence of malignancy.

Pituitary macroadenomas: Very rarely a macroadenoma is unresponsive to medical therapy and may require excision.

POLYCYSTIC OVARIAN SYNDROME

As an entity the polycystic ovarian syndrome (PCOS) deserves special consideration. Although first described in 1935 by Stein and Leventhal, with recent improvements in diagnosis it is now recognized as the most common cause of hyperandrogenic chronic anovulation. It often presents with menstrual disturbance in the form of oligo-amenorrhoea or anovulatory dysfunctional uterine bleeding.

Approximately 25 per cent of women in the UK will have ultrasound evidence of polycystic ovaries (PCO). However, not all of these women will have symptoms that constitute PCOS. In addition not all women with clinical features of PCOS will have ultrasound evidence of PCO. Figures 5.2 and 5.3 show the typical gross and ultrasound appearances of polycystic ovaries respectively.

Aetiology

The fundamental pathophysiological process underlying PCOS remains uncertain. However, increasing evidence points toward the role of both insulin hypersecretion and insulin resistance which are now recognized to be common features of PCOS, particularly in women who are overweight or have an associated menstrual disturbance. It is most likely that this insulin hypersecretion is responsible for the excessive androgen secretion from the ovary that is another feature of the syndrome. More recent evidence also points towards a genetic link among families with PCOS, possibly with variable levels of expression.

Diagnosis

There are a number of investigations useful to confirm a diagnosis of PCOS. The characteristic features of the ovaries seen on transvaginal ultrasound are:

- ten or more peripheral cysts of between 2–8 mm in diameter ('string of pearls' sign);
- increased ovarian stromal volume to >8 cm^3.

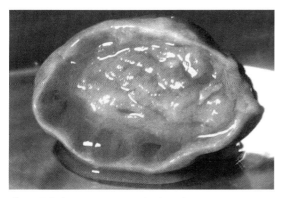

Figure 5.2 Gross appearance of polycystic ovary. (Photograph courtesy of Dr H Mason.)

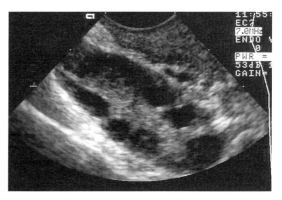

Figure 5.3 Ultrasound appearance of polycystic ovary. (Image courtesy of Dr P Sladkevicius.)

S Symptoms

The typical clinical features of a patient with PCOS are:

- Oligo-amenorrhoea: occurs in up to 80 per cent of patients with PCOS and is predominantly related to chronic anovulation
- Hyperandrogenism: patients may commonly present with hirsutism, acne and occasionally male pattern baldness
- Subfertility: PCOS is the commonest cause of anovulatory subfertility
- Obesity: at least 40 per cent of patients with PCOS are clinically obese. In addition, obese women with PCOS tend to be more symptomatic and weight loss can lead to significant improvements
- Recurrent miscarriage: PCOS is seen in around 50–60 per cent of cases of women with more than three early pregnancy losses

Laboratory investigations
The following blood tests are useful to aid diagnosis.

- LH:FSH ratio – normally 1:1 but in PCOS is often 2–3:1.
- Androgen – typically testosterone and androstenedione are elevated but it is not a universal finding. In addition there is a poor correlation between extent of hyperandrogenic features and serum levels of androgens. Sex-hormone-binding globulin levels may be reduced particularly in obese women with PCOS. This leads to elevated levels of active androgens.
- Insulin – serum levels may be elevated. In fact around 40 per cent of women with PCOS have a degree of glucose intolerance.

Management

The aims of treatment will largely depend on the main complaint of the individual patient. In the future it is most likely that treatment options will focus on treating the more causal elements of the condition, i.e hyperinsulinaemia.

Weight loss
In obese patients with PCOS significant improvements in symptoms can be achieved with a reduction in bodyweight. Regular menses and ovulation may return.

Menstrual disturbance
Menstrual disturbance can be managed with cyclic progestagens or a combined oral contraceptive pill for a limited period of time.

Hirsutism/acne
The primary aims of treatment are to reduce androgen levels, increase sex-hormone-binding globulin levels or reduce the activity of 5α-reductase enzyme at the level of the hair follicle. These methods of treatment may cause erratic bleeding so it is common practice to prescribe with an oral contraceptive to regulate bleeding. Options include:

- cyproterone acetate: an anti-androgen which competitively inhibits the androgen receptor;
- spironolactone: an anti-androgen and an anti-aldosterone diuretic;
- finasteride: a 5α-reductase enzyme inhibitor;
- cosmetic therapies such as waxing and bleaching should also be encouraged.

Subfertility

Ovulation may be induced using anti-oestrogens (clomiphene or tamoxifen) or gonadotrophins. Treatment should be monitored to avoid higher order multiple gestations.

Hyperinsulinaemia

Newer forms of therapy are aimed at reducing the elevated insulin levels seen in many patients with PCOS. Studies using the antidiabetic medication Metformin have shown encouraging results particularly in obese patients with chronic anovulation.

It is also essential that the patient is aware of the longer-term health implications of PCOS. Those with hyperinsulinaemia are at significant risk of developing type II diabetes and gestational diabetes during pregnancy. The hyperandrogenic state that is characteristic of PCOS places individuals at higher risk of arterial disease. These patients tend to be prone to hypertension and often have abnormal lipid profiles. In addition, patients with chronic anovulation are at risk of endometrial hyperplasia and carcinoma resulting from prolonged unopposed oestrogen stimulation.

DYSMENORRHOEA

Dysmenorrhoea is defined simply as painful menstruation. It is a very common complaint with at least 50 per cent of postmenarchal women experiencing some degree of dysmenorrhoea. In at least 10 per cent of women it is of such severity that it interferes with daily activities. Classification of dysmenorrhoea is either primary or secondary.

Primary dysmenorrhoea

This refers to the presence of painful menses where there is no underlying pathology that can account for the pain. There are a number of factors that may have an aetiological role in the presence of primary dysmenorrhoea.

Endocrine

By definition, ovulatory cycles are necessary for the development of primary dysmenorrhoea. This implicates a role for cyclic oestrogen and progesterone

and is backed up by the fact that oral contraceptives may alleviate dysmenorrhoea to some degree.

Abnormal uterine activity

Studies have shown that women with primary dysmenorrhoea have an elevated resting uterine tone or pressure. This may be mediated by increased prostaglandin levels or elevated levels of vasopressin. In addition, the pain is often improved with the use of antiprostaglandins.

Psychological

Although unlikely to be a primary cause of dysmenorrhoea, psychological factors may influence individual perception to painful stimuli.

Diagnosis

Primary dysmenorrhoea usually begins just prior to, or during menses and lasts for the duration of flow only. It is usually described as 'crampy' in nature and is most intense in the suprapubic region. It may occur in conjunction with other symptoms such as nausea, fatigue and headache.

Diagnosis is usually based on the history and normal findings on clinical examination. Further invasive tests are only indicated if there is a strong suspicion of underlying pathology (secondary dysmenorrhoea).

Management

A sympathetic approach to the patient, including consideration of psychological and behavioural elements, will enhance the likelihood of a positive outcome for the patient.

Currently there are two pharmacological treatments that are widely used for treating primary dysmenorrhoea.

- Oral contraceptives: these act by inhibiting ovulation and in doing so tend to reduce menstrual prostaglandin levels via a reduction in endometrial growth. At least 90 per cent of patients experience significant relief of symptoms.
- Antiprostaglandins (NSAIDs): these act via their suppression of menstrual fluid prostaglandins. They are usually taken only during the first few days of menstruation and may be used in conjunction with oral contraceptives.

Patients who remain unresponsive to medical therapy should be investigated further for a pathological cause. In general, laparoscopy is the diagnostic procedure of choice. In rare circumstances ablation of the uterine nerve or a presacral neurectomy may provide long-term relief in patients resistant to drug therapy.

Secondary dysmenorrhoea

Secondary dysmenorrhoea occurs in the presence of an identifiable pathologic cause. It is more common in older women and often the pain is more severe prior to menstruation. It may also be associated with uterine retroversion and is usually due to one of the following conditions.

Endometriosis
Endometriosis is the presence of functioning endometrium outside the uterine cavity. It is commonly associated with dysmenorrhoea, the severity of which is often not related to the extent of the disease. Other common features are dyspareunia and menorrhagia. Aetiology remains uncertain but theories include retrograde menstruation and metaplasia of coelomic epithelium. It appears that genetic and immune factors may also be important.

Adenomyosis
Adenomyosis is the presence of endometrium embedded within the myometrium. It is a difficult diagnosis to confirm although ultrasound and MRI may show typically diagnostic images in severe disease. At least one-third of hysterectomy specimens show evidence of adenomyosis. It is classically associated with severe dysmenorrhoea.

Pelvic inflammatory disease
This may be associated with dysmenorrhoea.

Intrauterine adhesions (Asherman's syndrome)
Intrauterine adhesions can develop after uterine instrumentation or infection.

Cervical stenosis
Narrowing of the endocervical canal may result from conization of chronic infection. Painful menses is a common association with this condition.

Management

Secondary dysmenorrhoea is easily diagnosed from the history. However, the underlying cause may not be readily identified from clinical examination.

Important investigations that may help identify the cause are:
- laparoscopy: generally the single most useful diagnostic procedure that can also provide an opportunity to treat certain conditions;
- pelvic ultrasound: this will show ovarian endometriosis and demonstrate fixity of the ovaries in pelvic inflammatory disease;
- hysterosalpingogram: useful at identifying intrauterine adhesions;
- microbiological cultures: from endocervix, from the peritoneal fluid if pelvic inflammatory disease is suspected.

Treatment of secondary dysmenorrhoea is generally aimed at the underlying cause. Supportive measures with analgesics in a similar manner to that used in primary dysmenorrhoea may also be used. Effective treatment for endometriosis may involve hormonal treatment or surgery. In patients with intractable dysmenorrhoea, hysterectomy (often with bilateral oophorectomy) may be the ultimate end result.

PREMENSTRUAL SYNDROME

Premenstrual syndrome (PMS) is defined as the cyclical presence of somatic, psychological and emotional symptoms that worsen as menses approaches and are ameliorated by the onset of menstrual flow. Nearly all women with regular cycles do experience some form of symptomatology in the premenstrual phase but in around 5 per cent of women these are severe and debilitating.

There have been many theories as to the exact aetiology of PMS. Most recent theories favour a relationship between variations in levels of ovarian sex steroids and changes in serotonin levels within the central nervous system.

The variety of symptoms that may be associated with PMS is broad. In fact, more than 150 different symptoms have been linked to PMS.

S Symptoms of PMS

The most common are:
- Bloating
- Cyclic weight gain
- Mastalgia
- Abdominal cramps
- Fatigue
- Headache
- Depression
- Irritability

Diagnosis

By definition PMS is a clinical diagnosis. In order to confirm the diagnosis there are a number of criteria that need to be met.
- Symptoms are cyclic and occur only during the luteal phase.

- Symptoms increase in severity as the cycle progresses.
- Symptoms are relieved with the onset of menses and are absent by day 3 of flow.
- There must be a postmenstrual symptom-free period of at least seven days.
- Symptoms must be present for at least three consecutive cycles.
- Symptoms should be of a severity to interfere with daily activities.

It is important that PMS is distinguished from any underlying psychiatric condition, such as depression. By using a symptoms chart in a prospective fashion the diagnosis may become more apparent.

Treatment

Many pharmacological preparations have been used for the treatment of PMS but very few have been tested by appropriate clinical trials. Vitamin B6 (pyridoxine)

CASE HISTORY

Ms J S

20-year-old nursing student presents with a five-year history of irregular periods and worsening facial hair.

Menarche aged 14 years, cycle always irregular, usually only 5–6 periods per year. Not currently using any contraception. Mother had hysterectomy aged 39 years for 'heavy periods'. Father has non-insulin-dependent diabetes. No other history of note.

Clinical examination reveals a BMI of 36. Blood pressure = 110/65, moderate degree of facial hirsutism and prominent facial acne. Abdominal and pelvic examination were normal.

Discussion
What is the most likely diagnosis?
Given the history of irregular menstrual periods and presence of hyperandrogenic symptoms (hirsutism and acne) the most likely diagnosis would be polycystic ovarian syndrome.

What investigations would help confirm the diagnosis?
Transvaginal ultrasound may demonstrate the classical appearances of polycystic ovaries, i.e. multiple peripheral ovarian cysts and increased ovarian stromal volume.

A blood test for gonadotrophins may show an elevated LH:FSH ratio. Levels of serum androgens may be elevated

and sex hormone binding globulin (SHBG) may be reduced. Insulin levels may also be elevated.

What treatment options should be discussed with the patient?
The patient should be encouraged to lose weight as symptoms may improve with weight loss alone.

The patient's menstrual irregularity may be controlled with either cyclic progestagens or the combined oral contraceptive pill. The addition of an anti-androgen may help control the hyperandrogenic features. The patient should be advised that an improvement in hirsutism might not be seen for several months. If the patient has hyperinsulinaemia then the use of an insulin-lowering medication can be discussed.

What other health issues should be discussed with the patient?
The patient should be counselled regarding the long-term health implications of polycystic ovarian syndrome. She should be informed of her increased risk of diabetes and coronary heart disease. In addition, the long-term effects of chronic anovulation on the endometrium and fertility issues (see Chapter 7) also need to be discussed.

is widely prescribed but its efficacy and safety have not been adequately studied. Therapies that have been shown to improve symptoms in many patients include:

- psychotherapy involving both behavioural and cognitive methods;
- suppression of ovulation using oral contraceptives, danazol, GnRH analogues;
- selective serotonin reuptake inhibitors, i.e. fluoxetine.

In addition, factors such as diet modification, exercise or stress relaxation techniques may improve many individual symptoms. In situations where PMS is refractory to pharmacological treatment, hysterectomy with oophorectomy may be considered as a last option and is generally curative.

References for further reading

Shaw RW, Soutter WP, Stanton SL, (eds). *Gynaecology*. Edinburgh: Churchill Livingstone,1992.

Jacobs AJ, Gast MJ, (eds). *Practical Gynaecology*. Norwalk, Connecticut: Appleton and Lange,1994.

Johnson MH, Everitt BJ, (eds). *Essential Reproduction*. Cambridge: Blackwell,1988.

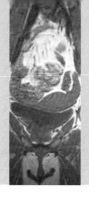

Fertility control

OVERVIEW

During the last two or three decades both professional and public attitudes towards fertility control have changed, and a significant proportion of gynaecological practice is now concerned with problems of contraception.

The ideal method of contraception would be reliable, inexpensive, easy to use and safe. When an individual has decided that they no longer wish to conceive then permanent and voluntary sterilization may be appropriate. When contraception is not used, or fails, then some women may consider termination of pregnancy, either medical or surgical.

Contraception

Men and women have used contraception, in one form or another, for thousands of years. There is no one method that will suit everyone and individuals may use different types of contraception at different stages in their lives. The characteristics of the ideal contraceptive are listed below.

- Highly effective.
- No side effects.
- Independent of intercourse.
- Rapidly reversible.
- Cheap.
- Widespread availability.
- Acceptable to all cultures and religions.
- Administration by healthcare personnel not required.
- Easily distributed.

There is enormous variation in uptake and usage of contraceptive techniques in different countries worldwide. Over 95 per cent of women in the UK who do not want to become pregnant will use contraception and current usage in the UK is detailed in Table 6.1. Some couples may use more than one method at the same time, such as taking the oral contraceptive pill in conjunction with using condoms. Some contraceptives can be prescribed only by a doctor whilst others can be used without ever having to seek medical advice.

All contraceptives will fail occasionally and some are much more effective than others. Failure rates are traditionally expressed as the number of failures per 100 women years (HWY), i.e. the number of pregnancies one would expect to occur if 100 women were to use the method for one year. Failure rates reported for some methods vary considerably, largely because of the potential for failure caused by

Table 6.1 – Current use of contraception in the UK

Method of contraception	% usage
Combined oral contraceptive pill	36
Condoms	25
Vasectomy	16
Female sterilization	10
IUDs	6
Diaphragms	2
Natural family planning	1.5

Classification

Hormonal contraception	Barrier methods
Combined oral contraceptive pills	Condoms
	Female barriers
Progestogen-only preparations	Coitus interruptus
Progestogen-only pills	Natural family planning
Injectables	Emergency contraception
Subdermal implants	
Intrauterine devices (IUDs)	Sterilization
Conventional IUDs	Female sterilization
Hormone-releasing intrauterine systems	Vasectomy

imperfect use (user failure) rather than an intrinsic failure of the method itself. The failure rates of contraceptive methods are listed in Table 6.2.

HORMONAL CONTRACEPTION

Combined oral contraceptive pills

The combined oral contraceptive pill (COC) or 'the pill' was first licensed in the UK in 1961. It contains a combination of two hormones: a synthetic oestrogen and a progestogen (a synthetic derivative of progesterone). Since COC was first introduced, the dose of both oestrogen and progestogen has been reduced dramatically and this has considerably improved its safety profile. It is estimated that at least 200 million women worldwide have taken COC since it was first developed and that there are currently around 3 million users in the UK alone.

COC is easy to use and offers a very high degree of protection against pregnancy with many other beneficial effects. It is used mainly by young, healthy women who wish to use a method of contraception that is independent of intercourse.

Formulations

There are many different formulations and brands of COC (Fig. 6.1). Most modern preparations contain the oestrogen ethinyl oestradiol in a daily dose of between 20–35 mg. However, those containing lower dosages are associated with slightly poorer cycle control. Pills containing a higher daily dosage of oestrogen, e.g. 50 mg ethinyl oestradiol are generally only now prescribed in the special situations discussed below. Higher dosages of oestrogen are strongly linked to an increased risk of both arterial and venous thrombosis (see below). Current COCs con-

Table 6.2 – Failure rates of contraceptive methods

Contraceptive method	Failure rate per 100 women years
Combined oral contraceptive pill	0.1–1
Progestogen-only pill	1–3
Depo Provera	0.1–2
Norplant	0.2–1
Copper-bearing IUD	1–2
Levonorgestrel-releasing IUD	0.5
Male condom	2–5

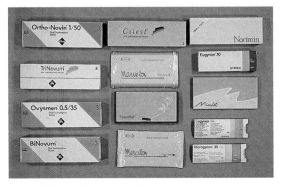

Figure 6.1 Combined oral contraceptive pill preparations

Contraindications to COC

Absolute contraindications

- circulatory diseases:
  - ischaemic heart disease
  - cerebro-vascular accident
  - significant hypertension
  - arterial or venous thrombosis
  - any acquired or inherited prothrombotic tendency
  - any significant risk factors for CV disease
- acute or severe liver disease
- oestrogen-dependent neoplasms particularly breast cancer
- focal migraine

Relative contraindications

- generalized migraine
- long-term immobilization
- irregular vaginal bleeding
- less severe risk factors for CV disease, e.g. obesity, heavy smoking, diabetes

tain progestogens that are classed as second or third generation. Commonly prescribed formulations are listed in Table 6.3.

Monophasic pills contain a standard daily dosage of both oestrogen and progestogen. Biphasic and triphasic pills have two or three incremental variations in hormone dose. Current thinking is that biphasic and triphasic preparations are more complicated for women to use and have few real advantages.

Most brands of COC in the UK contain 21 pills. One pill is taken daily, followed by a seven-day pill-free interval. There are also some every day (ED) preparations that include seven placebo pills that are taken instead of having a pill-free interval. For maximum effectiveness, COC should always be taken regularly at roughly the same time each day.

Mode of action

COC acts both centrally and peripherally.
- Inhibition of ovulation is by far the most important effect. Both the oestrogen and progestogen suppress the release of pituitary FSH and LH, which prevents follicular development within the ovary and therefore ovulation.
- Peripheral effects include making the endometrium atrophic and hostile to an

implanting embryo and altering cervical mucus to prevent sperm ascending into the uterine cavity.

Contraindications

There are lengthy lists of both absolute and relative contraindications to COC. The most important contraindications are summarized in the box. Most of these can be worked out quite logically and are mainly related to the side effects of sex steroid hormones on the cardiovascular and hepatic systems. Women should ideally discontinue COC at least two months before any pelvic or leg surgery.

Side effects
The vast majority of women tolerate COC well with few problems. However, a number of potential side effects exist, the most important relating to cardiovascular disease. Other side effects are listed in Table 6.4. Many minor side effects will settle within a few months of starting COC.

Venous thromboembolism
Oestrogens alter blood clotting and coagulation in a way that induces a pro-thrombotic tendency, although the exact mechanism of this is poorly understood. The higher the dose of oestrogen, the greater the risk of venous thromboembolism (VTE). Recent data suggest that the type of progestogen also affects the risk of VTE with users of COC containing third generation progestogens being twice as likely to sustain a VTE.

Table 6.3 – Hormonal content of commonly used monophasic COC preparations

Oestrogens	Progestogens
Ethinyl oestradiol: 20, 30, 35 and 50 mg	2nd generation: Norethisterone acetate 0.5, 1.0 and 1.5 mg Levonorgestrel 0.15, 0.25 mg
Mestranol 50 mg	3rd generation: Gestodene 0.075 mg Desogestrel 0.15 mg Norgestimate 0.25 mg

The risks of VTE are:

- 5 per 100,000 for normal population;
- 15 per 100,000 for users of second generation COC;
- 30 per 100,000 for users of third generation COC;
- 60 per 100,000 for pregnant women.

Arterial disease

The risk of myocardial infarction and thrombotic stroke in young, healthy women using low-dose COC is extremely small. Cigarette smoking will however increase the risk and any woman who smokes must be advised to stop COC at the age of 35 years. Around 1 per cent of women taking COC will become significantly hypertensive and they should be advised to cease taking COC.

Breast cancer

Advising women on the association between breast cancer and COC is very difficult. A recent large review of all the data did show a slight increase in the risk of developing breast cancer among current COC users (relative risk of 1.24). This is not of great significance to young women as the background rate of breast cancer is very low at their age. However for a woman in her 40s these are more relevent data as the background rate of breast cancer is higher. The same review also showed that beyond ten years after stopping COC there was no increase in breast cancer risk for former COC users.

Drug interaction

This can occur with enzyme-inducing agents such as some anti-epileptic drugs. Higher dose oestrogen pills containing 50 mg ethinyl oestradiol may need to be prescribed (see Table 6.3). Some broad-spectrum antibiotics can alter intestinal absorption of COC and reduce efficacy. Additional contraceptive measures should therefore be recommended during antibiotic therapy and for one week thereafter.

Positive health benefits of COC

Not all side effects are undesirable. Users of COC generally have light, pain-free, regular bleeds and therefore COC can be used to treat heavy or painful periods. It will also improve pre-menstrual syndrome (PMS) and reduce the risk of pelvic inflammatory disease. COC offers long-term protection against both ovarian and endometrial cancers. It can also be used as treatment for acne.

Table 6.4 – Other potential side effects of COC

System	Side effect
Central nervous system	depression
	headaches
	loss of libido
Gastrointestinal system	nausea and vomiting
	weight gain
	bloatedness
	gall stones
	cholestatic jaundice
Genitourinary system	cystitis
	irregular bleeding
	vaginal discharge
	growth of fibroids
Breast	breast pain
Miscellaneous	chloasma (facial pigmentation)
	leg cramps

Patient management

For a woman to take COC successfully there must be careful teaching and explanation of the method, supplemented by information leaflets. Before the pill is prescribed, a detailed past medical and family history should be taken and blood pressure checked (Fig. 6.3). Routine weighing, breast and pelvic examination are not mandatory and should not be forced on a young woman requesting COC. Most women are given a three-month supply of COC in the first instance and six-monthly reviews thereafter. Women need clear advice about what to do in the event of missing pills (Fig. 6.2).

Progestogen-only contraception

All other types of hormonal contraception in current use are progestogen-only and share many similar features in terms of mode of action and side effects. Because they do not contain oestrogen, they are extremely safe and can be used if a woman has cardiovascular risk factors. The dose of progestogen within them varies from very low to high.

Current methods of progestogen-only contraception are:

- progestogen-only pill or 'mini-pill';

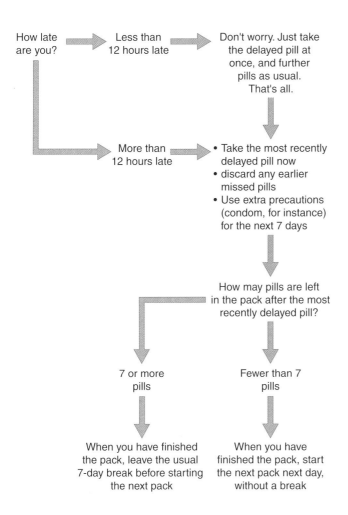

How late are you?

→ Less than 12 hours late → Don't worry. Just take the delayed pill at once, and further pills as usual. That's all.

→ More than 12 hours late →
• Take the most recently delayed pill now
• discard any earlier missed pills
• Use extra precautions (condom, for instance) for the next 7 days

How may pills are left in the pack after the most recently delayed pill?

7 or more pills

Fewer than 7 pills

When you have finished the pack, leave the usual 7-day break before starting the next pack

When you have finished the pack, start the next pack next day, without a break

Figure 6.2 Management of missed pills (algorithm). Reproduced with permission from Handbook of Family Planning and Reproductive Health Care 3rd Edition Eds Loudon N, Glasier A, Gebbie A. Churchill Livingstone.

• injectable;
• subdermal implant 'Norplant';
• hormone-releasing intrauterine system (see IUDs).

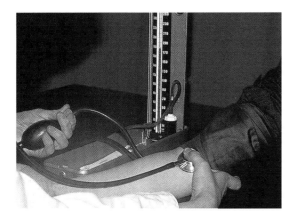

Figure 6.3 Monitoring blood pressure in women taking COC.

All progestogen-only methods work by a local effect on cervical mucus, making it hostile to ascending sperm, and on the endometrium, making it thin and atrophic thereby preventing implantation and sperm transport. Higher dose progestogen-only methods will also act centrally and inhibit ovulation.

Common side effects of progestogen-only methods:
• erratic or absent menstrual bleeding;
• functional ovarian cysts;
• breast tenderness;
• acne.

Progestogen-only pills (POP)

The POP is ideal for women who like the convenience of the pill but cannot take COC. Although the failure rate of POP is greater than that of COC (see Table 6.2), it is ideal for women at times of lower fertility. If the POP fails, there is a slightly higher risk of ectopic pregnancy. There is a small selection of brands on the market (Fig. 6.4) and all contain the second generation progestogens, norethisterone or norgestrel (or their derivatives). The POP is taken every day without a break.

Particular indications for POP:
- breastfeeding;
- older women;
- presence of cardiovascular risk factors;
- diabetes.

Injectable progestogens

Two injectable progestogens are marketed:
1 Depot medroxyprogesterone acetate 150 mg (Depo Provera);
2 Norethisterone enanthate 200 mg.

Most women choose Depo Provera and each injection lasts around 12 13 weeks. Norethisterone enanthate only lasts for eight weeks and is not nearly so widely used.

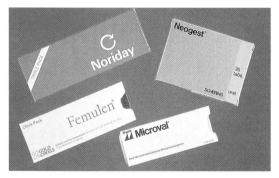

Figure 6.4 Progestogen-only pill preparations.

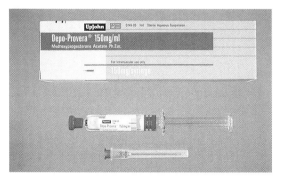

Figure 6.5 Injection of Depo Provera.

Depo Provera is a highly effective method of contraception and is given by deep intramuscular injection (Fig. 6.5). Most women who use it develop very light or absent menstrual bleeding and it can be used to treat menstrual problems.

Particular indications for Depo Provera are difficulty in remembering to take a pill, painful periods or PMS.

Particular side effects of Depo Provera include:
- weight gain of around 6 lb in the first year;
- delay in return of fertility – it may take about six months longer to conceive than after stopping COC;
- persistent menstrual irregularity;
- very long-term use may slightly increase the risk of osteoporosis (because of low oestrogen levels).

Subdermal implants

Norplant has been available in the UK since 1993. It consists of six silastic rods inserted subdermally in the upper arm, which release the progestogen levonogestrel, and lasts for five years (Fig. 6.6). Insertion and removal of Norplant must be done by a trained healthcare professional. It is extremely effective but is relatively expensive. Although Norplant was very popular when it was first introduced, many women have not been happy with the menstrual pattern and other side effects and it has now been withdrawn.

Intrauterine contraception

Modern intrauterine devices (IUDs) are highly effective contraceptives but are not widely used in the UK. Fitting of an IUD should be carried out by trained

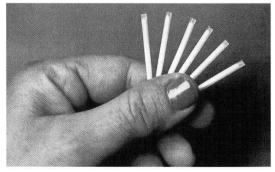

Figure 6.6 Norplant.

healthcare personnel only and is a brief procedure associated with minimal discomfort. A fine thread is left protruding from the cervix into the vagina and the IUD can be removed in due course by traction on this thread. An IUD is ideal for women who want a long-term method of contraception independent of intercourse and where regular compliance is not required. IUDs protect against both intrauterine and ectopic pregnancy, however, if pregnancy does occurs, there is a higher chance than normal that it will be ectopic.

Types

Original IUDs were large plastic inert devices (Lippes Loop or Saf-T coil) which often caused heavy and painful menstrual periods (Fig. 6.7). These are no longer available although some women may still have them *in situ*. Once fitted, they could be left in place until the menopause.

Most women nowadays will use the smaller copper-bearing IUDs that are available in various shapes and sizes (Fig. 6.8). They cause much less menstrual disruption than the older plastic devices. Most copper-bearing IUDs are licensed for 3–5 years of use but many will last longer, possibly up to 10 years. The more copper a device has, the more effective it is, and some IUDs have silver-cored copper for added efficacy.

Hormone-releasing IUDs are also available (Fig. 6.9). The relatively new levonorgestrel-releasing intrauterine system (IUS) has the advantages (and disadvantages) of both hormonal and intrauterine contraception (Table 6.5). It is associated with a dramatic reduction in menstrual blood loss and although currently licensed for contraception only, many women request an IUS to help improve heavy periods alone.

Mode of action

All IUDs induce an inflammatory response in the endometrium that prevents implantation. However, copper-bearing IUDs work primarily by a toxic effect on sperm that prevents fertilization. The hormone-releasing IUS prevents pregnancy by a local hormone effect on the cervical mucus and endometrium.

Although IUDs increase the risk of pelvic inflammatory disease (PID) during the first few

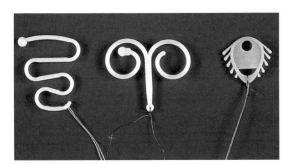

Figure 6.7 Plastic intrauterine devices: Lippes loop, Saf-T coil, Dalkon shield.

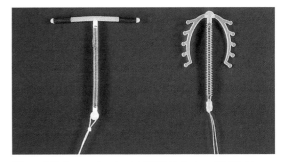

Figure 6.8 Copper-bearing intrauterine devices: Multiload, Copper T 380.

Table 6.5 – Levonorgestrel-releasing IUS

Advantages	Disadvantages
Highly effective Dramatic reduction in menstrual blood loss Protection against PID	Persistent spotting and irregular bleeding in the first few months of use Progestogenic side effects, e.g. acne, breast tenderness

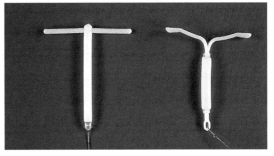

Figure 6.9 Hormone-releasing intrauterine devices: Progestogen-releasing IUD, levonorgestrel-releasing IUD.

IUDs

Contraindications to IUDs
- previous pelvic inflammatory disease
- previous ectopic pregnancy
- known malformation of the uterus
- copper allergy (would be suitable instead for hormone-releasing IUS)

Side effects of IUDs
- increased menstrual blood loss
- increased dysmenorrhoea
- increased risk of pelvic infection following insertion

weeks after insertion, the long-term risk is the same as for women using no method of contraception at all. In a mutually monogamous relationship, an IUD user has no increased risk of PID. If an IUD user has a partner with a sexually transmitted infection, such as chlamydia or gonorrhoea, the IUD will not protect against these infections in contrast to condoms or hormonal methods, which do.

BARRIER METHODS OF CONTRACEPTION

Condoms

Male condoms are usually made of latex rubber, pre-lubricated with spermicide. They are cheap and are widely available for purchase or are even free from many clinics. They have been heavily promoted in the Safe Sex campaign to prevent spread of sexually transmitted diseases particularly HIV and AIDS. Condoms of varying sizes are now available. It is important to use condoms that reach British Standards Institute requirements and are within their 'sell-by' date. Couples using condoms should be aware of the availability of emergency contraception in the event of a condom bursting or slipping off during intercourse. Some men and women may be allergic to latex condoms or spermicide and hypoallergenic latex condoms and plastic male condoms are now available. Men must be instructed to put on condoms before any genital contact and to withdraw the erect penis from the vagina immediately after ejaculation.

Female barriers

The diaphragm, or Dutch cap, is the female barrier used most commonly in the UK. Other female barriers include vault caps, vimules and cervical caps. They should all be used in conjunction with a spermicidal cream or gel. Diaphragms are inserted prior to intercourse and should be removed no earlier than six hours later. Effective use of a diaphragm involves careful fitting and teaching. Female barriers offer protection against ascending pelvic infection but can increase risk of urinary tract infection and vaginal irritation.

Female condoms made of plastic are also available. They offer particularly good protection against infection as they cover the whole of the vulva and vagina and, being plastic, are less likely to burst. Many couples however, find them unaesthetic and they have not achieved widespread popularity.

Coitus interruptus

Coitus interruptus, or withdrawal, is widely practised and obviously does not require any medical supervision. It involves removal of the penis from the vagina immediately before ejaculation takes place. Unfortunately, it is not reliable as pre-ejaculatory secretions may contain millions of sperm and young men often find it hard to judge timing of withdrawal. Use of emergency contraception should be considered if coitus interruptus has taken place (see below).

Natural family planning

This is an extremely important method of contraception worldwide and may be the only one acceptable to some couples because of cultural and religious reasons. It requires abstinence from intercourse during the fertile period of the month.

The fertile period is calculated by various techniques such as:
- changes in basal body temperature;
- changes in cervical mucus;
- changes in the cervix;
- multiple indices.

Some commercially available kits are now available, such as Persona, and use quite complex technology to define fertile periods when abstinence is required. The failure rates of natural methods of family planning are quite high, largely because couples find it difficult to abstain from intercourse when required.

The lactational amenorrhoea method (LAM) is when fully breastfeeding mothers who are amenorrhoeic rely on this alone for contraception. During the first six months after birth, full breastfeeding gives over 98 per cent contraceptive protection.

Emergency contraception

The terms 'morning-after pill' or postcoital contraception have now been replaced simply by the term 'emergency contraception' (EC). EC is used after intercourse has taken place and before implantation has occurred. There is considerable interest in increasing provision and uptake of EC particularly among young women as it is thought to have significant potential in the reduction of unplanned pregnancies. EC should be considered if unprotected intercourse has occurred, if there has been failure of a barrier method, e.g. a burst condom or if a COC has been forgotten. There are two types of emergency contraception in general usage.

Hormonal emergency contraception

A combination of 100 mg ethinyl oestradiol and 500 mg levonorgestrel is taken twice, the two doses being 12 hours apart and started within 72 hours of unprotected intercourse. Nausea and vomiting are common side effects and there are very few contraindications to its use. Hormonal EC is not 100 per cent effective but will prevent three-quarters of pregnancies that would otherwise have occurred. It is currently a prescription-only medicine but there are proposals to make it available over the counter in the UK. The mechanism of action is believed to be prevention of implantation due to endometrial shedding.

An IUD for emergency contraception

A copper-bearing IUD can be inserted for EC. It is effective up to five days following the anticipated day of ovulation and can be used to cover multiple episodes of intercourse. The IUD prevents implantation and the copper ions exert an embryotoxic effect. The normal contraindications to an IUD apply and if there is a risk of sexually transmitted infection, antibiotic cover should be given.

STERILIZATION

Female sterilization and male vasectomy are permanent methods of contraception. They are generally chosen by relatively older individuals who are sure that they have completed their families. Occasionally, individuals who have no children or who, for example, carry a genetic disorder may choose to be sterilized. The uptake of female sterilization and vasectomy in the UK is relatively high compared to many other European countries with around 50 per cent of couples over the age of 40 relying on one partner being sterilized. Both female sterilization and vasectomy can technically be reversed with subsequent pregnancy rates of up to 60 per cent, but reversals are not available on the NHS in many parts of the UK.

Consent

It is of vital importance that individuals are very carefully counselled before sterilization and give written consent to having the procedure performed. Nowadays, most consent forms do not ask for the partner's written consent. The consent form should clearly indicate that sterilization is a permanent procedure but also acknowledge that occasionally it can fail. Failure of female sterilization and vasectomy is a major area of medical litigation.

Female sterilization

This involves the mechanical blockage of both Fallopian tubes to prevent sperm reaching and fertilizing the oocyte (Fig. 6.10). Sterilization can also be achieved by hysterectomy or total removal of both Fallopian tubes. Female sterilization should not alter the menstrual pattern per se but if a woman stops the combined pill to be sterilized, she may find her subsequent menstrual periods heavier. Alternatively, if she had an IUD removed at the time of sterilization, she may find her subsequent menstrual periods are lighter.

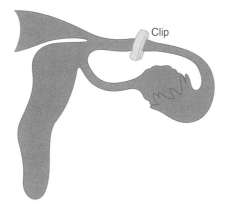

Figure 6.10 Female sterilization.

Sterilization in the UK is most commonly performed by laparoscopy under general anaesthesia, which enables women to be admitted to hospital as a day-case. Alternative techniques are mini-laparotomy with a small transverse supra-pubic incision or through the posterior vaginal fornix (colpotomy). Mini-laparotomy is the technique of choice when the procedure is done postnatally (the uterus is enlarged and more vascular) and in developing countries where laparoscopic equipment is not available. Different ways of occluding the Fallopian tubes are described in Table 6.6.

Complications of female sterilization

Very occasionally, a woman may experience anaesthetic problems or there may be damage to intra-abdominal organs during the procedure. Sometimes,

it is not possible to visualize the pelvic organs at laparoscopy due to adhesions or obesity. It may then be necessary to proceed to mini-laparotomy.

Female sterilization is highly effective. Ectopic pregnancy can be a late complication and any sterilized woman who misses her period and has symptoms of pregnancy should seek immediate medical advice.

Vasectomy

Vasectomy involves the division of the vas deferens on each side to prevent the release of sperm during ejaculation (Fig. 6.11). It is technically an easier,

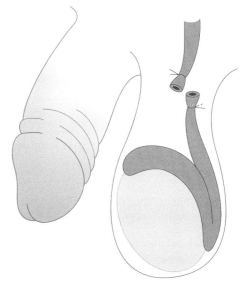

Figure 6.11 Vasectomy.

Table 6.6 – Techniques of female sterilization

Technique of tubal occlusion	Special features
Ligation	used at postpartum mini-laparotomy
Electrocautery /diathermy	may damage surrounding structures, e.g. bowel, bladder, blood vessels
	relatively higher late failure rate
Falope rings	easy to apply
	damages 2–3 cm of tube thereby making subsequent reversal more difficult
Clips	technique of choice
	small and simple to use
	occasionally may not occlude whole of the Fallopian tube
Laser	not widely used
	very expensive technique

more straightforward and quicker procedure than female sterilization and is usually performed under local anaesthesia. Various techniques exist to block the vas and their effectiveness is related primarily to the skill and experience of the operator (Table 6.7).

Vasectomy differs from female sterilization in that it is not effective immediately. Sperm will still be present higher in the genital tract and azoospermia is therefore achieved more quickly if there is frequent ejaculation. Men should be advised to hand in a sample of semen after 12 weeks and then 16 weeks to check for the presence of sperm. If two consecutive samples are free of sperm then the vasectomy can be considered complete. An alternative form of contraception must be used until that time.

Complications

Immediate complications such as wound infection, bleeding and haematoma may occur. Occasionally small lumps appear at the cut ends of the vas as a result of a local inflammatory response. These so-called 'sperm granulomas' may need surgical excision. Some men develop antisperm antibodies following vasectomy. These do not cause symptoms but if the vasectomy is reversed, pregnancy may not occur because the autoantibodies inactivate sperm.

Concerns have been raised about a possible association between vasectomy and the development of both prostatic and testicular cancer. Although this issue has received widespread media interest, there is currently insufficient evidence to support it.

Table 6.7 – Vasectomy techniques

Techniques	Special considerations
Ligation or clips Unipolar diathermy	most common techniques
Excision	allows histological confirmation
No-scalpel vasectomy	widely used in China special instruments used which puncture the skin low incidence of complications
Silicone plugs/ sclerosing agents	also used in China avoids a skin incision

ABORTION

For centuries, women have attempted to end unwanted pregnancies by a variety of methods and illegal abortion has been the source of considerable morbidity and mortality. Abortion is a subject that attracts very strong opinions and there is a widespread divergence of views on the subject mainly relating to religious and cultural background.

The UK Abortion Act was passed in 1967. It allowed the lawful termination of pregnancy under certain criteria, which are very widely interpreted. As a result, illegal abortion in the UK has virtually disappeared. Under the terms of the 1967 Abortion Act, a woman may have a pregnancy terminated if two medical practitioners acting in good faith are willing to certify to one or more of the following criteria.

- The continuance of the pregnancy would involve risk to the life of the pregnant woman greater than if the pregnancy were terminated.
- The termination is necessary to prevent grave permanent injury to the physical or mental health of the pregnant woman.
- The pregnancy has not exceeded its 24th week and that the continuance of the pregnancy would involve risk, greater than if the pregnancy were terminated, of injury to the physical or mental health of the pregnant woman.
- The pregnancy has not exceeded its 24th week and that the continuance of the pregnancy would involve risk, greater than if the pregnancy were terminated, of injury to the physical or mental health of any existing child(ren) of the family of the pregnant woman.
- There is a substantial risk that if the child were born it would suffer from such physical or mental abnormalities as to be seriously handicapped.

The form must be signed by both medical practitioners prior to the abortion being performed and posted to the Chief Medical Officer of the Department of Health, or of the Scottish Office (Fig. 6.12). If the abortion is undertaken in order to save a woman's life then only one signature is required.

Any medical practitioner who has an objection to abortion is not required to participate in abortion services unless the treatment is necessary to save the life of the pregnant woman. However, a medical practitioner who conscientiously objects to abortion

IN CONFIDENCE   Certificate A

Not to be destroyed within three
years of the date of the operation

ABORTION ACT 1967
Certificate to be completed in relation to an abortion
under Section 1(1) of the Act

I   ....
        (Name and qualifications of practitioner : in Block Capitals)

of   ....

        ....
        (Full address of practitioner)

Have/have not* seen/examined* the pregnant woman to whom this certificate relates at

*(*delete as
appropriate)*

        ....

        ....
        (Full address of place at which patient was seen or examined)

on   ....

and I ....
        (Name and qualifications of practitioner : in Block Capitals)

of   ....

        ....
        (Full address of practitioner)

Have/have not* seen/and examined* the pregnant woman to whom this certificate relates at

        ....

        ....
        (Full address of place at which patient was seen or examined)

on   ....

We hereby certify that we are of the opinion, formed in good faith, that in the case of

        ....
        (Full name of pregnant woman : in Block Capitals)

of   ....

        ....
        (Usual place of residence of pregnant woman : in Block Capitals)

☐ A   the continuance of the pregnancy would involve risk to the life of the pregnant woman greater than if
        the pregnancy were terminated.

☐ B   the termination is necessary to prevent grave permanent injury to the physical or mental health of the
        pregnant woman.

*Tick
appropriate
box*

☐ C   the pregnancy has NOT exceeded its 24th week and that the continuance of the pregnancy would
        involve risk, greater than if the pregnancy were terminated, of injury to the physical or mental health
        of the pregnant woman.

☐ D   the pregnancy has NOT exceeded its 24th week and that the continuance of the pregnancy would
        involve risk, greater than if the pregnancy were terminated, of injury to the physical or mental health
        of the existing child(ren) of the family of the pregnant woman.

☐ E   there is a substantial risk that if the child were born it would suffer from such physical or mental
        abnormalities as to be seriously handicapped.

This certificate of opinion is given before the commencement of treatment for the termination of pregnancy
to which it refers.

Signed   ....   Date   ....

Signed   ....   Date   ....

Figure 6.12 UK Abortion Act form.

should still be prepared to refer a woman seeking abortion to a colleague who would be willing to consider her request sympathetically and arrange termination if appropriate.

Incidence of legal abortion

Approximately 190,000 abortions are carried out each year in England, Wales and Scotland. Abortion is only permitted in Northern Ireland when it is undertaken to save the life of the pregnant woman. The current abortion rate is around 9–14 per 1000 women aged 15–45 years which represents a lifetime chance of abortion of around 1 in 40. The number of abortions undertaken in the UK includes women who travel from other countries where abortion is illegal, particularly from the Republic of Ireland. The UK has a significantly lower abortion rate than the US but it is still considerably higher than some western European countries such as The Netherlands.

Provision of abortion services

In the UK, abortions are carried out within NHS hospitals, in private hospitals and clinics run by charitable organizations. Many NHS regions have set up abortion services to allow rapid referral and the efficient management of women seeking abortion with dedicated units, staffed by individuals who are particularly sensitive and sympathetic. It is particularly important that women seeking abortion should not be subject to unnecessary delays in their referral as increasing gestation increases the risks and complexity of the abortion procedure.

Assessment and counselling

Prior to an abortion, a woman should have:
- Confirmation of the pregnancy by a pregnancy test.
- Assessment of the gestation – the date of the last menstrual period should be documented. Abdominal and pelvic examination should be performed. If the gestation is uncertain, refer for ultrasound scan.
- Infection screen – all women should be screened for *Chlamydia*. Consider the need for further STD screening (including HIV and Hepatitis B) if the woman has a vaginal discharge, is a rape victim or in a high-risk category.
- Haemoglobin and blood grouping – give anti-D at the time of the procedure if Rhesus negative.
- Cervical smear if this is due.
- Medical history to determine if there is any contraindication to surgery or anaesthetic or a history of allergies or drug reactions.

Pre-abortion counselling is extremely important. It should be non-judgemental and offer adequate information and explanation to allow the woman to make an informed choice. Obtaining the partner's consent should be encouraged but is not mandatory. The following areas should be discussed in the counselling process:
- Alternatives to abortion – continuing the pregnancy and either keeping the baby or having it adopted.
- The way in which the abortion will be carried out.
- The risks of the procedure.
- Her relationship with the partner and his attitude to the pregnancy.
- Ensuring adequate support for the woman both before and after the abortion
- Offer of post-termination support counselling.
- Contraception after the abortion.
- Arrangements for follow-up.

Abortion techniques

The technique of inducing abortion is determined primarily by gestation. Newer methods now allow women the choice of either a surgical or medical procedure when the pregnancy is under 9 weeks' gestation. Ideally, an abortion should always be performed at the earliest possible gestation as both morbidity and mortality rates rise with increasing gestation. The risk of death from an early surgical termination of pregnancy is less than 1 per 100,000, which is lower than the maternal mortality associated with a full-term pregnancy.

1st Trimester

Surgical

The contents of the uterus are removed by suction using a small catheter inserted through the cervix and attached to an electrical pump. A general anaesthetic is generally given. Dilatation of the cervix is required to allow the catheter to pass into the uterine cavity and the greater the gestation of the pregnancy, the greater the amount of dilatation necessary. Priming of the cervix with agents such as prostaglandin (given three hours prior to surgery) reduces risk of cervical trauma and haemorrhage.

Surgical abortions under 6 weeks' gestation have a higher failure rate and the procedure should probably not be performed until the woman has reached 6 weeks' gestation.

Medical

The discovery in 1980 of the antiprogestogenic agent, mifepristone or RU 486 has made early medical

abortion possible. The action of RU 486 blocks progestogen receptors in the uterus and as a result induces abortion. RU 486 on its own will only induce complete abortion in around 60 per cent of women although when given in combination with prostaglandin, the rate of complete abortion increases to over 95 per cent. The commonly used schedule is 600 mg of oral RU 486 followed 48 hours later by insertion of 1 mg gemeprost vaginal pessary. Lower dose regimens may be equally effective. The woman stays in hospital for 4–6 hours after insertion of the pessary during which time most women will abort the pregnancy. Medical and surgical methods of early termination are compared in Table 6.8.

Mid-trimester (14 weeks)

Although only around 10–15 per cent of all abortions in the UK are done at this stage, mid-trimester abortions are associated with many more complications. Major fetal abnormality detected on ultrasound may necessitate a termination even beyond 24 weeks. Not infrequently, women who present for abortion at later gestations are the very young, or older women who attribute amenorrhoea to being menopausal.

Surgical

Surgical techniques involve dilatation of the cervix and evacuation of the uterus (D&E) under general anaesthetic. D&E is widely used in North America and although often preferred by women this

Table 6.8 – Early medical and surgical abortion

	Surgical	Medical
Anaesthesia /analgesia	usually general anaesthetic	oral or IM analgesia may be required
Average blood loss	80 mL	80 mL
Completeness	95%	95%
Number of visits required for procedure	1	2
Availability in the UK	widespread	regional variation so may not be available locally
Contraindications	nil	asthma, cardiac disease, adrenocortico-insufficiency
Patient preference	equal	equal
Reason for choice	unaware of events	in control of situation
Gestation	up to 14 weeks	up to 9 weeks

procedure is generally disliked by many members of staff as fetal parts may have to be removed piecemeal from the uterus.

Medical

Most mid-trimester terminations in the UK involve the pre-treatment administration of RU 486 followed 36 hours later by vaginal prostaglandin pessaries. A gemeprost pessary is inserted into the vagina every 3–6 hours until the fetus is aborted. Opiate analgesia is usually required and around 10 per cent of women will need a subsequent surgical evacuation of the uterus. Older techniques involved the intra-amniotic injection of urea or hypertonic saline combined with intravenous infusions of oxytocin or prostaglandins. These older methods were relatively inefficient and it often took women many days to abort. Use of the current combination of RU 486 and vaginal prostaglandins has significantly shortened the time taken to abort the pregnancy to around 6–8 hours.

Complications

Incomplete abortion

Placental and/or fetal tissue may remain in the uterus after both medical and surgical abortion. Many women will pass the remaining tissue spontaneously but surgical evacuation of the uterus may be required if there is heavy bleeding or the cervix is still dilated. Very occasionally, the entire gestational sac remains within the uterus after an abortion technique and the pregnancy is still ongoing.

Infection and infertility

Pelvic infection following an abortion will present with a febrile illness, offensive vaginal discharge, lower abdominal pain and tenderness of the pelvic organs on vaginal examination. Antibiotic therapy should be instituted as soon as possible. Postabortion infection may cause tubal damage and subsequent infertility. With modern abortion techniques and screening for pelvic infections such as *Chlamydia* and gonorrhoea in high-risk women, the risk of subsequent infertility is very low.

Traumatic injuries

Risk of trauma to the genital tract during an abortion is minimal where there is a high standard of gynaecological practice. During surgical abortion, perforation of the uterus can occur or there may be damage to the cervix, which can predispose to the risk of pre-term labour in subsequent pregnancies (cervical incompetence).

Psychological problems

These can be minimized if the woman has been well counselled prior to the abortion. Many women feel quite emotionally vulnerable in the following weeks although for most it is an enormous relief to have the ordeal over. It is quite normal for women to experience feelings of regret and guilt after an abortion although there is no evidence of a subsequent increase in serious psychiatric disease. Many abortion units will offer a post-termination support service to which women may refer themselves in the months and even years following an abortion.

Follow-up

All women who have had an abortion should be seen for follow-up around two weeks later. As most hospitals do not arrange follow-up visits, this should be done in the general practice setting or Family Planning Clinic. This visit is essential to:

- ensure that the abortion is complete;
- exclude an ongoing pregnancy – the woman should always be examined vaginally;
- check for possible pelvic infection;
- offer advice on contraception and sexual health;
- assess the woman's emotional state.

Contraception

Ovulation may occur within a few weeks of an abortion. It is therefore very important that contraception is instituted as soon as possible to avoid the chance of a further unplanned pregnancy.

The COC, POP or Depo Provera should be started on the day of the abortion. An IUD can be inserted at that time or preferably at the follow-up visit. Barrier methods of contraception can be used immediately although it may be necessary to refit a new size of diaphragm. Female sterilization is usually performed 6–8 weeks after an abortion as it has a higher failure rate when undertaken at the time of surgical abortion.

New developments

Contraception for women
- Hormonal transdermal patches and vaginal rings
- Contraceptive vaccines (anti-HCG, anti-zona pellucida)
- Once a month pill (RU 486)
- Emergency contraception with progestogen only

Contraception for men
- Contraceptive vaccines (anti-sperm)
- Long-acting testosterone preparations

CASE HISTORY

Miss X
Aged 19 years, single
Smokes 20 cigarettes per day

Miss X recently had an abortion having conceived following a burst condom. She tried the combined pill a few years ago but kept forgetting to take it. She is not in a regular relationship but has had several recent partners.
Her past medical history includes migraine and severe pre-menstrual syndrome. Her mother had a deep vein thrombosis during pregnancy.

Discussion
As compliance seems to be an important issue here, the injectable progestogen Depo Provera would be very suitable. It will not trigger migraine and may well help her pre-menstrual syndrome. Miss X should be warned about the possibility of irregular bleeding and slight weight gain with Depo. When she has a new sexual partner, she should be advised to use condoms in combination with Depo Provera for personal protection against sexually transmitted infections.

She could also consider restarting the COC in combination with condoms. Prior to this, she should have a thrombophilia screen performed in view of her mother's history of venous thrombo-embolism.

If she decides to continue with condoms alone, she must be given information about use and availability of emergency contraception in case another condom bursts.

Key Points

- There has been a significant rise in the use of contraception worldwide over the last 40 years
- The combined oral contraceptive pill is a method primarily used by young, healthy women and it is estimated that there are around 3 million current users in the UK
- Progestogen-only contraception can be used by women with cardiovascular disease and is ideal for breastfeeding or older women
- The modern copper-bearing intrauterine devices are highly effective and their main mode of action is a toxic effect on the gametes
- Condoms should always be recommended in new relationships for personal protection against sexually transmitted infections
- Natural family planning is an extremely important method worldwide and, for cultural or religious reasons, may be the only method acceptable to some couples
- Emergency contraception can prevent unplanned pregnancy and there is considerable current interest in making it more available and accessible particularly to teenagers
- Before sterilization, men and women should give written consent to the procedure, which states that they are aware it is permanent and also that it has a very small failure rate
- Vasectomy is generally an easier, quicker and safer procedure than female sterilization and is usually performed under local anaesthetic

- Provision of abortion service varies but many regions in the UK have dedicated abortion units allowing for the rapid referral and specialist care of women seeking termination of pregnancy
- Women under 9 weeks' gestation will have the choice of having either a medical or surgical termination procedure in many regions of the UK
- The morbidity and mortality associated with legal abortion is very low but complication rates rise as gestation of the pregnancy increases

References for further reading

Loudon N, Glasier A, Gebbie A (eds). *The Handbook of Family Planning*, 3rd Edition. Churchill Livingstone, 1995.

Guillebaud J (ed.). *Contraception – Your Questions Answered*, 2nd Edition. Churchill Livingstone, 1993.

Drife JO, Baird DT (eds). Contraception. *British Medical Bulletin* 1993; **49**(1), 1–258.

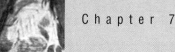

Infertility

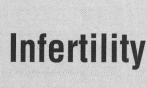

OVERVIEW

Approximately 10–15 per cent of couples are affected by infertility. The single most important factor in determining prognosis is the age of the female partner. Although advanced assisted conception techniques have significantly improved prospects for subfertile couples, simple cost-effective evidence-based treatments should always be considered as the first option.

Definition

Infertility is the inability of a couple to obtain a clinically recognizable pregnancy after 12 months of unprotected intercourse. Infecundity is the inability of a couple to achieve a live birth after 12 months of regular, unprotected intercourse.

Most couples seeking help are in fact subfertile rather than infertile. Some may have normal fertilizing potential. Infertility is classified as primary, secondary or voluntary.

- Primary infertility – Those who have never conceived in the past and who have regular, unprotected intercourse for 12 months.
- Secondary infertility – Those who have conceived in the past and who have regular, unprotected intercourse for 12 months.
- Voluntary infertility – Those who have never tried for a pregnancy and have taken contraception to avoid pregnancy.

The chances of conception should be expressed in terms of fertility of the couple rather than the individual partner. In Table 7.1 the principal factors affecting fertility are listed. For a young couple with no adverse factors the chance of conception per cycle per couple is around 20 per cent. The particular combination of adverse factors will determine the altered probability of conception per cycle per couple.

EPIDEMIOLOGY

Approximately 60 per cent of healthy women up to the age of 25 years conceive after six months of unprotected intercourse and 85 per cent conceive after 12 months. The single most important factor in determining fertility is the age of the female partner. If the female partner is 35 years or above, fertility is halved. Fertility declines sharply after the age of 37. For many couples it is customary to defer

Table 7.1 – Factors adversely affecting conception rates

Female factors	Male factors	Combined factors
Age (>37 years)	Low numbers of motile, healthy sperm	Duration of infertility (>2 years)
Menstrual FSH level (>10 u/L)	Drug intake	No previous conception in current relationship

investigation until after one year of unprotected intercourse, but it is essential to start early investigation (i.e. after six months after unprotected intercourse) in women above 35 years of age.

Although the evidence is limited, the prevalence of infertility is said to be increasing globally. Certainly the number of couples attending infertility clinics in the UK is rising, although this may be due to the fact that couples are more aware of the importance of early investigation.

It is difficult to determine the true cause of infertility because there are numerous factors that bias studies. The cause is established only after investigation and therefore can be affected by referral policies, special interests of the clinic, types of couples seeking investigation, resources available and investigations instituted. Unexplained infertility of a couple in one centre may be explained in another that has facilities for more detailed investigations. For example, the use of simple seminal microscopy in a general microbiological laboratory is less likely to identify sperm dysfunction than a dedicated andrology clinic and male factor problems may be missed leading to inappropriate treatment.

Causes of female infertility

The main causes of infertility are disorders of oocyte production and ovulation, sperm production and delivery, fallopian tube function and implantation of the embryo. The causes of infertility vary from one geographical area to another. Social factors have an influence on the cause. For example, in Africa, most infertile women have tubal infertility whereas in the Western world, it is either male factor infertility or ovulation disorders. An algorithm for management of the infertile couple is shown at the end of this chapter (Fig. 7.11).

Total ovarian failure

Premature ovarian failure is a condition where women aged 40 and below cease to have menses due to total

P **Understanding the pathophysiology**

Oogenesis
Oogenesis (Fig. 7.1) is the process of formation and maturation of oocyte. It is initiated with the growth of primordial follicle and completed with the final maturation of preovulation follicle. In humans, growth of primordial follicle to preantral follicle takes approximately 85 days. Final maturation of follicle from preantral stage to preovulatory stage takes approximately 14 days, which is the follicular phase of a 28-day menstrual cycle. Figure 7.2 shows a preovulatory follicle with blood flow.

Disorders of ovulation
Ovulation is the event in the ovarian cycle when a secondary oocyte is released from the follicle, and marks the time of onset of formation of the corpus luteum. An intact hypothalamic–pituitary–ovarian axis is essential for normal ovarian function. Pulsatile release of gonadotrophin-releasing hormone (GnRH) from the hypothalamus controls gonadotrophin (follicle-stimulating hormone [FSH] and luteinizing hormone [LH]) secretion from the pituitary. Both FSH and LH are necessary for complete follicle maturation through their effects on follicular (granulosa and theca) cells. A number of follicles start the recruitment process during the early follicular phase but normally only one follicle continues to mature to become a dominant follicle. The remainder of the follicles become atretic. The dominant follicle reaches 20–26 mm in mean diameter when LH surge (Fig. 7.3) occurs, resulting in luteinization of granulosa cells, follicular rupture and release of the oocyte. The presence of a regular menstrual cycle does not imply that ovulation is occurring.

ovarian failure. It is associated with autoimmune disease and may be hereditary. The term 'resistant ovary syndrome' is used when primordial follicles have failed to mature due to lack of gonadotrophin receptor antibodies. Infrequent or irregular ovulation is more common than total ovarian failure.

Ovarian Folliculogenesis

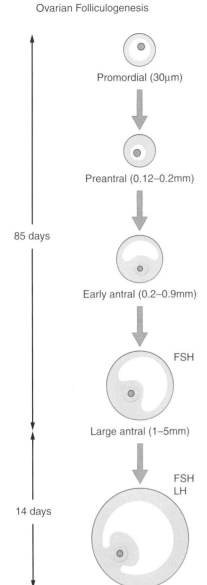

Figure 7.1 Ovarian folliculogenesis.

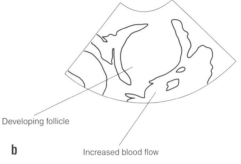

Figure 7.2a and b Ultrasound of preovulatory follicle with blood flow.

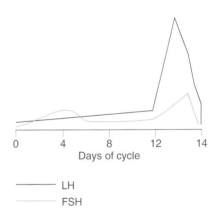

Figure 7.3 The luteinizing hormone (LH) surge that precedes ovulation.

Disorders of ovulation

Hypothalamic causes

Abnormal release of GnRH results in altered dopaminergic or endorphenergic tone and leads to anovulation. It may be mediated by external factors such as stress, weight loss or may be drug induced. It is often reversible when induced by exogenous factors.

Pituitary disorders

Anterior pituitary macro- or microadenomas may alter prolactin secretion and lead to amenorrhoea and anovulation. A transient rise in prolactin may be stress related. Prolactin levels higher than 1000 mL/L may suggest an adenoma and further evaluation with magnetic resonance imaging (MRI) of the pituitary fossa is indicated.

Ovarian causes

Polycystic ovarian syndrome (PCOS) is thought to be the commonest cause of anovulatory infertility. This condition is associated with oligoamenorrhoea, obesity and hirsutism. Women with PCOS have raised LH levels, altered LH:FSH ratio and may have increased peripheral androgens. About one in five normally menstruating women have polycystic ovaries. The condition is more common in Asian women. A typical appearance of a polycystic ovary on ultrasound scan suggests an enlarged ovary with ten or more peripheral small cysts and thickened stroma with increased stromal blood flow (Fig. 7.4). Elevated LH secretions during mid and late follicular phase may lead to impaired fertilization and early pregnancy failure.

Luteinized unruptured follicle (LUF)

In this condition the dominant follicle is luteinized but remains unruptured. Occasional LUF cycles are not infrequent in normally menstruating women. They may be drug induced (prostaglandin synthetase inhibitors) or may be associated with endometriosis. Circulating progesterone levels may be raised in the luteal phase and the diagnosis can only be made with the use of ultrasound scan or laparoscopy.

Thyroid and adrenal system

Disorders of thyroid function, either hypothyroidism or hyperthyroidism, may lead to menstrual disorders and ovulatory dysfunction. Adrenal conditions such as Cushing's syndrome or congenital adrenal hyperplasia also cause anovulation.

Chromosome abnormalities

The age-related decline in fertility in women is associated with an increase in chromosomal abnormalities in oocytes.

Abnormalities in the sex chromosomes may also lead to infertility. Women with Turner's syndrome and other variants may have an absent or defective X-chromosome.

Tubal dysfunction

Tubo-peritoneal factors affect the normal transport of oocyte and embryo. Tubal dysfunction may either be due to impaired oocyte pick-up mechanism (peritubal adhesions, damaged fimbriae) or damaged tubal epithelium. Pelvic inflammatory disease (PID) is the major cause of tubal infertility. Sexually transmitted disease with chlamydia, trachomatis, gonococci or other microorganisms may lead to tubal damage; chlamydia is the most common. Peritoneal adhesions associated with endometriosis or peritonitis following appendicitis or sepsis following pelvic or abdominal surgery may cause tubal dysfunction.

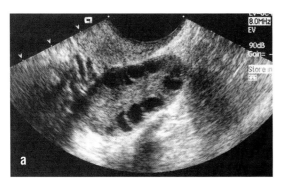
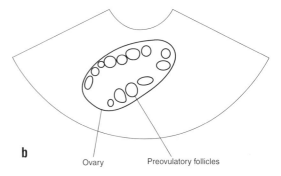

Figure 7.4 (a) Ultrasound of polycystic ovary showing dense stroma and peripheral cysts. (b) Schematic representation.

Disorders of implantation

Luteal insufficiency with impaired secretion of progesterone may adversely affect the endometrium thereby affecting implantation. A number of growth factors or adhesion molecules produced by the blastocyst and endometrium are known to affect implantation although a deficiency of these factors has got to be implicated in implantation failure. Submucus fibroids may distort the endometrial cavity and impair implantation.

Other factors

Smoking, alcohol, drugs, psychological and environmental factors can also affect the fertility of a couple.

 Key Points

Causes of female infertility
- Disorders of ovulation
- Impaired oocyte production (oocyte factors)
- Tubal dysfunction
- Disorders of implantation

CAUSES OF MALE INFERTILITY

Disorders of spermatogenesis

Impaired spermatogenesis could result from defects in any of the above mechanisms. The normal scrotal temperature is 1 degree lower than the rest of the body temperature and a rise in scrotal temperature is found in undescended testes and varicocele wherein increased scrotal temperature may impair spermatogenesis. Other factors, such as hot baths, tight underwear, etc, will also raise the scrotal temperature. Microdeletions of Y chromosomes may lead to defective spermatogenesis. Impaired sperm production and sexual function may result from the intake of certain drugs such as some psychotropic drugs, anti-epileptic and antihypertensive agents, antibiotics and chemotherapeutic agents which adversely affect sperm production and sexual function.

P **Understanding the pathophysiology**

Spermatogenesis
Spermatogenesis requires testicular growth and differentiation and it is under endocrine control by FSH and paracrine control by androgens produced by LH-stimulated Leydig cells. A man's testes can produce up to 2×10^{12} spermatozoa in a lifetime. Spermatogenesis comprises the mitotic division of spermatogonia and the meiotic division of spermatocytes. Transformation of spermatids into mature spermatozoa is called spermiogenesis. In humans this takes about 74 days.

Male fertility depends upon the endocrine and paracrine functions of the testes. The androgen-producing cells of the testes are called Leydig cells. Sertoli cells (homologous of ovarian granulosa cells) are embedded in the terminal epithelium of the seminiferous tubules and secrete inhibin, which controls FSH release from the pituitary with a negative feedback (Fig. 7.5). Transformation of spermatids into spermatozoa is a unique process involving germ cell-specific gene expression. Genes involved in spermatogenesis are expressed on the Y chromosome.

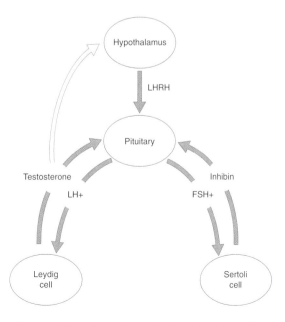

Figure 7.5 Flow diagram illustrating the relationships of the hypothalamus–pituitary–testicular axis.

Sperm transport

Immotile spermatozoa are released into the lumen of the seminiferous tubules and travel to the ampulla of the vas deferens where they acquire motility. During ejaculation the semen is released by adrenergically mediated contractions of the distal epididymis and vas deferens. Spermatozoa are then mixed with the secretions of the accessory glands, prostate seminal vesicles, Cowpers and urethral glands.

Impairment of sperm transport can be seen in men with epididymal malformation, obstruction due to inflammation, enlargement or absence of vas deferens or immobile cilia syndrome. Sperm transport is blocked or impaired after vasectomy.

Ejaculatory dysfunction

Ejaculatory dysfunction only occurs in 1–2 per cent of males with infertility. It could be due to anejaculation, premature ejaculation or retrograde ejaculation and could be drug induced or idiopathic. Metabolic and systemic conditions like diabetes and multiple sclerosis may lead to impotence.

Other causes

Immunological factors such as antisperm antibodies (IgG or IgA) and general infections may affect sperm function and lead to infertility.

HISTORY AND EXAMINATION

History from both partners must include details about general health, previous surgery, drug history, family history and lifestyle including smoking and alcohol intake. The female partner must be questioned about her knowledge of her menstrual cycle, when she is most fertile and details of her coital and menstrual history. Preconception counselling must be part of the initial consultation. Assessment of the female's general health including cervical smear, rubella status, body weight and breast examination must not be forgotten. Women with irregular menstruation must be asked about symptoms suggestive of PCOS, thyroid disorders and hyperprolactinaemia and they should have a full general and pelvic examination. Male partners should be examined to rule out testicular masses, congenital absence of vas deferens and varicocele. Small testes may be associated with primary testicular failure.

Examination of partners separately provides an opportunity to ask any confidential history regarding sexually transmitted diseases or previous pregnancies.

INVESTIGATIONS

Investigations must be aimed at individual couples. Modern evidence-based investigations are cost effective and likely to achieve better results. Specialist units should draw up protocols if general practitioners are involved with the initial management of infertile couples. Women above 35 years of age who have irregular menstruation are best managed by specialist units.

Investigations are aimed to assess the hypothalamus–pituitary–ovarian (HPO) axis, transport of gametes and implantation. An early follicular (day 1–3) gonadotrophins (FSH and LH) level is essential to assess ovarian reserve and an LH:FSH ratio of 2:1 or more would indicate underlying PCOS. Assessment of thyroid function, prolactin level and androgen profile is necessary for women with irregular menstruation. The day of the menstrual cycle that the blood test was taken, and the normal values for local laboratory should be noted to avoid misinterpretation of results. Mid-luteal serum progesterone levels assay (>30 nmol/L) in women with regular cycles usually indicate that ovulation has occurred but occasionally unruptured luteinized follicles may give normal luteal progesterone levels. A low progesterone level confirms anovulation in the menstrual cycle but a high level does not necessarily confirm ovulation. A detailed (pivotal) ultrasound scan performed between days 10 and 12 will establish follicular and endometrial maturity and will help to identify polycystic ovaries and uterine abnormalities. Confirmation of ovulation can only be established with serial scans.

Assessment of tubal patency

An outpatient hysterosalpingogram (HSG) (Fig. 7.7) is adequate to assess tubal patency. A radio-opaque aqueous solution is injected through the cervix under X-ray control to assess the uterine cavity and the patency of the fallopian tubes. The test is normally carried out within the first ten days of menstruation in order to avoid inadvertent exposure of the early embryo to ionizing radiation. Free spill of dye from both fallopian tubes confirms patency. Loculated spill may indicate peritubal adhesions and a club-shaped, dilated appearance of the tubes on X-ray may suggest hydrosalpinges. Filling defects in the uterine cavity are likely to be due to submucous fibroids, polyps or adhesions. Further evaluation of tubes with laparoscopy and dye intubation is indicated if the woman has symptoms of pelvic pain and if HSG is inconclusive. Hysteroscopy may be necessary to treat intrauterine pathology if the cavity is distorted. Hysterocontrast sonography (HyCoSy) (Fig. 7.6) is a modern, ultrasound-based investigation using a negative (normal saline) and positive (Echovist) contrast media to outline the uterine cavity and fallopian tubes. It is a simple test to assess the uterine cavity and tubal patency and avoids exposure to X-rays (Figs 7.6 and 7.7).

Laparoscopy and dye intubation

Routine diagnostic laparoscopy in the investigation of all infertile women is no longer justifiable. Women with pelvic pain and those with inconclusive findings with HSG or HyCoSy need further evaluation with laparoscopy. In those cases, therapeutic intervention with laparoscopy (e.g. adhesiolysis or ovarian cystectomy) should be performed at the same time. Tubal patency is tested by injection of methylene blue through the cervix and observing spillage of dye from fimbrial ends. Assessment of the uterine shape and ovaries is done during the procedure.

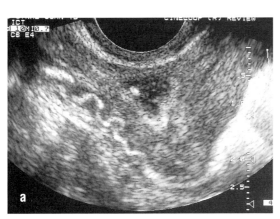
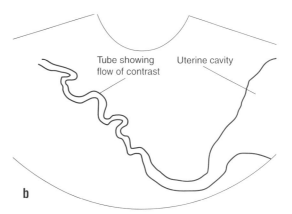

Figure 7.6 (a) Hysterocontrast sonography (HyCoSy) showing fallopian tube. (b) Schematic representation.

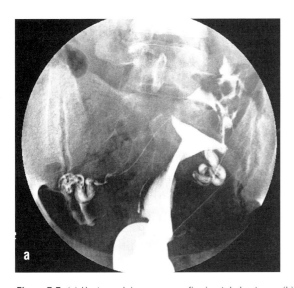
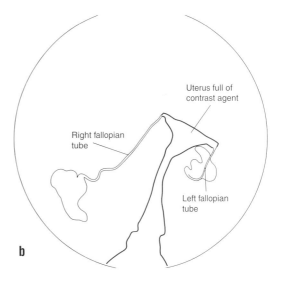

Figure 7.7 (a) Hysterosalpingogram confirming tubal patency. (b) Schematic representation.

Semen analysis

A motile, healthy population of sperm in a semen sample is more important than the total number of sperm in semen. Progressive motility, morphology and agglutination of sperm are more indicative of fertilizing ability rather than sperm numbers.

One detailed semen analysis is adequate if performed after 2–3 days of sexual abstinence. A second sample should be requested if the first sample shows suboptimal results. In men with oligo- or azoospermia, a blood sample for gonadotrophins, testosterone and prolactin may be necessary to identify where the problem lies.

Postcoital test

The postcoital test is performed around ovulation and it is aimed at evaluating periovulatory cervical mucus and sperm survival. The couple is asked to abstain from intercourse for two days prior to the test. The standard test is performed 6–10 hours after intercourse. Accurate timing of the test is important to avoid misinterpretation of results. A recent study has shown that this test has limited prognostic value.

🔧 Key Points

Causes of male infertility
- Disorders of spermatogenesis
- Impaired sperm transport
- Ejaculatory dysfunction
- Immunological and infective factors

Semen analysis

Semen analysis (World Health Organization reference values)
Volume: 2–5 mL
Liquification time: Within 30 minutes
Concentration: 20 million/mL
Motility: >50% progressive motility
Morphology: >30% normal forms
White blood cells: <1 million/mL

TREATMENT OF FEMALE INFERTILITY

With the advent and increasing need for expensive assisted conception technologies it is necessary to adopt a 'cost per conception' or 'cost per baby' policy while planning management of an infertile couple. Any test or treatment planned must take into account whether the outcome is measured with conception and the cost is justified, for example, the treatment of minor endometriosis or the medical management of oligospermia increases the cost without necessarily increasing conception rates. Treatment policies must be individualized to a couple's chances of success. Many factors affecting conception rates would include female partner's age, (as fertility declines after the age of 35 years), baseline FSH level, previous conception and associated sperm dysfunction. Fast-track management is essential in women over 35 years of age. Women with a baseline FSH greater than 10 U/L have a poor prognosis.

Counselling is an essential part of infertility management. Men with sperm abnormalities tend to suffer from low self-esteem and may need counselling. A recent survey of infertile women in the UK has shown that one in 20 has had suicidal tendencies. Advice regarding adoption and gamete donation should be available in infertility clinics and given early if indicated.

Nomenclature for some semen variables

Normozoospermia	Normal ejaculate as defined by the reference values
Oligozoospermia	Sperm concentration less than the reference value
Asthenozoospermia	Less than the reference value for motility
Teratozoospermia	Less than the reference value for morphology
Oligoasthenoterato-zoospermia	Signifies disturbance of all three variables (combinations of only two prefixes may also be used)
Azoospermia	No spermatozoa in the ejaculate
Aspermia	No ejaculate

Ovulation induction

Ovulation induction is aimed at the development of more than one mature follicle in a woman who is anovulatory so that more oocytes are available for fertilization. The term 'superovulation' is applied when used in women who may be already ovulating but irregularly. This treatment should be performed in a specialist clinic. The most appropriate method is selected after identifying where the defect lies in the HPO axis. Before starting therapy, the male partner's semen must be analysed.

Clomiphene citrate has been used widely since the early 1960s for induction of ovulation. It is a non-steroidal agent with both oestrogenic and non-oestrogenic properties. It stimulates the release of FSH by blocking oestradiol receptors. A rise in endogenous FSH through negative feedback results in follicle stimulation. Clomiphene can be prescribed up to a maximum of six cycles if ovulation is occurring. The dose depends upon the cause of anovulation, the female partner's age and history of previous response or ovarian surgery. Usually Clomiphene is started at 50 mg daily from day 2–6 of the menstrual cycle and increased up to 150 mg daily if there is no response. Women with PCOS respond to 25 mg daily from day 2–6 of cycle.

Tamoxifen (20–40 mg, day 2-6) is a similar drug, a triphenylethylene derivative, and has anti-oestrogenic properties. The clinical effectiveness of anti-oestrogen therapy is measured in conception rates per cycle and cumulative conception rates after six cycles of therapy. Monitoring of treatment cycles with serial ultrasound scans is recommended. Women undergoing ovulation induction must be counselled about the risks of multiple gestation, ovarian hyperstimulation and the possibility of fetal reduction. Protocols must be aimed at reducing ovarian hyperstimulation syndrome and the risks of multiple gestation. An ovulatory trigger dose (5000 IU) of hCG may be required if there is evidence of an unruptured luteinized follicle.

In women with Clomiphene-resistant PCOS, gonadotrophin therapy with either follicle-stimulating hormone (FSH, urinary or recombinant) or human menopausal gonadotrophin (HMG, a combination of FSH and LH, derived from postmenopausal urine) is used. Either FSH (subcutaneously) or HMG (intramuscularly) is given as daily or alternate daily injections from early follicular phase until follicular maturation is confirmed. Treatment cycles are monitored with serial ultrasound scans. An ovulatory trigger with hCG may be required. If more than three follicles are mature, hCG is withheld and the couple are asked to avoid pregnancy in that cycle; a 'low-dose, step-up' regime is preferred with a starting dose of 37.5 IU daily. The risk of multiple gestation (up to 20 per cent) and ovarian hyperstimulation syndrome must be explained prior to commencing therapy. Laparoscopic ovarian drilling either with laser or diathermy is effective in selected cases of Clomiphene resistance.

Ovarian hyperstimulation syndrome

Ovarian hyperstimulation syndrome (OHSS) is an iatrogenic condition following ovarian stimulation and can be potentially life-threatening. It can present in mild, moderate or severe forms. In all forms, it complicates up to 5 per cent of cycles with ovarian stimulation, severe cases occur in 0.5–2 per cent of all IVF cycles. The exact pathophysiology is uncertain, but the release of vascular endothelial growth factor (VEGF) from luteinized granulosa cells seems to trigger the events. hCG, either endogenous or exogenous, is necessary for the development of OHSS. Women with PCOS and aged under 35 are at an increased risk of developing severe OHSS. Clinical features include abdominal distension due to ovarian cystic enlargement and ascites as a result of extravascular accumulation of exudate. There is excessive ovarian response with multiple follicles and the condition is characterized by intravascular volume depletion and haemoconcentration.

Anovulation due to hyperprolactinaemia

Anovulation due hyperprolactinaemia is effectively treated with dopamine agonists. Bromocriptine is an ergot alkaloid with dopamimetic properties. It is administered in a daily dose of 1.25–7.5 mg. Cabergoline and Quinagolide are D2 receptor agonists with longer half-life. Cabogorline is administered in a dose of 0.25–1 mg twice weekly and Quinagolide in a dose of 25–150 mg daily. Cabogerline is more effective and better tolerated than Bromocriptine, which not uncommonly causes gastrointestinal side-effects.

Hypothalamic anovulation

This condition is diagnosed with gonadotrophin assessment and oestrogen deficiency. Gonadotrophin (FSH and LH) levels are low (< 5 u/L). An

MRI scan of the pituitary and hypothalamus is useful to rule out pituitary tumours. Hypothalamic anovulation can be effectively treated with pulsatile GnRH, administered with an infusion pump either subcutaneously or intravenously. If the patient is not competent in using a pump, gonadotrophin therapy is indicated.

Superovulation and intrauterine insemination

Intrauterine insemination (IUI) of a prepared sperm is carried out together with superovulation in couples where the sperm motility is suboptimal and in women with unexplained infertility. There is some evidence that IUI in stimulated cycles is better than no treatment in couples with unexplained infertility. Sperm preparation is carried out with sperm washing gradient separation or swim up techniques. Superovulation and IUI is intended to:

1 optimize chances of conception by ensuring that there is at least one mature follicle;
2 decrease the distance sperm has to travel by injecting it into the fundus of the uterus;
3 time the insemination at ovulation.

Treatment of tubal disease

The aim of tubal surgery is to restore normal anatomy. Tubal damage has been graded depending upon severity of disease, with grade 1 being the least damaged and grades 3 and 4 being severely damaged. Surgery is only indicated in grades 1 and 2. The status of tubal mucosa is correlated with conception rates and sites.

Tubal surgery or *in vitro* fertilization (IVF) and embryo transfer (ET) are the options available. The outcome of tubal surgery is influenced by the expertise of the surgeon, the facilities available and the extent of tubal damage. If the female partner is older or if there is a male factor problem, the outcome is poor. With the increasing availability and success of assisted conception technologies, the role for tubal surgery is diminishing.

Salpingo-ovariolysis
Removal of peritubal and periovarian adhesions is performed either at laparotomy or by video laparoscopy.

Fimbrial surgery
This includes division of fimbrial adhesions or repair of fimbrial disease (fimbrioplasty) in trained hands. The conception rates could be up to 30 per cent per cycle and 50 per cent after six months. Ectopic pregnancy occurs in 5 per cent of women treated.

The aim of tubal surgery is to restore normal anatomy tubal damage and has been graded depending upon the severity of the disease, grades I and II being the least damaged and grades III and IV being severely damaged. Surgery is only indicated in grades I and II. The status of tubal mucosa is correlated with conception sites and rates.

Salpingoneostomy
In this procedure, a new uterine tubal orifice is established at laparotomy or laparoscopy. Transcervical cannulation of the tube is performed either with falloposcopy or selective salpingography. There are no randomized studies establishing success rates. Reversal of sterilization achieves good results as the tubal damage is limited, mucosal damage is unlikely and the woman has proven fertility. IVF-ET provides the only chance of conception in women with blocked fallopian tubes that cannot be opened by tubal surgery. Recent evidence suggests that the presence of hydrosalpinges adversely affects implantation in women undergoing IVF-ET treatment and therefore removal of such tubes is recommended prior to IVF treatment.

TREATMENT OF MALE INFERTILITY

While considering treatment of male factor infertility, one should take into account the female partner's age, history of previous conception and duration of infertility. Male fertility depends on sperm quality rather than numbers. Hormonal treatment is not effective unless a diagnosis of hypogonadotrophic hypogonadism is the cause. Exogenous gonadotrophins, hCG and sometimes pulsatile GnRH therapy for 12 months is likely to restore testicular volume and spermatogenesis. Intrauterine insemination with ovarian stimulation will give higher conception rates in couples with poor sperm motility compared to no treatment.

Antioxidant therapy (vitamin E and vitamin C) and the use of antibiotics in the presence of infection help to improve fertility. In men with antisperm antibodies, systemic steroids have been used but the benefit is conflicting and there can be severe side effects.

Approximately 25 per cent of men with abnormal sperm parameters have varicoceles. Varicocele ligation is indicated in symptomatic cases but improvement in fertility following surgery is not confirmed. Assisted conception technologies such as intracytoplasmic sperm injection (ICSI) (Fig. 7.8) achieve better results than other treatments. Men with azoospermia can be offered sperm aspiration treatments followed by ICSI. Chromosomal testing for cystic fibrosis, karyotyping and Y microdeletions is essential prior to treatment.

ASSISTED CONCEPTION TECHNIQUES

The birth of Louise Brown on July 25th 1978 was a landmark in the treatment of infertility. Initially, women with tubal damage were considered for IVF-ET during spontaneous cycles. The technique is now offered for a number of other indications and generally carried out in cycles with ovarian stimulation. Hundreds of thousands of babies have been born worldwide as a result of assisted conception technologies.

In vitro fertilization and embryo transfer (IVF-ET) involves the fertilization of gametes in the laboratory and transfer of embryos to the uterus. There are a number of related techniques that are carried out to overcome barriers to enhance fertilization. The commonly used techniques are listed below.

IVF   *in vitro* fertilization
DI   donor insemination

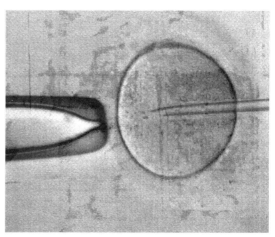

Figure 7.8 Intracytoplasmic sperm injection (ICSI).

GIFT   gamete intrafallopian transfer
ZIFT   zygote intrafallopian transfer
SUZI   subzonal insemination
ICSI   intracytoplasmic sperm injection
TESA   testicular sperm aspiration
PESA   percutaneous sperm aspiration
MESA micro-epididymal sperm aspiration

Of all the techniques described above, IVF and ICSI are the most commonly used techniques (Table 7.2).

A typical IVF-ET cycle

Initial consultation and tests
It is an important event with the couple to assess the cause of infertility, choose the most appropriate technique, explain the procedure, side effects, complica-

Table 7.2 – Indications for assisted conception techniques

Female	Male	Technique indicated
1. Tubal damage Unexplained Endometriosis PCOS	normal	IVF-ET
2. Unexplained	normal	IVF-ET, GIFT, ZIFT
3. Any of the above	sperm disorder	ICSI, SUZI
4. Any of the above	non-obstructive azoospermia	TESA, DI
	obstructive azoospermia	PESA, MESA
5. Ovarian failure	normal	donor oocyte treatment

tions and success rates. An assessment of the most recent baseline FSH level, semen analysis, tubal patency test and ultrasound scans are essential before commencing treatment.

Pituitary downregulation

In spontaneous cycles and cycles with ovarian stimulation only, there is a risk of spontaneous LH surge necessitating unplanned oocyte collection. Oocytes may not be collected due to rupture of follicles prior to the procedure. Pre-treatment with gonadotrophin-releasing hormone analogues (GnRH analogues) has helped to simplify the treatment and to achieve more embryos from one treatment cycle.

GnRH analogues are used either subcutaneously or intranasally from day 1 or day 21 of the menstrual cycle for two weeks. Pituitary downregulation is confirmed with low serum oestradiol levels (less than 100 pmol/L) or quiescent ovaries and thin endometrium as seen on ultrasound scan. In some cases, the analogue is used prior to (short protocol) or in conjunction with (ultrashort protocol) ovarian stimulation. In all cases, the analogue is continued until the administration of hCG.

Ovarian stimulation

FSH (either recombinant or urinary) or MG injections are used daily until the leading follicles have reached 18–20 mm in diameter. This process takes normally 12–14 days (Fig. 7.9a and b).

Ovulation trigger with hCG

An injection (5000 or 10,000 IU) of hCG is administered which acts as a surrogate for LH surge. Oocyte

A typical IVF-ET cycle

Initial consultation

Pituitary downregulation

Superovulation

hCG trigger

Oocyte collection

Insemination of oocytes

Embryo transfer

Luteal support

Pregnancy test

collection is carried out 34–36 hours after hCG administration.

Oocyte collection

This procedure is normally carried out under transvaginal ultrasound guidance as an outpatient under intravenous sedation. Once the follicular contents are aspirated, the cumulus oocyte complex is identified under microscope and incubated at 37°C in culture medium (Fig. 7.10).

Semen preparation

The main aim is to separate motile healthy sperma-

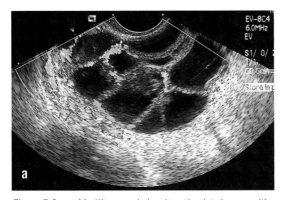
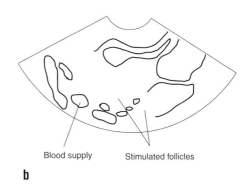

Blood supply   Stimulated follicles

a   **b**

Figure 7.9a and b Ultrasound showing stimulated ovary with multiple follicles and associated blood supply.

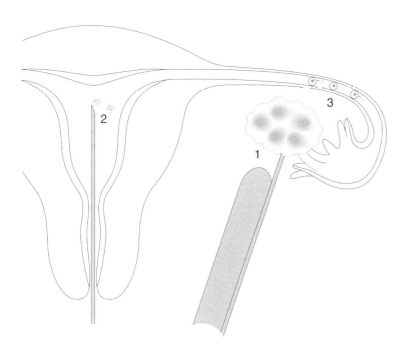

Figure 7.10 Techniques used in assisted conception.

1. Transvaginal oocyte collection
2. Embryo transfer
3. GIFT

tozoa from the seminal fluid so that they can be used for fertilization. Semen is produced by masturbation, allowed to liquefy, then diluted with culture medium and centrifuged to sediment spermatozoa. Motile sperm are separated either with 'swim up' or with 'Percoll gradient' technique, washed and kept in culture medium for insemination.

Insemination

In 'conventional' IVF, prepared sperm (between 100,000 and 200,000) are added to each oocyte approximately 4–6 hours after they are collected (metaphase II stage). In cases of ICSI, sperm is injected directly into the cytoplasm of the oocyte through the zona pellucida.

Fertilization and embryo cleavage

Cumulus cells are removed from each oocyte using a glass pipette approximately 16–18 hours after insemination. The oocytes are then transferred to a fresh culture medium and examined for fertilization. The presence of two pronuclei and two polar bodies indicates normal fertilization. Fertilized oocytes are re-examined to check for embryo cleavage. Embryos are graded microscopically from I to IV, with I being excellent and IV being poor, depending on the presence of a number of fragments.

Embryo transfer

Embryos are normally transferred to the uterus 2–3 days after oocyte collection (i.e. 2–8 cell stage) transcervically. The maximum number of embryos replaced at any one time is three, according to the Human Fertilization and Embryology Authority (HFEA).

Embryo cryopreservation

Spare embryos are cryopreserved for future use. Cryopreservation and thawing techniques, embryo quality at freezing and after thawing and clinical protocols for replacement influence the success.

Luteal support and establishment of pregnancy

Luteal phase is supported with low dose hCG or by administration of progesterone. A urine pregnancy test or a blood test for hCG is performed 14 days after embryo transfer.

Sperm aspiration techniques

In men with azoospermia, sperm can be aspirated either from the testes or the epididymis and used for ICSI. Sperm aspiration is a simple technique performed under local anaesthetic on the day of the partner's egg collection.

Donor gamete treatment

Assisted conception techniques are used to help couples to conceive donor gametes if they are unable to conceive with their own gametes. Oocyte donation is used in women with genetic disorders involving X chromosomes, premature ovarian failure, Turner's syndrome and in those whose ovaries do not respond to ovarian stimulation. Sperm donation is used in couples where the male partner is azoospermic and if no sperm are obtained with sperm aspiration techniques.

The HFEA provides a legal framework to protect the interests of donors, recipients and children born as a result of donor gamete treatment.

GIFT or ZIFT

In GIFT procedure, the oocytes are collected under laparoscopic control, mixed with prepared sperm and transferred back to the fallopian tube (see Fig. 7.10). Fertilization occurs *in vivo*. In ZIFT, fertilized oocytes (zygotes) are transferred into the fallopian tube. The procedures are normally performed under general anaesthetic with the use of laparoscopy. In GIFT, fertilization cannot be confirmed in case of failure. IVF has therefore been a procedure of choice as it offers a diagnosis of fertilization.

Complications of IVF treatment

Ovarian hyperstimulation syndrome and multiple gestation remain to be the major concerns. Possible long-term effects of ovarian stimulation such as development of ovarian tumours and early menopause need further evaluation.

Human Fertilization and Embryology Authority (HFEA)

The Human Fertilization and Embryology Authority was established for the regulation of all assisted conception treatments, storage of gametes and research involving fertilization of human oocytes *in vitro*. All centres are licensed by the authority and have a legal obligation to inform the HFEA of every treatment cycle including the outcome of treatment and pregnancy. This information is kept confidentially and analysed annually. The centres are required to take

History and examination of
both partners

Advice regarding
• Smoking and alcohol intake
• Fertile period and regular intercourse
• Weight loss if female BMI>30
• Folic acid intake
• Drugs affecting fertility
• Age-related decline in fertility

• Day 1–5 FSH and LH
• Mid luteal progesterone
• Prolactin and thyroid profile
  (if regular cycles)
• Pivotal scan (day 8–12)
• Hysterosalpingogram
• Chlamydia screen
• Semen analysis

Discuss results and plan treatment

Figure 7.11 The management of an infertile couple.

necessary steps to ensure that account has been taken of the welfare of children who may be born as a result of treatment or of any children who may be affected by the birth.

New developments

Preimplantation diagnosis of genetic disease (PGD)
Embryos created with IVF technique can be tested for genetic disease. A single blastomere can be removed from an embryo by micromanipulation for genetic analysis. A single gene defect (e.g. cystic fibrosis, Tay Sachs disease, Duchene muscular dystrophy) can be detected. Embryos unaffected are transferred into the uterus.

In vitro culture
In vitro culture (IVC) of primordial follicles obtained from ovarian cortex through to mature graafian follicles containing oocytes at metaphase II phase. This technique is not likely to be available in the near future.

In vitro maturation

The term '*In vitro* maturation (IVM)' is used when immature oocytes from antral follicles are matured to metaphase 2 oocytes capable of fertilization. This technique is currently under evaluation. The clinical application of IVM is likely to reduce short-term and long-term risks of ovarian stimulation .

GnRH antagonists

GnRH antagonists bind to receptors competitively and prevent the endogenous GnRH release by exerting its stimulatory effects on the pituitary cells. These compounds can be administered for a short period during mid and late follicular phases of a superovulation cycle to prevent spontaneous LH surge. This has recently been licensed for use in IVF cycles.

⚿ Key Points

- History, examination and investigations and counselling must include both partners
- Advice should be given regarding the effects of smoking, alcohol, lifestyle and spontaneous conception rates
- Treatment should be initiated taking into account the duration of infertility, female partner's age, previous conception history and success rates
- Women aged 35 years and above and those with irregular cycles should be referred to specialist clinics
- Total motile, normal sperm population is more important than the sperm count but sperm morphology is a more stable indicator of fertilization than motility
- Men with abnormal sperm analysis should have endocrine assessment, those with low (<5 million/mL) or no sperm must be offered chromosomal analyses
- Couples must be given written information regarding risks of OHSS, multiple gestation and ovarian tumors
- FSH and HMG should be used in low dose in clomiphene-resistant women, clomiphene is an effective treatment in anovulatory women
- All ovulation induction cycles should be monitored
- The welfare of the child born as a result of treatment, or any existing children must be taken into account

CASE HISTORY

Mrs S williams

39 year old lawyer
Regular periods. Non-smoker. No significant medical or gynaecological history.

Partner: Mr A Smith
38 year old electrical engineer
No significant medical or surgical history. Non-smoker and consumes less than 10 units of alcohol per week.

Investigations
Female partner: FSH, LH, rubella status, pelvic ultrasound scan
Male partner: Semen analysis

Results
Female partner: FSH – 6.5 u/l, LH 5.0 u/l. Immune to rubella. Late follicular pelvic scan showed dominant follicle in right ovary; endomatrial changes consistent with ovarian activity; normal left ovary.
Male partner: Sperm count – 2 million/ml; motility – 10% with low progression; morphology – 85% abnormality.

They were offered counselling for male factor cause. In view of severe oligospermia, testing for cystic fibrosis mutations and Y chromosome deletion was requested and the results were normal. IVF and intracytoplastic sperm injection (ICSI) was offered after full discussion. The couple achieved a successful conception after the second attempt of IVF/ICSI.

CASE HISTORY

Mrs J Patel

27 year old housewife.

Wt 84 kg – Ht 5' 1".

Irregular periods. Previously diagnosed to have polycystic ovary syndrome. Trying to conceive for 6 months.

Mr Patel's semen analysis shows normal sperm parameters.

Mrs Patel was advised to lose weight. No treatment was offered. 8 months later Mrs Patel managed to lose 12 kilos. Her menstrual cycle was regular. She conceived spontaneously 3 months later.

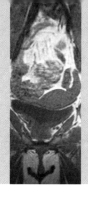

Chapter 8

Disorders of early pregnancy (ectopic, miscarriage, GTD)

OVERVIEW

Early pregnancy disorders currently account for approximately three-quarters of emergency gynaecological admissions in Europe and are an important cause of maternal morbidity and mortality throughout the world.

Pregnancy loss may have a profound effect on a woman and, in addition to the medical management, appropriate counselling and support should be made available.

Introduction

The three main categories of early pregnancy disorders are:
1. spontaneous miscarriages;
2. ectopic pregnancies;
3. gestational trophoblastic disease.

Gynaecological complications, such as cervical or vaginal cancer and infections, may present with similar symptoms and should be considered in the differential diagnosis.

The normal early pregnancy

Implantation and subsequent placental development in the human requires complex adaptive changes of the uterine wall constituents.

Development of the blastocyst

At the beginning of the fourth week after the last menstrual period, the implanted blastocyst is composed, from outside to inside, of the trophoblastic ring, the extra-embryonic mesoderm and the amniotic cavity and the primary yolk sac, separated by the bilaminar embryonic disk (Fig. 8.1). The extra-embryonic mesoderm progressively increases and 12 days after ovulation (around the 26th menstrual day)

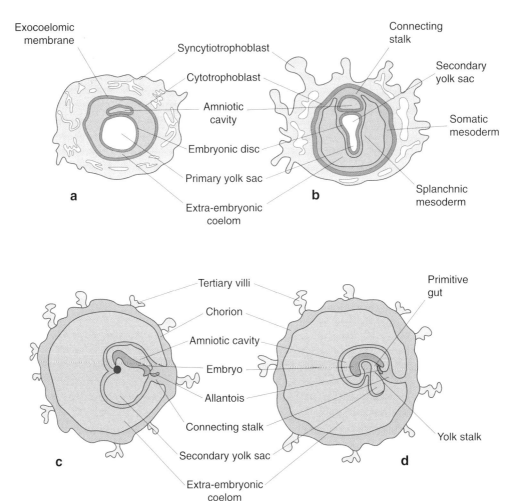

Figure 8.1 Schematic representations of human pregnancies at the beginning (a) and at the end (b) of the 4th menstrual week and during the 5th (c) and 6th (d) menstrual weeks.

it contains isolated spaces that rapidly fuse to form the extra-embryonic coelom. As the latter forms, the primary yolk sac decreases in size and the secondary yolk sac arises from cells growing from the embryonic disk inside the primary yolk sac.

Formation of the placenta

Primary chorionic villi develop between 13 and 15 days after ovulation (end of 4th week of gestation). Simultaneously, blood vessels start in the extra-embryonic mesoderm of the yolk sac, the connecting stalk and the chorion. The primary villi are composed of a central mass of cytotrophoblast

surrounded by a thick layer of syncytiotrophoblast. During the 5th week of gestation, they acquire a central mesenchymal core from the extra-embryonic mesoderm and become branched, forming the secondary villi. The appearance of embryonic blood vessels within their mesenchymal cores transforms the secondary villi into tertiary villi. Up to 10 weeks' gestation, which corresponds to the last week of the embryonic period (stages 19 to 23), villi cover the entire surface of the chorionic sac (see Fig. 8.1).

As the gestational sac grows during fetal life, the villi associated with the decidua capsularis, surrounding the amniotic sac, become compressed and degenerate forming an avascular shell known as the chorion laeve, or smooth chorion. Conversely, the villi

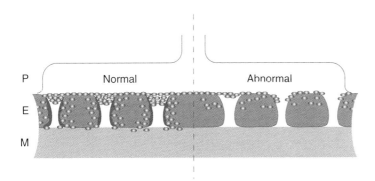

P   Normal   Abnormal

E

M

Figure 8.2 Diagram comparing the histological features of the placental bed (P, placenta; E, endometrium; M, myometrium) in normal and abnormal pregnancies. In normal pregnancies the extravillous trophoblast infiltrates the endometrium down to the myometrium and forms a continuous shell obliterating the tip of the transformed spiral arteries. In spontaneous abortions there is a reduced trophoblastic infiltration, a fragmented or absent trophoblastic shell and defective transformation of the spiral arteries.

associated with the decidua basalis proliferate forming the chorion frondosum or definitive placenta.

Normal placentation

As soon as the blastocyst has hatched, the trophoectoderm layer attaches to the cell surface of the endometrium and by simple displacement, early trophoblastic penetration within the endometrial stroma occurs. Progressively, the entire blastocyst will sink into maternal decidua and the migrating trophoblastic cells will encounter venous channels of increasing size, then superficial arterioles and, during the 4th week, the spiral arteries (Fig. 8.2). The trophoblastic cells infiltrate deeply the decidua and attain the deciduo-myometrial junction between 8 and 12 weeks' gestation. This extravillous trophoblast penetrates the inner third of the myometrium via the interstitial ground substance and affects its mechanical and electrophysiological properties by increasing its expansile capacity. The trophoblastic infiltration of the myometrium is progressive and achieved before 18 weeks' gestation in normal pregnancies.

Ultrasound imaging

The gestational sac representing the deciduoplacental interface and the chorionic cavity are the first sonographic evidence of a pregnancy (Fig. 8.3). The gestational sac can be visualized with transvaginal ultrasound around 4.4–4.6 weeks (32–34 days) following the onset of the last menstruation when it reaches a size of 2–4 mm. By contrast, the gestational sac can only be observed by means of abdominal ultrasound imaging during the 5th week postmenstruation.

The first embryonic structure that will become visible inside the chorionic cavity will be the secondary yolk sac, when the gestational sac reaches 8 mm. The demonstration of the yolk sac (Fig. 8.4) reliably indicates that an intrauterine fluid collection represents a true gestational sac, thus excluding the possibility of a pseudosac or an ectopic pregnancy (see below).

Symptomatology

The classical symptom triad for early pregnancy disorders is amenorrhea, pelvic or low abdominal pain and vaginal bleeding. Pregnancy symptoms are often non-specific and many women of reproductive age have irregular menstrual cycles. Therefore, the first test to perform to confirm the existence of a

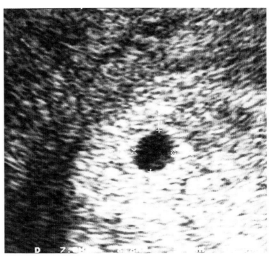

Figure 8.3 Transvaginal ultrasound of a gestational sac at 4 weeks' gestation.

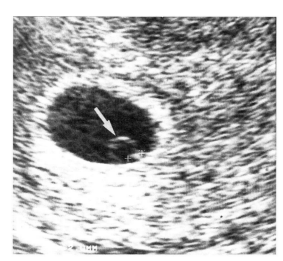

Figure 8.4 Transvaginal ultrasound of a normal 5 week pregnancy showing from outside to inside the placental echogenic ring, the chorionic or exocoelomic cavity the embryo (CRL = 2 mm) and the secondary yolk sac (arrow).

pregnancy is to demonstrate the presence of human chorionic gonadotrophin (hCG) in the patient's urine or plasma.

Pregnancy tests

hCG is a placental-derived glycoprotein, composed of two subunits, α and β, which maintains the corpus luteum for the first seven weeks of gestation. Extremely small quantities of hCG are produced by the pituitary gland and thus plasma hCG is almost exclusively produced by the placenta. hCG has a half life of 6–24 hours and rises to a peak in pregnancy at 9–11 weeks' gestation.

Urine testing

It is possible to detect low levels of hCG in urine by rapid (1–2 min) dipstick tests. The sensitivity of these tests is high (detection limit of around 50 iu/L) and they produce positive results around 14 days after ovulation.

Plasma testing

Measurement of hCG in plasma is more accurate (detection limit around 0.1–0.3 iu/L) and is able to detect a pregnancy 6–7 days after ovulation which corresponds to the time of implantation. They also allow quantification of the hCG level which may be required to determine whether a pregnancy is normal or abnormal and is of pivotal importance in the follow-up of some pregnancy disorders.

Miscarriage

Definition

The miscarriage of an early pregnancy is the commonest medical complication in humans with one in two conceptions lost before the end of the first trimester. Most conceptions are lost during the first month after the last menstrual period and are often ignored, particularly if they occur around the time of an expected menstrual period.

Epidemiology and risk factors

The rate of clinical pregnancy loss is known to decrease with gestational age from 25 per cent at 5–6 weeks to 2 per cent after 14 weeks (Table 8.1).

Table 8.1 – Epidemiology of early pregnancy disorders

Variable	%
Total loss of conception	50–70
Total rate of clinical miscarriage	25–30
Before 6 weeks	18
Between 6 and 9 weeks	4
After 9 weeks	3
After 14 weeks	2
Rate of chromosomal defect in miscarriage	50–70
Rate of miscarriage in primigravidas	6–10
Rate of miscarriage in primigravidas 40+-year-old women	30–40
Rate of recurrent miscarriages	1–2
Risk of recurrent miscarriage after three miscarriages	25–30
Ectopic pregnancies per live births	2
Complete hydatidiform mole	0.1

Chromosomal abnormalities and maternal age

The incidence of chromosomal abnormality increases with maternal age. Approximately 50–60 per cent of chromosomal abnormalities are associated with a chromosomal defect of the conceptus and the frequency of abnormal chromosomal complement increases when embryonic demise occurs earlier in gestation (up to 90 per cent). The risk of pregnancy loss also increases with maternal age, i.e a 40-year-old woman carries twice the risk of a 20-year-old woman. The past obstetric history also influences the risk. The pregnancy loss rate among primigravidas is 6–10 per cent whereas the recurrent rate after three or more losses is 25–30 per cent (Table 8.1).

Autosomal trisomies are the most common with an incidence of 30–35 per cent followed by triploidies and monosomies X. Triploidy and tetraploidy are frequent but extremely lethal chromosomal abnormalities and are therefore rarely found in late abortuses. Structural chromosomal rearrangements such as translocation or inversions are present in only 1.5 per cent of abortuses in the general population but are a significant cause of recurrent miscarriages.

Rare causes of miscarriage

The other causes of miscarriage include endocrine diseases, anatomic abnormalities of the female genital tract, infections, immune factors, chemical agents, hereditary disorders, trauma, maternal diseases and psychological factors (Table 8.2). Prospective epidemiological surveys suggest that the attributable risk of most of these factors to first trimester spontaneous abortion is small. Aetiologies, such as exposure to certain toxins, are rare in the general population but this may become an important issue in the context of ecological disasters. Some other causes, such as translocations or thrombophilia, may be found more frequently in cases of recurrent miscarriages.

Müllerian tract fusion and cervical abnormalities are well-accepted causes of second trimester losses, but are not associated with a higher rate of first trimester miscarriages.

P | Understanding the pathophysiology

Disturbance of placentation

In most cases of early pregnancy failure there is an inadequate placentation. In particular, there is a defective transformation of the spiral arteries and a reduced trophoblastic penetration into the decidua and into the spiral arteries (see Fig. 8.2). This defect of placentation is more pronounced in chromosomal abnormalities.

In pregnancies complicated by hypertension, there is a probable relationship between the severity of the disease and the degree of inadequate placentation. If this concept is extrapolated to the first trimester, some forms of recurrent, early spontaneous abortions related to medical disorders associated with a defect of placentation, such as the systemic lupus erythematosus disease, could represent the earliest form of this phenomenon.

Differential diagnosis

There are four different clinical forms of miscarriages.

Threatened miscarriage

A threatened miscarriage is defined as a painless vaginal bleeding occurring any time between implantation and 24 weeks' gestation. Probably one-quarter of all pregnancies are complicated by threatened miscarriage, although many patients may be unaware of their pregnancy at the time they present with vaginal bleeding.

Threatened miscarriage is one of the most common indications (together with suspected ectopic pregnancy) for emergency referral of young women to a casualty department. The bleeding may resolve spontaneously in a few days, never to recur. It may also continue, or stop and start over several days or weeks. It is only when abdominal cramps supervene that the process may move in the direction of inevitability, in particular if the cervix opens. It usually occurs between 6 and 9 weeks' gestation when the definitive placenta forms (Fig. 8.5).

The diagnosis is usually based on clinical examination. The role of ultrasound and endocrinology in predicting this type of early pregnancy complication remains controversial. Nevertheless, the evaluation of the size of the gestational sac or the embryo and demonstration of embryonic heart action are

Table 8.2 – Aetiological factors of early pregnancy disorders

Miscarriages

Chromosomal abnormalities (Maternal age >35 years)	Trisomies (Down's syndrome)
	Triploidies and tetraploidies
	Monosomy X (Turner's syndrome)
	Translocation (hereditary)
Endocrine disorders	Diabetes, hypothyroidism, luteal phase deficiency, polycystic ovarian syndrome
Abnormalities of the uterus	Uterine septa (bicornuate uterus)
	Endometrial adhesions (post-curettage or Asherman's syndrome)
Infections	*Salmonella typhi*, malaria, cytomegalovirus, *Brucella*, toxoplasmosis, *Mycoplasma hominis*, *Chlamydia trachomatis*, and *Ureaplasma urealyticum*.
Chemical agents	Tobacco, anaesthetic gases, arsenic, benzene, solvents, ethylene oxide, formaldehyde, pesticides, lead, mercury, and cadmium
Psychological disorders	
Immunological disorders	Antiphospholipid syndrome
	Thrombophilia (hereditary)

Ectopic pregnancies

Maternal age	> 35 years old
Contraception	Intrauterine device
Pelvic inflammatory disease	Gonorrhoea, *chlamydia*
Pelvic surgery	Tubal surgery
	Myomectomy, Caesarean Section

Complete hydatidiform mole

Maternal age	> 35 years old
Racial/dietary factor	Asia

important in the management of this common pregnancy complication. Within this context, ultrasound probably plays its most important role in reassuring the patient that the fetus is alive and developing normally.

Missed abortion

A missed abortion is a gestational sac containing a dead embryo/fetus before 20 weeks' gestation without clinical symptoms of expulsion. The diagnosis is usually made by failure to identify a fetal heart action on ultrasound (Fig. 8.5). Within this context, the mother often complains of chronic but light vaginal bleeding. With the introduction of transvaginal ultrasound, the diagnosis can now be made from as early as 6 weeks' gestation. When the gestational sac is more than 25 mm in diameter and no embryonic/fetal part can be seen, the terms 'blighted ovum' or 'anembryonic pregnancy' have often been used by pathologists and more commonly by obstetricians, suggesting wrongly that the sac may have developed without an embryo. The explanation for this feature is the early death and resorption of the embryo with persistence of the placental tissue rather than a pregnancy originally without an embryo.

Inevitable miscarriage

An inevitable miscarriage can be complete or incomplete depending on whether or not all fetal and placental tissues have been expelled from the uterus (Fig. 8.5). The typical features of incomplete abortion are heavy, sometimes intermittent, bleeding with passage of clots and tissue, together with lower abdominal cramps. If these symptoms improve spontaneously, a complete abortion is more likely. Ultrasound examination is important in determining the absence or persistence of conception products inside the uterine cavity.

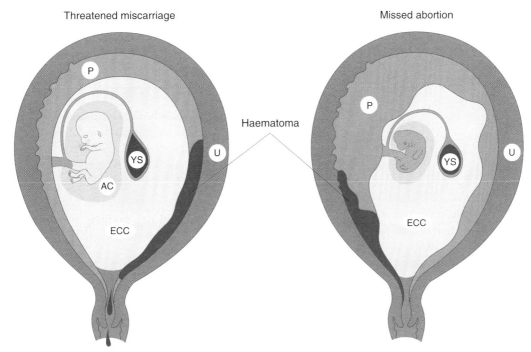

Threatened miscarriage

Missed abortion

Haematoma

Figure 8.5 Diagram showing the different types of miscarriage. (P, placenta; U, uterus; AC, amniotic cavity; YS, yolk sac; ECC, extra-coloemic cavity)

Recurrent miscarriage

A recurrent miscarriage is defined as three or more consecutive spontaneous abortions. The aetiologies of recurrent pregnancy failure are diverse and are not well-understood. They may present clinically as any of the previously described forms of miscarriages.

Clinical features

History

A history of amenorrhea followed by vaginal bleeding with low abdominal pain and a positive pregnancy test is fundamental. Other factors pertinent to the history are maternal age, medical disorders and a previous history of miscarriage.

General examination

This must include a record of pulse rate and blood pressure and assessment of hand palm and conjunctive colour will give an idea about secondary anaemia.

Speculum examination

When a patient is seen during the first trimester with vaginal bleeding, a history of abdominal pain and passage of clots or tissue through an open cervix, the diagnosis of abortion is usually conspicuous. But when the cervix is closed and the bleeding is not heavy, distinguishing between complete or incomplete miscarriage and threatened or missed abortions can be difficult on clinical findings only.

Ultrasound examination

Ultrasound will confirm the intrauterine location of the gestational sac and establish the viability of the pregnancy. If the gestational sac is smaller than expected for gestational age, the possibility of incorrect dates should always be considered, especially in the absence of clinical features suggestive of threatened abortion. Under these circumstances a repeat scan should be arranged after a period of at least seven days and be performed by an experienced operator.

Laboratory investigations

These must include a full blood count and blood group. Patients who are Rhesus negative must systematically receive a dose of anti-D in case of bleeding during pregnancy.

hCG, progesterone and other placental hormones are of limited use in predicting a miscarriage. The correlations of ultrasound and circulating placental protein measurements indicate that the diagnostic value of ultrasound in threatened miscarriage is often better than that of biochemical tests. As a clinical predictive tool, measurement of placental proteins is often unnecessary if fetal life can be demonstrated by ultrasound.

Management

Surgical

The mechanical dilatation and curettage of the uterus for the evacuation of retained products of conception is usually a simple procedure. Complications are uncommon and include cervical tears, uterine perforation and the creation of false passage. Some of these complications can be prevented by cervical preparation, using prostaglandins.

Medical

Includes surveillance, drug therapy and psychological support. Women with minimal residual tissue in the uterine cavity on ultrasound can be treated expectantly safely. Prostaglandin analogues have been used within the context of missed abortion but so far the results have been disappointing. This is because when they are administered vaginally, complete evacuation of the uterus was achieved in only half the cases because of the long interval required. Mifepristone (RU486) is a progesterone competitive antagonist, which, used in combination with prostaglandin analogues, has been shown to be effective in about 90 per cent of cases.

Follow-up

Although the majority of miscarriages is not treatable, the prognosis for future pregnancies is directly dependent on the type of abnormality and on whether the mother or her partner carries it. Counselling the parents regarding the diagnostic evaluation processes, treatments required, prognosis and risks for the future pregnancies should always be offered in case of early pregnancy failure.

In couples with recurrent miscarriages (more than three consecutive miscarriages) investigation should include parental and fetal karyotype to exclude a translocation, gynaecological examination to exclude a uterine abnormality and blood tests (glucose level, thyroid functional tests, antiphospholipid and anticardiolipin antibodies, lupus anticoagulant) (Table 8.3).

Ectopic pregnancy

Definition

An ectopic pregnancy is when the conceptus implants either outside the uterus (fallopian tube, ovary and abdominal cavity) or in an abnormal position within the uterus (cornua, cervix). Combined tubal and uterine (heterotopic) pregnancies are uncommon.

Epidemiology and risk factors

The incidence of ectopic pregnancy is 22 per 1000 live births and 16 per 1000 pregnancies. A dramatic increase in incidence over time has been reported in several countries. In the USA, in 1970–1992, the overall increase has been almost five-fold, from 4 to 19 per 1000 pregnancies. Between 95 and 98 per cent of ectopic pregnancies occur in the fallopian tube. Over 50 per cent of tubal pregnancies are situated in the ampulla, approximately 20 per cent occur in the isthmus, around 12 per cent are fimbrial and approximately 10 per cent are interstitial (Fig. 8.6).

Risk factors

There is a strong tendency for the risk of ectopic pregnancy to increase with maternal age, the number of sexual partners, the use of an intrauterine device, after a proven pelvic inflammatory disease (gonorrhoea, *Chlamydia*) and after pelvic surgery. The various risk factors for ectopic pregnancy are highly interrelated. For example, smoking is associated with sexual promiscuity and thus with a higher exposure risk to sexually transmitted infectious agents. The risk of recurrence is around 10 per cent and is increased in those who have had a previous miscarriage or who have suffered tubal damage.

Mortality rate

In England and Wales, the mortality rate due to ectopic pregnancy has fallen from 17 per million deliveries in 1961–63 to 4 per million in 1982–84. Despite this decline in case-fatality rates, mortality from ectopic pregnancy remains high, representing 13 per cent of all maternal deaths in 1989. The fatality rate of ectopic pregnancy is about four times higher than the chance of dying in childbirth.

Table 8.3 – Diagnosis and management of early pregnancy disorders

Miscarriage	**Features**
Threatened miscarriage	Normal hCG for gestational age.
	Intrauterine gestational sac.
	Embryonic/fetal heart activity.
	Intrauterine bleeding/haematoma.

Management => Clinical surveillance including weekly ultrasound examination

Missed abortion	Low hCG for gestational age.
	Intrauterine gestational sac (>20 mm in diameter) with no embryo or with 6 mm embryo with no heart activity on TVS.

Management => Surgical evacuation (ERPC) or medical induction (RU486 + Pgs).

Incomplete miscarriage	Persistence of conception products inside the uterine cavity on TVS.

Management => Surgical evacuation (ERPC) or medical induction (RU486 + Pgs).

Ectopic pregnancies	Normal to low hCG for gestational age (discriminatory level).
	Small uterus for gestational age with no gestational sac or small pseudosac (decidual reaction) on TVS.
	Adnexal gestational sac or mass with or without pelvic fluid on TVS.

Management => Salpingectomy (removal of the tube and gestational sac) or sapingostomy (opening of the tube and removal of the gestational sac, only) via laparoscopy or laparotomy.

Complete hydatidiform mole	Very high hCG for gestational age.
	Uterine enlargement greater than expected for gestational age.
	Uterine cavity filled with multiple sonolucent areas of varying size and shape without associated embryo/fetus.

Management => Surgical evacuation (ERPC) and weekly hCG level monitoring until undetectable followed by monthly monitoring for 6–24 months.

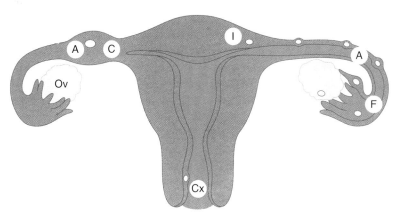

Figure 8.6 Diagram showing the different possible locations of an ectopic pregnancy.

A = Ampulla
Cx = Cervix
F = Fimbrial
I = Interstitial
Ov = Ovary

Ectopic pregnancy

In theory any mechanical or functional factors that prevent or interfere with the passage of the fertilized egg to the uterine cavity may be an etiological factor for an ectopic pregnancy.

It is believed that the main cause for a tubal implantation of the gestational sac is a low-grade infection as approximately 50 per cent of women operated on for an ectopic pregnancy have evidence of chronic pelvic inflammatory disease. A high proportion of women with a tubal pregnancy miscarry during the early stages of gestation. The products of conception may persist for a considerable period of time within the tube as one form of 'chronic ectopic pregnancy', or they may be gradually absorbed.

If implantation occurs into a site of the tube which offers a sufficient area for placentation, the process is very similar to that of an intrauterine pregnancy, for the conceptus penetrates the tubal mucosa and becomes embedded in the tissues of the tubal wall (Fig. 8.6). The extravillous trophoblast will penetrate the full thickness of the muscular layer of the tube to reach the subserosa and the tubo-ovarian circulation. Due to its limited distensibility, the tube will rupture. Although this event is usually accompanied by fetal death, occasionally, the fetus, following the rupture, retains sufficient attachment to its blood supply to maintain viability and secondary abdominal pregnancy can proceed to term.

In an ectopic pregnancy, the uterine endometrium usually responds to the hormonal changes of pregnancy and undergoes focal decidua changes (Arias–Stella reaction). If the ectopic pregnancy miscarries, the uterine decidua may slough off as a cast but more commonly as fragments mixed with small blood clots.

Clinical features

Compared to the other forms of early pregnancy disorders, there is no pathognomonic pain of findings on clinical examination that are diagnostic of a developing extrauterine pregnancy. Vaginal bleeding (usually old blood in small amounts) and chronic pelvic pain (iliac fossa, sometimes bilateral) are the most commonly reported symptoms.

General examination

This must include a record of pulse rate and blood pressure. Shoulder pain, which may occur secondary to blood irritating the diaphragm and vascular instability characterized by low blood pressure, fainting, dizziness and rapid heart rate may be noted. These symptoms are present in about 59 per cent of patients and are most typical of patients whose ectopic pregnancy has ruptured (intra-abdominal bleeding).

Gynaecological examination

Speculum or bimanual examination must be performed in an environment where facilities for resuscitation are available as this examination may provoke the rupture of the tube.

Laparoscopy and uterine curettage

These have traditionally been the gold standard by which to establish the diagnosis of extrauterine pregnancy. The mere absence of placental villi in the curettage does not necessarily indicate an ectopic pregnancy. Conversely, the presence of placental villi in the curettage does not invalidate completely a diagnosis of ectopic pregnancy for an ectopic pregnancy in a tube, cornua or in the cervix may partially abort.

Culdocentesis

To exclude hemoperitoneum has also been a routine investigation in the emergency room for the rule out 'ectopic patient'. Because this test is based on late development in the natural history of the ectopic pregnancy, it is easy to imagine that it is not useful in detecting an early ectopic pregnancy.

hCG and transvaginal ultrasound

Screening algorithms incorporating plasma hCG and transvaginal sonography have allowed for a less invasive evaluation of the patient with a suspected ectopic pregnancy. hCG levels and ultrasound findings must be interpreted together. One of the most important parameters is the discriminatory hCG level above which the gestational sac of an intrauterine pregnancy should be detectable by ultrasonography (usually 1000 iu/L).

The presence or absence of an intrauterine gestational sac is the principle point of distinction between intrauterine and tubal pregnancy. The sonographic finding of an extrauterine sac with an embryo or embryonic remnants is the most reliable diagnosis of ectopic pregnancy. An empty ectopic sac or a heterogeneous adnexal mass are more common ultrasound features. The presence of fluid in the pouch of Douglas is a non-specific sign of ectopic pregnancy. In 10–20 per cent of ectopic pregnancies, a pseudogestational sac is seen as a small, centrally located endometrial fluid collection surrounded by a single echogenic rim of endometrial tissue undergoing decidual reaction.

A laparoscopy should be considered in women with hCG above the discriminatory level and absence of an intrauterine gestational sac on ultrasound.

Management

The classical approach to the treatment of ectopic pregnancy has always been surgical (salpingectomy or salpingotomy) either by laparotomy or laparoscopy.

With the wider use of ultrasound, an early diagnosis is now possible in many cases before the onset of symptoms. Non-surgical (medical) therapeutic approaches have been introduced, such as puncture and aspiration of ectopic sac, local injections of prostaglandins, potassium chloride, hyperosmolar glucose or methotrexate. Advantages of treatment that does not involve surgery or the use of potentially toxic drugs are obvious. With earlier diagnosis it has also become apparent that spontaneous regression of tubal pregnancies is more common than previously thought. This has led to non-interventional expectant management, which is based on the assumption that a significant proportion of all tubal pregnancies will resolve without any treatment. Unfortunately, not all patients will be suitable for this type of treatment or for a simple follow-up and strict criteria must be observed in the selection of patients. Ultrasound examinations combined with serial hCG assessments are prerequisites for successful expectant management or in the follow-up of the patient treated medically.

Gestational trophoblastic disorders

Definitions

Gestational trophoblastic disease (GTD) is a term commonly applied to a spectrum of inter-related diseases originating from the placental trophoblast. The main categories of GTD are complete hydatidiform mole, partial hydatidiform mole and choriocarcinoma. Complete or classical hydatidiform moles are described as a generalized swelling of the villous tissue, diffuse trophoblastic hyperplasia and no embryonic or fetal tissue. Partial hydatidiform mole is characterized by focal swelling of the villous tissue, focal trophoblastic hyperplasia and embryonic or fetal tissue. The abnormal villi are scattered within macroscopically normal placental tissue that tends to retain its shape.

Epidemiology and risk factors

Incidence rate
Estimates of the incidence of the various forms of GTD vary, mainly because few countries have registries and complete and partial mole have often been treated as a single entity in epidemiological study. The estimated incidence of complete mole is 1 per 1000–2000 pregnancies (Table 8.1) whereas the incidence of partial mole is around 1 per 700 pregnancies. The vast majority of complete and partial mole abort spontaneously during the first trimester and the incidence of molar pregnancies has been estimated to be 2 per cent of all miscarriages. The incidence of choriocarcinoma varies from 1 in 10,000 to 1 in 50,000 pregnancies, or, expressed as a percentage of hydatidiform mole, 3 to 10 per cent.

Risk factors
Maternal age and a previous history of molar pregnancy have consistently been shown to influence the risk of hydatidiform mole and choriocarcinoma, whereas the evidence that the rate of molar pregnancies varies according to the dietary habits of some ethnic groups remains controversial. The ABO blood groups of the parents appear to be a factor in choriocarcinoma development, i.e. women with blood group A have been shown to have a greater risk than blood group O women.

Clinical features

General and gynaecological examination
Patients with a complete mole present with vaginal bleeding, uterine enlargement greater than expected for gestational age and an abnormally high level of serum hCG. Medical complications include pregnancy-induced hypertension, hyperthyroidism, hyperemesis, anaemia and the development of ovarian theca lutein cysts. The ovarian hyperstimulation and

P Understanding the pathophysiology

Complete hydatidiform mole

These have a diploid chromosomal constitution totally derived from the paternal genome usually resulting from the fertilization of an oocyte by a diploid spermatozoon. The maternal chromosomes may be either inactivated or absent, remaining only inside the mitochondria.

Partial moles are usually triploid and of diandric origin, having two sets of chromosomes from paternal origin and one from maternal origin. Most have a 69XXX or 69XXY genotype derived from a haploid ovum with either reduplication of the paternal haploid set from a single sperm, or less frequently, from dispermic fertilization. Triploidy of digynic origin, due to a double maternal contribution is not associated with placental hydatidiform changes.

Choriocarcinoma is a highly malignant tumour that arises from the trophoblastic epithelium and metastasizes readily to the lungs, liver and brain. Around 50 per cent of choriocarcinomas follow a molar pregnancy, 30 per cent occur after a miscarriage and 20 per cent after an apparently normal pregnancy. Choriocarcinomas can occur after an extrauterine pregnancy and will present with signs and symptoms similar to those classically outlined for ectopic pregnancy. There have been a few well-documented examples of choriocarcinoma arising from villous tissue in an otherwise normally developed placenta, suggesting that most or possibly all choriocarcinomas that follow an apparently normal pregnancy are in reality metastases from a small intraplacental choriocarcinoma.

enlargement of both ovaries may subsequently lead to ovarian torsion or rupture of theca lutein cysts.

The primary symptoms of choriocarcinoma are gynaecological, i.e. vaginal bleeding, in only 50–60 per cent of the cases. Many women will present with dyspnoea, neurological symptoms and abdominal pain, a few weeks or months and sometimes up to 10–15 years after their last pregnancy.

Arteriograpy

Arteriography was first used in the *in utero* diagnosis of molar pregnancy. Because of cost, maternal discomfort and morbidity it was rapidly replaced by ultrasound imaging in the 1960s. In women with persistent GTD or with chemotherapy-resistant disease, angiography has proved to be of great value in the diagnostic work-up of myometrial invasion and surgical management.

Ultrasound examination

Molar changes can now be detected from the second month of pregnancy by ultrasound which typically reveals a uterine cavity filled with multiple sonolucent areas of varying size and shape ('snow storm appearance') without associated embryonic or fetal structure (Fig. 8.7).

Laboratory examinations

The measurement of plasma hCG is pivotal in the diagnosis and follow-up of GTD.

Other investigations

These must include a histological examination of the sample confirming the trophoblastic hyperplasia and a chest X-ray to exclude the presence of lung metastasis.

Management

Following uterine evacuation, 18–29 per cent of patients with a complete mole and 1–11 per cent of patients with a partial mole will develop a persistent trophoblastic tumour. Pulmonary complications due to trophoblastic embolization are frequently observed following the evacuation of a molar pregnancy and the prognosis for these patients depends on the severity of the symptoms. Thus early diagnosis reduces the risk of severe complications and in particular respiratory failure.

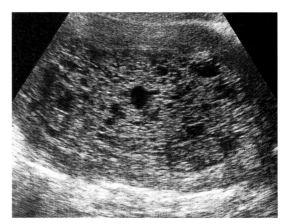

Figure 8.7 Ultrasound view of a complete hydatidiform mole at the end of the first trimester.

Serial hCG levels is the gold standard for the diagnosis and monitoring therapeutic response of GTD. After evacuation of a molar pregnancy, the hCG level should be monitored weekly until undetectable followed by monthly monitoring for 6–24 months.

New developments

Ultrasound imaging has improved the diagnostic capability of early pregnancy disorders. The diagnosis of suspected miscarriages and life-threatening ectopic pregnancies is now more accurate and less invasive than it has ever been in the past. Ultrasound and, in particular, transvaginal sonography combined with fast and accurate hCG testing are the best routine tools that obstetricians and gynaecologists can offer women with an abnormal early pregnancy.

Key Points

- The miscarriage of an early pregnancy is the commonest medical complication
- hCG is a placental-specific protein that can be detected in maternal plasma and urine seven and 14 days after ovulation, respectively
- Transvaginal ultrasound should demonstrate a gestational sac from 4.4–4.6 weeks (LMP).
- Mortality from ectopic pregnancy remains high as the incidence of ectopic pregnancy has increased over the last 15 years (1–2 per cent of pregnancies)
- Screening algorithms incorporating plasma hCG and transvaginal sonography should allow the diagnosis of most ectopic pregnancies before tubal rupture
- Complete and partial hydatidiform moles can be complicated by persistent trophoblastic disease and the patient should be offered a follow-up

CASE HISTORY

Mrs SP

Twenty-four, single, caucasian, 64 kilograms.

Presents with a 2-day history of right iliac fossa pain and some vaginal bleeding. Her last period was 6 weeks prior to the onset of pain and her periods have been regular. She has not been using regular contraception but has a regular partner. She admits to some breast tenderness and feeling nauseous first thing in the morning. She has no significant past medical history. She has never previously been pregnant.

She is otherwise fit and well.

On examination she looks well. She has some guarding and rebound tenderness in the right iliac fossa. She is afebrile. Vaginal examination confirms tenderness in the right iliac fossa and there is no unusual vaginal discharge.

Her pregnancy test is positive.

Discussion

What is the differential diagnosis?

There are several causes for bleeding in early pregnancy. She could have a threatened or incomplete miscarriage. It is unlikely that this is a complete miscarriage as she has only had a light bleed. It is also possible she might have had a missed miscarriage. **However, the most likely diagnosis is ectopic pregnancy and this must be excluded before assuming another cause.** It is also possible that she may have an early pregnancy that is intact with other pathology such as an ovarian cyst that may have ruptured, torted or haemorrhaged. She may even have accompanying appendicitis.

How would you make a diagnosis?

As the patient seems systemically well but the diagnosis of ectopic has not been excluded blood should be taken for blood count, grouping and saving and IV access must be maintained. An ultrasound scan will confirm whether the gestation is intrauterine or not and whether it is viable or not. Vaginal ultrasound would probably be of most benefit at this stage. If there is no intrauterine pregnancy and no obvious ectopic a laparoscopy is still indicated to exclude the ectopic pregnancy. The optimum management may include laparoscopic removal of the ectopic through a salpingotomy or even salpingectomy.

References for further reading

RCR/RCOG. *Guidance on ultrasound procedures in early pregnancy.* Royal College of Radiologists/Royal College of Obstetricians and Gynaecologists, 1995, 1–8.

Jurkovic D. *Ultrasound and early pregnancy.* Jauniaux E. (eds). Carforth: Parthenon Publishing, 1996.

O'Brian PMS, Grudzinskas JG. (eds). *Problems of early pregnancy – advances in diagnosis and management.* London: RCOG, 1997.

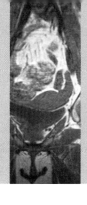

Benign disease of the uterus and cervix

OVERVIEW

Benign disease of the cervix and body of the uterus is extremely common. Cervical ectropion, fibroids and adenomyosis cause symptoms that women present with in almost every gynaecological out-patients clinic.

Benign disease of the uterus may conveniently be classified in terms of the tissue of origin: the uterine cervix, the endometrium or the myometrium.

Epithelium: the uterine cervix

The transformation zone is a special feature of the ectocervix, which is that portion of the uterine cervix visible during speculum examination. Within this zone the stratified squamous epithelium of the vagina meets the columnar epithelium of the cervical canal. The anatomical site of the squamocolumnar junction fluctuates under hormonal influence, and the high cell turnover of this tissue is important in the pathogenesis of cervical carcinoma, discussed in Chapter 12. The columnar epithelium is normally visible with the speculum during the ovulatory phase of the menstrual cycle, during pregnancy and in women taking the combined oral contraceptive pill,

where oestrogen levels are elevated. In contrast, only squamous epithelium is visible in a postmenopausal woman not taking hormone replacement therapy.

Cervical ectropion

The presence of a large area of columnar epithelium on the ectocervix can be associated with excessive mucus secretion, leading to a complaint of vaginal discharge. The appearance of the cervix is termed cervical ectropion or, very inappropriately, a cervical erosion. The latter term is best avoided as it conveys quite the wrong impression of what is really a normal phenomenon. Ectropion can be associated with excessive but non-purulent vaginal discharge, as the surface area of columnar epithelium containing mucus-secreting glands is increased. If the discharge associated with cervical ectropion becomes troublesome to the patient, discontinuing the oral contraceptive pill, or alternatively ablative treatment under local anaesthesia using a thermal probe can reduce it. This treatment involves a thermal probe which heats the tissue to around 100°C, destroying the epithelium to a depth of 3–4 mm. The technique is sometimes confusingly termed 'cold coagulation' to distinguish it from more destructive diathermy or laser treatment of the cervix. A less glandular epithelium regenerates after the procedure.

Cervical ectropion may also give rise to postcoital bleeding, as fine blood vessels present within the columnar epithelium are easily traumatized. This symptom may be very distressing as well as embarrassing, but should always be included as a direct question in the gynaecological history because of its association with cervical carcinoma. Reassurance about the cause and treatment as described above can be given after obtaining a normal cervical cytology result.

Nabothian follicles

Within the transformation zone of the ectocervix the exposed columnar epithelium undergoes squamous metaplasia. Glands contained within columnar epithelium may become roofed over with squamous cells, resulting in the formation of small (2–3 mm) mucus-filled cysts visible on the ectocervix. These are termed Nabothian follicles, and are of no pathological significance. Larger (up to 10 mm) Nabothian follicles are occasionally identified coincidentally during transvaginal ultrasound scanning, but do not require treatment.

Endometrium

The uterine endometrium comprises glands and stroma with a complex architecture including blood vessels and nerves. As discussed in detail in Chapter 4, during the follicular phase of the menstrual cycle proliferation of tissue from the basal layer occurs, followed by secretory changes under the influence of progesterone after ovulation and finally shedding as progesterone levels fall with corpus luteum regression. Disturbances of prostaglandin biosynthesis within the endometrium may give rise to menstrual disorders (see Chapter 5) but the increased use of endoscopy and ultrasound has provided a perspective on visible abnormalities of the endometrium.

Endometrial polyps

Historically, a diagnosis of 'dysfunctional uterine bleeding' was made in women with menstrual disturbance in whom curettage provided a histologically normal sample of endometrium. In current practice, hysteroscopy or ultrasound enable the identification of endometrial polyps that may be the cause of abnormal bleeding, especially intermenstrual bleeding. These typically occur in women aged over 40 years. Intermenstrual bleeding in younger women is more likely to be a consequence of combined or progestogen-only contraceptive pill use, or the wearing of an IUCD, and is less likely to require investigation. In peri- or postmenopausal women with abnormal bleeding the first priority is to exclude endometrial malignancy, but in many patients the cause will be a benign polyp that can be removed at hysteroscopy. Reflecting typical clinical experience, polyps were detected by out-patient hysteroscopy in 11 per cent of 2581 women referred for the investigation of menstrual symptoms.

After the menopause the endometrium is normally atrophic, but hormone replacement therapy does provide endometrial stimulation, leading to polyp formation. Women presenting special diagnostic problems are those taking tamoxifen for the treatment of breast cancer. This agent is a partial oestrogen agonist with inhibitory effects on breast tissue. However, the endometrium is stimulated, sometimes leading to polyp formation or even endometrial hyperplasia and malignancy. Ultrasound assessment is difficult because the drug affects the sonographic properties of the inner myometrium, giving the misleading impression of a greatly thickened endometrium.

Asherman's syndrome

When the endometrium has been damaged, in particular when it has been removed down to or beyond the basal layer, normal regeneration does not occur and instead fibrosis and adhesion formation occur, termed Asherman's syndrome. This phenomenon is exploited therapeutically in endometrial resection, a surgical treatment for menorrhagia where the endometrium is resected using a diathermy loop or is ablated with a laser, in each case beyond the basal layer into the myometrium so that regeneration cannot occur. The result is reduced, or absent, menstrual shedding.

Asherman's syndrome occurs as an adverse consequence of excessive curettage, especially at the time of evacuation of retained placental tissue after miscarriage or secondary postpartum haemorrhage. In a hysteroscopic follow-up study after surgical evacuation following retained placenta, the prevalence of adhesions within the endometrial cavity was 20 per cent, and these were strongly associated with menstrual symptoms. Treatment options for Asherman's syndrome include maintaining separation of the uterine walls by insertion of a large inert IUCD such as a Lippes loop, now obsolete other than for this purpose, or hysteroscopic lysis of intrauterine adhesions.

Other causes of Asherman's syndrome relevant in particular parts of the world are tuberculosis and schistosomiasis.

Complications of cervical stenosis

When premalignant disease of the cervix was treated by knife cone biopsy, rather than the currently preferred technique of diathermy loop excision (see Chapter 12), subsequent cervical stenosis was common. This is now less commonly seen, but it may give rise to haematometra as menstrual blood accumulates in the endometrial cavity. Suggestive features in the history are amenorrhoea associated with severe cyclical dysmenorrhoea-like pain, with a previous history of cervical surgery. In postmenopausal women cervical stenosis may give rise to pyometra, where accumulated secretions become a focus of infection. Underlying malignancy may also lead to pyometra. Treatment is by careful surgical dilatation of the cervix and endometrial biopsy under antibiotic cover. Finally, a cervix not completely stenosed but scarred from previous surgery may fail to dilate during labour (cervical dystocia), necessitating Caesarean Section.

Myometrium: uterine fibroids

Pathology

A fibroid is a benign tumour of uterine smooth muscle, termed a leiomyoma. The gross appearance is of a firm, whorled tumour located adjacent to and bulging into the endometrial cavity (submuccous fibroid), centrally within the myometrium (intramural fibroid), at the outer border of the myometrium (subserosal fibroid) or attached to the uterus by a narrow pedicle containing blood vessels (pedunculated fibroid) (Fig. 9.1). Fibroids can arise separately from the uterus, especially in the broad ligament, presumably from embryonal remnants. The typical whorled appearance may be altered following degeneration, three forms of which are recognized: red, hyaline and cystic.

Red degeneration follows an acute disruption of the blood supply to the fibroid during active growth, classically during pregnancy. This may present with the sudden onset of pain and tenderness localized to an area of the uterus, associated with a mild pyrexia and leucocytosis. The symptoms and signs typically resolve over a few days and surgical intervention is rarely required.

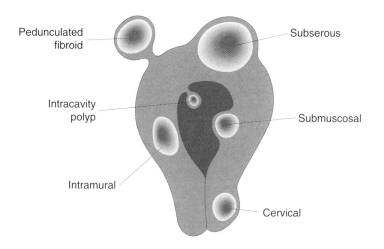

Figure 9.1 Typical location of uterine fibroids.

Pedunculated fibroid

Subserous

Intracavity polyp

Submuscosal

Intramural

Cervical

Hyaline degeneration occurs when the fibroid more gradually outgrows its blood supply, and may progress to central necrosis leaving cystic spaces at the centre, termed cystic degeneration. As the final stage in the natural history, calcification of a fibroid may be detected incidentally on an abdominal X-ray in a postmenopausal woman. Rarely malignant/sarcomatous degeneration may occur.

P Understanding the pathophysiology

Aetiology

A range of hypotheses accounting for the pathogenesis of fibroids has been explored. The key features of uterine leiomyomata are their occurrence during the reproductive years, where ovarian hormone levels are high, their diverse manifestation as either single or multiple tumours, and the existence of racial and familial predisposition. The possibility of abnormal oestrogen receptor expression has been explored and discounted; both main progesterone receptor subtypes are expressed similarly in myoma and normal myometrium. Thus myoma tissue is still influenced by ovarian hormones. Experimentally, progesterone has been shown to stimulate the production of both an apoptosis-inhibiting protein and epidermal growth factor (EGF) in cultured myoma tissue. Oestradiol has the effect of stimulating expression of EGF receptor.

Reduced expression of growth inhibitory factors such as monocyte chemotactic protein 1 (MCP-1) may play a part in the loss of inhibition required for fibroid growth. Treatment by ovarian suppression (see below) is associated with an increase in matrix metalloproteinase (MMP) expression and a decrease in metalloproteinase inhibitory (TIMP) activity, which suggests that ovarian hormones have a role in maintaining the architecture of a myoma once formed.

Cytogenetic studies have identified specific features of uterine myoma tissue compared to normal myometrium and to leiomyosarcoma. It appears that cells within an individual myoma are monoclonal in origin, but cells from different myomas within the same uterus are of independent origin. It is likely that the clonal expansion of tumour cells precedes the development of cytogenetic aberrations, but the latter may determine the clinical course depending on the extent to which control over growth is lost. Some evidence for this is provided by cytogenetic analysis, which showed a greater proportion of karyotypic abnormality in larger, compared to smaller, fibroids. The most common cytogenetic aberrations have been detected on chromosome 12, 6, 3 and 7, a ring chromosome 1, and translocation involving chromosomes 12 and 14. Relevant areas of chromosomes 12, 6 and 7 are thought to contain putative growth-regulating or tumour-suppressor genes. It is not yet clear to what extent the cytogenetic features can be correlated with the clinical picture.

The possibility of malignant transformation of a fibroid to a leiomyosarcoma has traditionally been cited as a reason to recommend surgery for fibroids, with a stated risk of up to 0.5 per cent. However, current opinion is that where a sarcoma develops in the presence of fibroids the association is coincidental, and that malignant transformation of a fibroid is unlikely. The cytogenetic evidence gives some basis for reassurance on this point as the typical findings in leiomyosarcoma tissue are of more extensive genetic instability, with frequent deletions especially involving chromosomes 1 and 10.

Clinical features

Fibroids are common, being detectable clinically in about 20 per cent of women over 30 years of age. Autopsy studies with systematic histology of the uterus show a prevalence of up to 50 per cent. Risk factors for clinically significant fibroids are nulliparity, obesity, a positive family history and African racial origin. The great majority do not cause symptoms but may be identified coincidentally, for example, at the time of taking a cervical smear or performing laparoscopic sterilization. Common presenting complaints are menstrual disturbance and pressure symptoms, especially urinary frequency. Pain is unusual except in the special circumstance of acute degeneration discussed above. Menorrhagia may occur coincidentally in a woman with fibroids: it is likely that only submucous fibroids distorting the endometrial cavity and increasing the surface area are truly causal.

Subfertility may result from mechanical distortion or occlusion of the fallopian tubes, and an endometrial cavity grossly distorted by submucous fibroids may prevent implantation of a fertilized ovum. Once a pregnancy is established, however, the risk of miscarriage is not increased. In late pregnancy, fibroids located in the cervix or lower uterine segment may be the cause of an abnormal lie. After delivery, post-partum haemorrhage may occur due to inefficient uterine contraction.

Abdominal examination might indicate the presence of a firm mass arising from the pelvis, and on bimanual examination the mass is felt to be part of the uterus, usually with some mobility.

Differential diagnosis

Other causes of an abdominopelvic mass in a woman in the reproductive years need to be considered. The uterus enlarged with fibroids is typically firm in contrast to that of a uterus enlarged with a pregnancy. An ovarian tumour, whether benign or malignant, primary or secondary, may enlarge to occupy the pelvis and be difficult clinically to differentiate from a uterine fibroid. Leiomyosarcomas typically present with a history of a rapidly enlarging abdominopelvic mass. There may be less mobility of the uterus than expected with a fibroid and general signs of cachexia.

Investigations

Often the clinical features alone will be sufficient to establish the diagnosis. A haemoglobin concentration will help to indicate anaemia if there is clinically significant menorrhagia. Ultrasonography is useful to distinguish a uterine from an ovarian mass. Imaging of the renal tract may be helpful in the presence of a large fibroid to exclude hydronephrosis due to pressure from the mass on the ureters. The clinical suspicion of sarcoma will be an indication for needle biopsy or, more likely, urgent laparotomy.

Treatment

Conservative management is appropriate where asymptomatic fibroids are detected incidentally. It may be useful to establish the growth rate of the fibroids by repeat clinical examination or ultrasound after a 6–12 month interval. Where treatment is required, the only practical currently available medical treatment is ovarian suppression using a GnRH agonist. Unfortunately, while very effective in shrinking fibroids, when ovarian function returns

the fibroids regrow to their previous dimensions. Mifepristone (an antiprogestogen) has been shown to be effective in shrinking fibroids at a low dose, but is not available for use in this indication. The optimal dose, duration of treatment and long-term effects have yet to be established.

The choice of surgical treatment is determined by the presenting complaint and the patient's aspirations for menstrual function and fertility. Menorrhagia associated with a submucous fibroid or fibroid polyp (Fig. 9.2) may be treated by hysteroscopic resection. Where a bulky fibroid uterus causes pressure symptoms, the options are myomectomy with uterine conservation, or hysterectomy. Myomectomy will be the preferred option where preservation of fertility is required, but care will be required in the management of a subsequent pregnancy as the uterus may be predisposed to rupture. It is traditionally held that uterine rupture during pregnancy is more likely when the endometrial cavity has been entered during myomectomy, but, not surprisingly, there are few data to confirm or refute this. In any event, the decision to undertake myomectomy in a woman who desires future fertility needs to be carefully considered and the benefits and risks fully discussed with the patient. An important point for the pre-operative discussion is that there is a small but significant risk of uncontrolled bleeding during myomectomy, which could lead to the need for hysterectomy.

Hysterectomy and myomectomy can be facilitated by GnRH agonist pretreatment over a two-month period to reduce the bulk and vascularity of the fibroids. Useful benefits of this approach are to enable a Pfannensteil (low transverse) rather than a midline abdominal incision, or to facilitate vaginal rather than abdominal hysterectomy, both of which are conducive to more rapid recovery and fewer

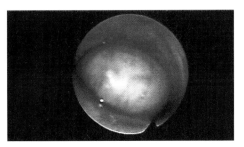

Figure 9.2 Hysteroscopic appearance of a fibroid polyp within the endometrial cavity. (Kindly supplied by Mr ED Alexopoulos.)

postoperative complications. A technical problem with myomectomy after GnRH agonist pretreatment is that the tissue planes around the fibroid are less easily defined, but on the positive side blood loss and the likely need for transfusion is reduced.

Adenomyosis

Adenomyosis is a condition in which functioning endometrial tissue has penetrated the myometrium by direct spread from the uterine lining.

P Understanding the pathophysiology

The majority of cells that invade the myometrium are from the basal layer of the endometrium. As they invade they cause a marked stromal reaction and form small nodules. These nodules contain some blood and cause proliferation of the myometrium and the 'tumour' enlarges progressively. Clinically it is difficult to distinguish between a myoma and adenomyosis and often both may co-exist. Adenomyosis causes slow growth of the uterus and therefore often occurs later in the reproductive years.

S Symptoms

- Women may be asymptomatic.
- Pain is often associated with menstruation. The pain tends to increase throughout menstruation reaching its peak towards the end of the bleeding.
- Regular menstruation, often with increased flow or more frequent periods.

Management

Pelvic examination often reveals an enlarged and tender uterus. If the woman has no symptoms and the uterus is not enlarged then no treatment is indicated. If the woman is symptomatic, hysterectomy is usually the preferred treatment since adenomyosis does not respond well to hormonal treatment.

New developments

Endoscopic surgical treatments for fibroids have proved disappointing: myolysis using a diathermy needle to destroy the tissue is followed by intense adhesion formation. Given the requirement for a substantial blood supply to support growth, interruption of the arterial supply to the tumour is a theoretically attractive concept. In practice this is feasible by the radiological technique of percutaneous selective catheterization of the uterine arteries. Microparticles are released into the vessels causing occlusion of both uterine arteries. Sufficient collateral circulation is present from the ovarian arteries to sustain normal uterine metabolic requirements and women experience a substantial reduction in fibroid bulk, together with improvement in menstrual symptoms over the following six months. Currently available follow-up data suggest that the symptomatic improvement be sustained. Figures 9.3 and 9.4 show contrast enhanced magnetic resonance imaging (MRI) of a fibroid uterus before and after embolization of the uterine arteries.

The prospect of more specific medical therapy with long-term benefit has moved closer with a recent report of sustained shrinkage of fibroids after systemic treatment with alpha-interferon, presumed to influence the expression of growth factors within myoma tissue.

Key Points

- Cervical ectropion is a very common finding and may be associated with chlamydial infection
- The aetiology of fibroids is unknown but growth is oestrogen dependent
- Fibroids are common being detectable clinically in about 20% of women over 30 years of age
- Risk factors for fibroids are nulliparity, obesity, a positive family history and African racial origin
- Factors contributing to menorrhagia may include a mechanical obstruction to venous drainage and also increased total surface area of the endometrium and disorders of prostaglandin synthesis and metabolism
- The mechanism whereby fibroids affect fertility is unclear
- Hysteroscopic techniques removal of submucous fibroids are becoming popular to avoid major surgery
- Hormone replacement therapy is not contraindicated in post-menopausal women with fibroids

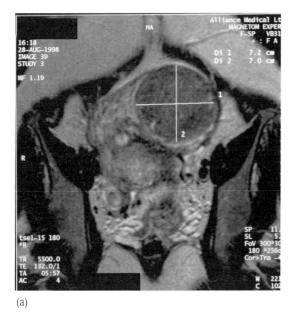
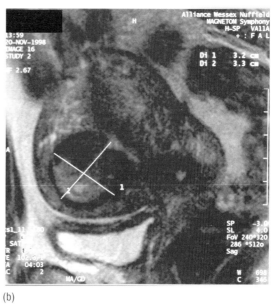

(a)   (b)

Figure 9.3 MRI appearances of uterine fibroids before (a) and after (b) uterine artery embolization. (Kindly supplied by Dr N Hacking.)

CASE HISTORY

Mrs AP

Thirty-seven year old African woman who works as a cleaner in a local hospital presents with a history of increasingly heavy regular painful periods. She also complains of increased urinary frequency especially on standing. There is no irregular bleeding and the smear history is normal. She has two children but still wishes to retain her fertility as she is planning a third. She is married. She is a non-smoker and is otherwise fit and well. On examination the abdomen is distended and there is a pelvic mass consistent with that of a 20-week size pregnancy. Vaginal examination confirms this and ultrasound scan shows two large fibroids which are intramyometrial but also subserous.

Discussion

How would you manage this lady?

The important factor here is that this lady has fibroids large enough to cause compression symptoms and menorrhagia. If fibroids do not cause symptoms they can be observed. The other important feature is she wishes to retain her fertility and therefore hysterectomy may be contraindicated.

Myomectomy can be attempted and obviously there is a risk of bleeding and a woman must be warned that she may lose the uterus if this is performed by laparotomy.

A more modern option is embolisation (i.e. obstructing the uterine artery by an injection of a variety of substances to cause necrosis of the fibroid).

References for further reading

Alexopoulos ED, Fay TN, Simonis CD. A review of 2581 outpatient diagnostic hysteroscopies in the management of abnormal uterine bleeding. *Gynaecological Endoscopy* 1999; **8**:105–10.

Lethaby A, Vollenhoven B, Sowter M. Pre-operative gonadotropin-releasing hormone analogue before hysterectomy or myomectomy for uterine fibroids (Cochrane Review). In: The Cochrane Library, Issue 2, 1999. Oxford: Update Software.

Minakuchi K, Kawamura N, Tsujimura A, Ogita S. Remarkable and persistent shrinkage of uterine leiomyoma associated with interferon alfa treatment for hepatitis. *Lancet* 1999; 353:2127–8.

Rein MS, *et al.* Cytogenetic abnormalities in uterine myomas are associated with myoma size. *Molecular Human Reproduction* 1998; **4**:83–86.

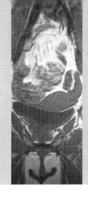

Endometriosis and adenomyosis

OVERVIEW

Endometriosis remains a challenging condition for clinicians and patients alike. Difficulties exist in relationship to explanation of its aetiology, pathophysiology, progression and to problems of its recognition, both from symptoms and at endoscopy. Similar problems exist in determining who, when and for how long to treat individuals once the diagnosis has been made.

Introduction

Endometriosis is most simply defined as the presence of endometrial surface epithelium and/or presence of endometrial gland and stroma outside the lining of the uterine cavity. One of the first definitive descriptions of endometriosis as a specific clinical condition was by Sampson in 1921.

Endometriosis is one of the commonest benign gynaecological conditions. It has been estimated that between 10 and 15 per cent of women presenting with gynaecological symptoms have the disease. This incidence is based on the finding of its presence in those who have undergone laparoscopy for diagnostic indications.

Clinical diagnosis is usually made following the laparoscopic observation of the small, but sometimes large, haemorrhagic or fibrotic lesions in the pelvic peritoneal or the serosal surface of various pelvic organs. These ectopic endometrial tissues respond in varying degrees to the clinical changes in ovarian hormones. Cyclical bleeding within, and from, the endometriotic deposits contributes to local inflammatory reaction and with healing the subsequent fibrosis and overlying peritoneal damage will lead to adhesions between associated organs. Ovarian implants lead to the formation of chocolate cysts or endometriomas.

Epidemiology

It is not known why some women acquire this disease. Its persistence and spread are dependent on the cyclical secretion of steroid hormones from the ovaries, since it is found almost exclusively in women in the reproductive age group with functioning ovaries. It can also be maintained in women who have undergone oophorectomy but are being administered exogenous hormone replacement treatment. It has been suggested that the frequency of this disease has increased in recent years. However one view is that this may reflect the greater use of diagnostic laparoscopy to investigate pain symptoms and the acceptance of the more subtle appearances of endometriosis as viewed endoscopically. There seems to be no association between the extent of the disease process with patient's age or symptomatology.

Histological sub-types

It is possible to link a number of histological sub-types of endometriotic deposits, specific appearances at laparoscopy and a variety of morphological components to the presence of steroid receptors and hormonal responsiveness in terms of proliferative and secretory change in relationship to ovarian steroid hormone stimulation. These are summarized in Table 10.1.

Free implants
These have a polypoidal cauliflower-like structure and grow along the surface or cover a cystic structure.

They are characterized by the presence of a surface epithelium supported by endometrial stroma. Endometrial glands may be present in an identifiable form or may be absent. Cyclical changes with both secretory differentiation and menstrual bleeding have been observed in such lesions (Fig. 10.1a and b). These lesions are highly responsive to alterations in oestrogen secretion, hence they are very sensitive to hormonal suppressive therapies.

Enclosed implants
At this next stage of development the implant has become covered with a surface layer of peritoneum and hence become located within tissue or within a part of a free growing lesion. These lesions will present as wedge-shaped extensions of stroma (ramification), often deep in local tissue planes connecting lesions with one another. In a minority of lesions there are clear-cut changes in response to the menstrual cycle with evidence of proliferative and secretory change and menstrual bleeding. However capillary and

---

P Understanding the pathophysiology

The precise aetiology of endometriosis remains unknown. Several theories exist to explain the process through which endometriosis develops and there is clinical evidence to support each of these concepts. However no single theory can explain the location of endometriotic deposits in all the sites reported.

Menstrual regurgitation and implantation
It has been suggested that endometriosis resulted from the retrograde menstrual regurgitation of viable endometrial glands and tissue within the menstrual fluid and subsequent implantation on the peritoneal surface. In animals, experimental endometriosis can be induced by placement of menstrual fluid or endometrial tissue in the peritoneal cavity. Endometriosis is also commonly found in women with associated abnormalities of the genital tract, causing obstruction to the vaginal outflow of menstrual fluid, lending credence to this theory.

Coelomic epithelium transformation
There is a common origin for the cells lining the Müllerian duct, the peritoneal cells and the cells of the ovary. It has been proposed that these cells undergo de-differentiation back to their primitive origin and then transform into

endometrial cells. This transformation into endometrial cells may be due to hormonal stimuli of ovarian origin by as yet unidentified chemical substances liberated from uterine endometrium or those produced from inflammatory irritation.

Genetic and immunological factors
It has been suggested that genetic and immunological factors may alter susceptibility of a woman and allow her to develop endometriosis. There appears to be an increased incidence in first degree relatives of patients with the disorder and racial differences with increased incidence amongst oriental women and a low prevalence in patients of Afro-Caribbean origin.

Vascular and lymphatic spread
Vascular and lymphatic embolization to distant sites have been demonstrated and explain the rare findings of endometriosis in sites outside the peritoneal cavity. This will explain foci in joints, skin, kidney and lung.

There is almost certainly an interaction between one or more of these theories to allow the development and subsequent growth of ectopic endometrial tissue to the fully developed endometriotic lesion.

venous dilatation is seen during the luteal phase of the ovarian cycle. They react in a similar way to basal endometrium and such lesions are only likely to be partly responsive to hormone treatment approach (Fig. 10.2a and b).

Healed lesions

These have the feature of cystically dilated glands containing a thin glandular epithelium supported by small numbers of stromal cells surrounded by connective tissue. This absence of functional stromal

Table 10.1 – Endometrial deposits – correlation between histological, morphological and functional activity

Histological subtype	Components	Hormonal response	Laparoscopic appearance
Free	Surface epithelium glands and stroma	Proliferative, secretory and menstrual changes	Haemorrhagic vesicle/bleb
Enclosed	Glands and stroma	Proliferative, variable Secretory change No menstruation	Papule and (later) nodule
Healed	Glands only	No response	White nodule or flattened fibrotic scar

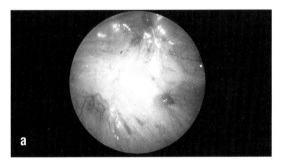 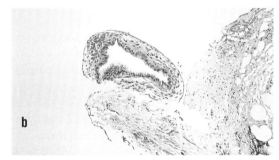

Figure 10.1 a) Red lesion on peritoneum. b) High power section of peritoneum with red lesions. Gland lined with endometrial-like epithelium and surrounded by stroma. Secretory activity not seen (biopsy taken on day 15 of cycle). Source: An Atlas of Endometriosis. Shaw, Robert W. © 1993 Parthenon Publishing Group.

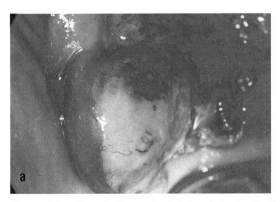 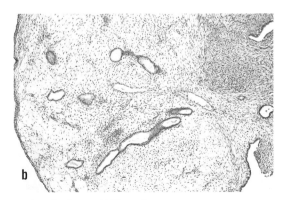

Figure 10.2 a) Extensive haemorrhagic lesions indicative of active, symptomatic disease. b) Biopsy from active lesions on day 24 of cycle. Histology shows oedematous connective tissue, haemosiderin-laden macrophages and complex glandular structures with secretory activity. Source: An Atlas of Endometriosis. Shaw, Robert W. © 1993 Parthenon Publishing Group.

tissue and the enclosure of the implant by increasing the amounts of scar tissue make the lesions insensitive to hormonal stimuli.

Ovarian endometriosis

Endometriosis involving the ovary may present either as a superficial form with haemorrhagic lesions or in a more severe form as an enclosed haemorrhagic cyst.

The superficial lesions have the varying appearances as seen with involvement of the peritoneum. They commonly present as superficial haemorrhagic lesions and red vesicles or blue–black powder burn lesions (Fig. 10.3a and b). Such haemorrhagic lesions are commonly associated with adhesion formation. Adhesions are of particular relevance when they involve the posterior aspect of the ovaries since they then rapidly lead to fixation within the ovarian fossa (Fig. 10.4).

The word endometrioma is used to describe endometriotic (or chocolate) cysts of the ovary. The name arises from the characteristic dark brown chocolate-coloured content of the cyst. Histological evaluation of an endometrioma shows there is a wide variation in the presence of endometriotic tissue. The cyst wall can be lined by free endometrial tissue, histologically and functionally similar to that of endometrial lining. However in many instances of a long-standing presence of an endometrioma, the cyst wall becomes covered only by thickened fibrotic reactive tissue with no specific features of glandular or stromal tissue.

Endometriomas are thought to be formed from lesions that commence on the outer surface of the ovary. As they grow larger there is inversion of the ovarian cortex and with increasing inflammatory reaction at the site of inversion this becomes occluded. The inverted ovarian cortex slowly becomes distended and filled with the 'chocolate' fluid from repeated 'menstrual bleeds'. Leakage from the cyst wall leads commonly to adhesion formation around the endometriomas, particularly on the posterior surface of the ovary within the ovarian fossa or to the posterior aspect of the broad ligament.

Symptoms

Patients with endometriosis have extremely variable symptoms. Some symptoms may vary depending on the site of the ectopic endometrial lesion but there is a lack of correlation between the apparent extent of the disease, as judged laparoscopically, and the intensity of symptoms. Indeed the disease may be a coincidental finding during open surgery or during investigation of a patient complaining of infertility. It may be possible to relate the variety of symptoms in patients with endometriosis to the siting of the deposits (summarized in Table 10.2) but often there is little direct correlation to more specific siting of lesions.

It can be seen that many of these symptoms are shared by a number of other common gynaecological conditions, or disorders of urogenital or gastrointestinal system origin. This cross-over of symptoms means that many patients with endometriosis have a delay from time of onset of symptoms to the time of diagnosis of the disorder. They may well have been treated for other conditions prior to its definitive

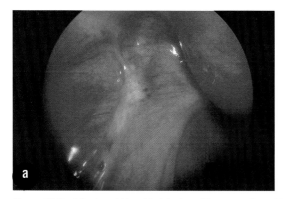
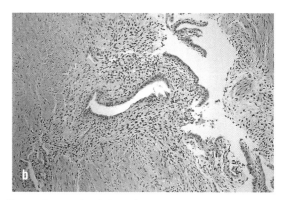

Figure 10.3 a) Puckered blue–black lesion with surrounding white fibrous plaque – classical powder-burn lesion but may represent a less active form of disease. b) High power biopsy of lesion showing fibrous tissue and endometriotic glands, which are inactive with no active bleeding (biopsy taken on day 21 of cycle). Source: An Atlas of Endometriosis. Shaw, Robert W. © 1993 Parthenon Publishing Group.

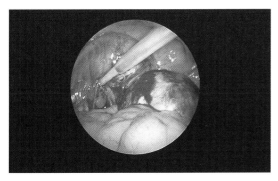

Figure 10.4 Endometrioma on left ovary with adhesions to descending colon. Source: An Atlas of Endometriosis. Shaw, Robert W. © 1993 Parthenon Publishing Group.

diagnosis or labelled as having significant psychosomatic components to their symptomatology. No one symptom is pathognomic of endometriosis but one symptom is highly predictive, that of spasmodic dysmenorrhoea, particularly if severe enough to warrant time off work and if unresponsive to normal analgesics. If this symptom is also associated with pain on postmenstrual days, pelvic pain throughout the cycle or deep pain at intercourse

Table 10.2 – Symptoms of endometriosis in relationship with site of lesion

Site	Symptoms
Female reproductive tract	Dsymenorrhoea Lower abdominal and pelvic pain Dyspareunia Rupture/torsion endometrioma Low back pain Infertility
Urinary tract	Cyclical haematuria/dysuria Ureteric obstruction
Gastrointestinal tract	Dyschezia Cyclical rectal bleeding Obstruction
Surgical scars/ umbilicus	Cyclical pain and bleeding
Lung	Cyclical haemoptysis Haemopneumothorax

(deep dyspareunia), this should further heighten the suspicion of endometriosis. The occurrence of abnormal cyclical bleeding at the time of menstruation, from the rectum, bladder or umbilicus is virtually pathognomic of the presence of the disease.

Endometriosis and infertility

Endometriosis in infertility

It is estimated that between 30 and 40 per cent of patients with endometriosis complain of difficulty in conceiving. In many patients there is a multifactorial pathogenesis to this infertility. It has yet to be shown how the presence of a few small endometriotic deposits render a patient infertile. In the more severe stages of endometriosis there is commonly anatomical distortion with periadnexal adhesions and destruction of ovarian tissue when endometriomas develop, hence a more readily explainable relationship is apparent. A number of possible and variable mechanisms have been postulated to connect mild endometriosis with infertility. These vary from endocrine disorders including anovulation, altered prolactin secretion and luteinized unruptured follicle syndrome, to disorders of sperm or oocyte function (Table 10.3).

Currently there is no simple explanation of how mild endometriosis may prevent conception occurring. For these reasons many investigators would question the benefit of any form of medical or surgical treatment in such cases. Clearly if the patient, apart from her infertility, also has symptoms associated with endometriosis, then appropriate therapy is indicated. However, it is accepted that endometriosis is a disease that tends to persist and often progress with time. There is an argument that offering therapy at an early stage may prevent further progression of the disease, the end result of which may well be mechanical disruption to tubal-ovarian function. For these reasons, endometriosis involving the posterior aspect of the ovary and the ovarian fossa is often treated at an early stage, whilst endometriosis occurring only on the uterosacral ligaments may well be left untreated. From the balance of evidence conclusions have been drawn that apart from mechanical damage, endometriosis does not cause infertility. This view has been substantiated from failure of

Table 10.3 – Infertility and endometriosis – possible mechanisms.

Ovarian function	Luteolysis caused by prosaglandins
	Oocyte maturation defects
	Endocrinopathies
	Luteinized unruptured follicle syndrome
	Altered prolactin release
	Anovulation
Tubal function	Impaired fimbrial oocyte pickup
	Altered tubal mobility
Coital function	Deep dyspareunia – reduced coital frequency
Sperm function	Antibodies causing inactivation
	Macrophage phagocytosis
Early pregnancy failure	Prostaglandin induced
	Immune reaction
	Luteal phase deficiency

medical therapies in placebo-controlled trials to improve conception rates. However this widely held viewpoint may well be brought into question following the data from a recent Canadian multicentre study in which surgical (laparoscopic) ablation of deposits was compared with no intervention. Surgical destruction did improve cumulative pregnancy rates in this study but further confirmatory trials are awaited.

Diagnosis

Clinical findings

On clinical grounds endometriosis is suggested by the clinical findings of thickening or nodularity of the uterosacral ligaments, tenderness in the Pouch of Douglas, an ovarian mass or masses and a fixed retroverted uterus. However a specific diagnosis requires visualization and in uncertain cases, biopsy of lesions, either at laparoscopy or laparotomy.

Non-invasive tests

Ca_{125} levels

Ca_{125} is a glycoprotein expressed by some epithelial cells of coelomic origin. Serum levels are known to be raised in a significant proportion of patients with ovarian epithelial carcinoma. It is noted that patients with severe endometriosis may also have elevated Ca_{125} levels but not to comparable levels in patients with ovarian cancer. In these individuals, levels of Ca_{125} often fall during treatment and rises in Ca_{125} correlate well with recurrence of disease. However in the majority of individuals measurement of Ca_{125} alone cannot be diagnostic of the presence of endometriosis.

Ultrasound

Ultrasound is of limited value in the diagnosis of endometriosis. It is particularly helpful when there are ovarian cysts present. A characteristic feature of an endometrioma is a homogeneous hypoechoic collection of low level echoes with an ovarian cyst.

Magnetic resonance imaging

Magnetic resonance imaging (MRI) potentially offers significant gains in imaging of endometriosis compared with ultrasound when there are ovarian cysts or invasion of surrounding organs (bowel, bladder, rectovaginal septum). However in the majority of patients MRI is of little benefit since peritoneal deposits are but a few millimetres in diameter and cannot be detected.

Laparoscopy

Laparoscopy remains the gold standard means of diagnosing this condition. As shown earlier in Figs. 10.1 and 10.2 the laparoscopic features of endometriotic deposits are quite variable and inexperienced laparoscopists may miss lesions unless very extensive, fail to recognize atypical lesions, and in many because of a failure to do an adequate visualization of the whole of the pelvis, particularly the ovarian fossa. The role of laparoscopy is vital since it provides direct visualization of endometriotic lesions, the possibility to biopsy suspected areas and allows staging of the disease in terms of extent of adhesions and number and size of lesions. It could also allow concurrent therapy at the time of laparoscopy in the form of cautery or laser treatment in selected cases.

Treatment

Patients with endometriosis are often difficult to treat, not only from a physical point of view, but often because of associated psychological issues. For some patients the label of endometriosis in itself may create its own problems since it is known by most patients to be a recurrent disorder throughout the whole of reproductive life. Whilst there is no standard formula for treatment, nor indeed a cure, it is important to tailor treatment for the individual according to her age, symptoms, extent of the disease and her desire for future childbearing.

Drug therapy

Non-steroidal inflammatory agents
Non-steroidal inflammatory drugs are potent analgesics and are helpful in reducing the severity of dysmenorrhoea and pelvic pain. However they have no specific impact on the disease and its progression and hence their use is as adjunctive treatment only.

Combined oral contraceptive agents
Oral contraceptive agents are known to reduce the severity of dysmenorrhoea and menstrual blood loss in many patients. They may be of some benefit but are often of little help when given in the standard manner of regular monthly withdrawal bleeds. Three packs of pills taken continuously may be beneficial for a small proportion of patients, particularly in those who have recently had a more definitive medical/surgical treatment. Such an approach may symptomatically at least have further benefits to the treatment reducing the number and frequency of menses and potentially extending the time to recurrence.

Danazol/Gestrinone
Danazol and Gestrinone are hormonal, ovarian suppressive, medical treatments comparable in their effect in reducing the severity of symptoms for endometriosis. Danazol is given in a dose of between 400 and 800 mg daily and Gestrinone at a dose of 2.5 mg twice weekly. In most instances the drugs are well-tolerated but many women do experience androgenic side effects, e.g. weight gain, greasy skin and acne. The drugs are normally given in courses of between three and six months. In longer-term administration of the drugs there may be alterations in lipid profiles or liver function, which need to be monitored.

Progestogens
Synthetic progestogens such as medroxyprogesterone acetate and dydrogesterone have been given on a continuous basis to produce pseudo-decidualization of the endometrium and comparable changes in endometriotic lesions. The dose of agents required to be effective is quite high and side effects, including breakthrough bleeding, weight gain, fluid retention and weight changes, are not uncommon.

Gonadotrophin-releasing hormone agonists
Gonadotrophin-releasing hormone agonists (GnRH-A) are equally as effective as Danazol in relieving the severity and symptoms of endometriosis and differ only in their side effects. These drugs induce a state of hypogonadotrophic-hypogonadism or pseudomenopause with low circulating levels of oestrogen. Side effects include symptoms seen at the menopause, in particular hot flushes and night sweats. Despite these side effects the drugs are well-tolerated and are gaining popularity in the treatment of endometriosis. They are available as multiple, daily-administered intranasal sprays or as slow-release depot formulations each lasting for one month or more. Apart from the symptomatic side effects described above, the low circulating oestrogen levels can affect bone metabolism in ways comparable to those seen at the natural menopause. Therefore, with continuing long-term use there can be reduction in bone mineral density, most acutely seen in the trabecular bone of the lumbar spine. Bone loss of some 5 per cent can occur over a six-month course of treatment but for the majority of patients this is readily replaced as ovarian function returns on ceasing the drug therapy. Administration of low dose hormone replacement therapy (HRT) along with the GnRH-A analogues, the so-called add back therapy, is being investigated in a large number of centres to allow long-term use of these effective drugs for the management of recurrent disease.

Surgical treatment

Conservative surgery

Development of new laparoscopic surgical techniques and intra-abdominal lasers has led to changes in recent years in the approach to surgical management of endometriosis. It is now much simpler and safer to eradicate visible endometriotic lesions with diathermy CO_2 or KTP lasers. Likewise, endometriotic cysts can be drained, opened and the inner cyst wall or lining destroyed and vaporized with laser. In many instances, because of the severe adhesive disease found with endometriomas, open surgery may still be necessary. Conservative approaches have reduced the need for open surgery with its long recovery times, and this allows patients to delay the time to when more definitive surgery may become necessary.

Definitive surgery

Where there is severe symptomatology, progressive disease or in women whose families are complete, definitive surgery for relief of dysmenorrhoea and pain is often necessary. This takes the form of hysterectomy and bilateral salpingo-oophorectomy. The removal of the ovaries and subsequent ovarian hormone production is beneficial in achieving long-term symptom relief.

Paradoxically such patients can receive hormone replacement treatment subsequent to surgery. To minimize the risk of recurrence the commencement of HRT is often deferred for a period of time following surgery, particularly when active disease was found to be present at the time of laparotomy and this delay is typically a period of six months or more.

Definitive surgery is also required for large adherent endometriotic cysts and for the small proportion of patients who have deep-seated endometriosis involving the bowel or bladder. Histologically and morphologically this deep-seated endometriosis differs considerably from that of peritoneal endometriosis. These lesions contain fibrosis of smooth muscle hypertrophy and reduced numbers of endometriotic glands with little stroma tissue. Whilst symptomatically these patients are rendered amenorrhoeic on medical treatment and have good symptom response, these symptoms rapidly recur on cessation of the drugs and surgery is virtually always necessary in due course.

Endometriosis thus remains a disorder of which we still have little understanding and, at present, little hope of a permanent cure other than definitive surgery in the form of pelvic clearance. New treatment options, both medical and laparoscopic surgery, have expanded the potential for delay in surgery but for most sufferers the disease remains one of repeat recurrences throughout their reproductive life.

Adenomyosis

Adenomyosis is often incorrectly termed internal endometriosis because of the histological features of the disorder in which endometrial glands are found deep within the myometrium. Adenomyosis is increasingly being viewed as a separate pathological entity affecting a different population of patients with an as yet unknown and different aetiology.

Patients with adenomyosis are usually multiparous and diagnosed in their late thirties or early forties. They present with increasingly severe secondary spasmodic dysmenorrhoea and increased menstrual blood loss (menorrhagia). Examination of patients may be contributory with the findings most often of a bulky and sometimes tender uterus, particularly if examined perimenstrually. Ultrasound examination of the uterus may be contributory on occasions when adenomyosis is particularly marked or localized to one area. Then ultrasound may show alterations of ecogenicity within the myometrium from the localized haemorrhage-filled distended endometrial glands. In some instances where there is a very localized area of adenomyosis this may give an irregular nodular development within the uterus, very similar to that of uterine fibroids. MRI, whilst less commonly available, may be more specific at identifying adenomyosis than ultrasound.

Clinically suspected adenomyosis is still most commonly diagnosed by pathologists on examination of the hysterectomy specimen performed for symptomatic reasons.

The difficulty then is in diagnosing adenomyosis preoperatively. Conservative surgery and medical treatments have been poorly developed. Treatments that induce amenorrhoea are clearly helpful since they relieve pain and excessive bleeding. Effective agents such as Danazol, Gestrinone and GnRH-A used in the treatment of endometriosis may also be beneficial for this condition. On ceasing treatment however the symptoms rapidly return in the majority of patients and, to date, hysterectomy is the only definitive treatment.

Key Points

- Endometriosis is one of the commonest gynaecological conditions and at present affects between 10% and 25% of women with symptoms of gynaecological origin
- Growth of endometriosis is oestrogen dependent. Endometriosis is associated with tubal and ovarian damage and the formation of adhesions and can compromise fertility
- The commonest presenting symptoms other than infertility are painful periods and dyspareunia
- The typical peritoneal lesion is described as a powder burn. The medical treatment of endometriosis involves suppressing oestrogen–progestogen levels to prevent cyclical changes and includes treatment with progestogens, Gestrinone, Danazol and GnRH analogues
- The surgical treatment of endometriosis is either minimally invasive using laparoscopic techniques or radical with total abdominal hysterectomy and bilateral salpingo-oophorectomy
- Adenomyosis is a common condition presenting with painful periods and is common in women in their late thirties or early forties

References for further reading

Dmowski WP, Steele RW, Baker GF. Deficient cellular immunity in endometriosis. *American Journal of Obstetrics and Gynecology* 1981; **141**: 377–83.

Fabraeus L, Larsson-Cohn U, Ljunbeg S, Wallentin I. Profound alterations in the lipoprotein metabolism during danazol treatment in premenopausal women. *Fertility and Sterility* 1984; **42**: 52–7.

Ingamells D, Thomas Ed. Infertility and endometriosis. In: Shaw RW (Ed). *Endometriosis – current understanding and management*. Oxford: Blackwell Science, 1995, 147–67.

Meyer R. Veberden stand der frage der adenomyositis, adenomyoma in allgemeinen (insbesundere ueber), adenomyosis und ademomyometritis sarcomatosa. *Zentralblatt für Gynakologie* 1919; **36**: 745–59.

Sampson JA. Perforating haemorrhagic (chocolate) cysts of the ovary. *Archives of Surgery* 1921; **3**: 245–323.

Sampson JA. Peritoneal endometriosis due to menstrual dissemination of endometrial tissue into the peritoneal cavity. *American Journal of Obstetrics and Gynaecology* 1927; **14**: 422–69.

Schrifin BS, Erez S, Moore JG. Teenage endometriosis. *American Journal of Obstetrics and Gynaecology* 1973; **116**: 973–80.

Shaw RW. Evaluation of treatment with gonadotrophin-releasing hormone analogues. In: Shaw RW (Ed.). *Endometriosis – current understanding and management*. Oxford: Blackwell Science, 1995, 206–34.

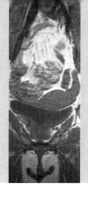

Benign disease of the ovary

OVERVIEW

Benign ovarian cysts are common, frequently asymptomatic and often resolve spontaneously. They are the fourth commonest gynaecological cause of hospital admission. By the age of 65 years, 4 per cent of all women will have been admitted to hospital for this reason.

Ninety per cent of all ovarian tumours are benign, although this varies with age. Amongst those that require surgery, 13 per cent are malignant in premenopausal women but 45 per cent are malignant in postmenopausal women. The main objectives of management are to exclude malignancy and to avoid cyst accidents, without causing undue morbidity or impairing future fertility in younger women.

Ovarian tumours may be physiological or pathological, and may arise from any tissue in the ovary. Most benign ovarian tumours are cystic. The finding of solid elements makes malignancy more likely. However, fibromas, thecomas, dermoids and Brenner tumours usually have solid elements.

Pathology

Physiological cysts

Physiological cysts are simply large versions of the cysts that form in the ovary during the normal ovarian cycle. Most are asymptomatic incidental findings at pelvic examination or ultrasound scan. Although they may occur in any premenopausal woman, they are most common in young women. They are an occasional complication of ovulation induction when they are commonly multiple. They may also occur in premature female infants and in women with trophoblastic disease.

Follicular cyst

Lined by granulosa cells, this is the commonest benign ovarian tumour and is most often found incidentally. It results from the non-rupture of a dominant follicle or the failure of atresia in a non-dominant follicle. A follicular cyst can persist for several menstrual cycles and may achieve a diameter of up to 10 cm. Smaller cysts are more likely to resolve but may require intervention if symptoms develop or if they do not resolve after 8–16 weeks. Occasionally, they may continue to produce oestrogen, causing menstrual disturbances and endometrial hyperplasia.

Luteal cyst

Less common than follicular cysts, luteal cysts are more likely to present with intraperitoneal bleeding. This is more common on the right side, possibly as a result of increased intraluminal pressure secondary to ovarian vein anatomy. They may also rupture. This usually happens on days 20–26 of the cycle. Corpora lutea are not called luteal cysts unless they are more than 3 cm in diameter.

Benign germ cell tumours

Germ cell tumours are among the commonest ovarian tumours seen in women of less than 30 years of age. Overall, only 2–3 per cent are malignant but in the under-20s this proportion may rise to a third.

Malignant tumours are usually solid, although commonly benign forms also have a solid element. Thus the traditional classification into solid or cystic germ cell tumours, signifying malignant or benign respectively, may be misleading. As the name suggests, they arise from totipotential germ cells, and may therefore contain elements of all three germ layers (embryonic differentiation). Differentiation into extra-embryonic tissues results in ovarian choriocarcinoma or endodermal sinus tumour. When neither embryonic nor extra-embryonic differentiation occurs, a dysgerminoma results.

Dermoid cyst (mature cystic teratoma)

The benign dermoid cyst is the only benign germ cell tumour that is common. It results from differentiation into embryonic tissues. It accounts for around 40 per cent of all ovarian neoplasms and is most common in young women and the median age of presentation is 30 years. It is bilateral in about 11 per cent of cases. However, if the contralateral ovary is macroscopically normal, the chance of a concealed second dermoid is very low (1–2 per cent), particularly if preoperative ultrasound is normal.

A dermoid is usually a unilocular cyst less than 15 cm in diameter, in which ectodermal structures are predominant. Thus it is often lined with epithelium like the epidermis and contains skin appendages, teeth, sebaceous material, hair and nervous tissue. Endodermal derivatives include thyroid,

<table>
<tr><td>**P**</td><td>**Understanding the pathophysiology**</td></tr>
</table>

Pathology of benign ovarian tumours

Physiological cysts
- Follicular cyst
- Luteal cyst

Benign germ cell tumours
- Dermoid cyst
- Mature teratoma

Benign epithelial tumours
- Serous cystadenoma
- Mucinous cystadenoma
- Endometrioid cystadenoma
- Brenner tumour
- Clear cell tumour

Benign sex cord stromal tumours
- Granulosa cell tumour
- Theca cell tumour
- Fibroma
- Sertoli–Leydig cell tumour

bronchus and intestine, and the mesoderm may be represented by bone, cartilage and smooth muscle.

Occasionally only a single tissue may be present, in which case the term monodermal teratoma is used. The classic examples are carcinoid and struma ovarii, which contain hormonally active thyroid tissue. Primary carcinoid tumours of the ovary rarely metastasize but 30 per cent may give rise to typical carcinoid. Thyroid tissue is found in 5–20 per cent of cystic teratomas. The term 'struma ovarii' should be reserved for tumours composed predominantly of thyroid tissue and as such comprise only 1.4 per cent of cystic teratomas. Only 5–6 per cent of struma ovarii produce sufficient thyroid hormone to cause hyperthyroidism. Some 5–10% of struma ovarii develop into carcinoma.

The majority (60 per cent) of dermoid cysts are asymptomatic. However, 3.5–10 per cent may undergo torsion. Less commonly (1–4 per cent of cases), they may rupture spontaneously: either suddenly causing an acute abdomen and a chemical peritonitis; or slowly causing chronic granulomatous peritonitis. As the latter may also arise following intraoperative spillage, great care should be taken to avoid this, and thorough peritoneal lavage must be performed if it does occur. During pregnancy, rupture is more common due to external pressure from the expanding gravid uterus or to trauma during delivery.

About 2 per cent of dermoid cysts are said to contain a malignant component, usually a squamous carcinoma in women over 40 years old. A poor prognosis is indicated by non-squamous histology and capsular rupture. Amongst women aged under 20 years, up to 80 per cent of ovarian malignancies are due to germ cell tumours (see Chapter 13).

Mature solid teratoma

These rare tumours contain mature tissues just like the dermoid cyst, but there are few cystic areas. They must be differentiated from immature teratomas, which are malignant (see Chapter 13).

Benign epithelial tumours

The majority of ovarian neoplasia, both benign and malignant, arise from the ovarian surface epithelium. They are therefore essentially mesothelial in nature, deriving from the coelomic epithelium overlying the embryonic gonadal ridge, from which develop Müllerian and Wolffian structures. Therefore, this may result in development along endocervical (mucinous cystadenomata), endometrial (endometrioid) or tubal (serous) pathways, or uroepithelial (Brenner) lines respectively.

Although benign epithelial tumours tend to occur at a slightly younger age than their malignant counterparts, they are most common in women over 40 years.

Serous cystadenoma

These are the most common benign epithelial tumours and is bilateral in about 10 per cent of cases. It is usually a unilocular cyst with papilliferous processes on the inner surface and occasionally on the outer surface. The epithelium on the inner surface is cuboidal or columnar and may be ciliated. Psammoma bodies are concentric calcified bodies that occasionally occur in these cysts, but are more frequent in their malignant counterparts. The cyst fluid is thin and serous. They are seldom as large as mucinous tumours.

Mucinous cystadenoma

These constitute 15–25 per cent of all ovarian tumours and are the second most common epithelial tumour. They are typically large, unilateral, multilocular cysts with a smooth inner surface. A recent specimen at the Hammersmith Hospital weighed over 14 kg. The lining epithelium consists of columnar mucus-secreting cells and the cyst fluid is generally thick and glutinous.

A rare complication is pseudomyxoma peritonei, which is more often present before the cyst is removed rather than following intraoperative rupture. Pseudomyxoma peritonei is more commonly associated with mucinous tumours of the appendix. Synchronous tumours of the ovary and appendix are common. These are usually well-differentiated carcinomas or borderline tumours. They result in seedling growths that continue to secrete mucin, causing matting together and consequent obstruction of bowel loops. The five-year survival rate is approximately 50 per cent, but by ten years as few as 18 per cent of patients are still alive.

Endometrioid cystadenoma

Benign endometrioid cysts are difficult to differentiate from ovarian endometriosis. They may be associated with pelvic pain and deep dyspareunia due to adhesions. They present a typical appearance on transvaginal sonography with an absence of pupillae and typical 'ground glass' contents of unclotted blood.

Brenner tumours

These account for only 1–2 per cent of all ovarian tumours, and are bilateral in 10–15 per cent of cases. They probably arise from Wolffian metaplasia of the surface epithelium. The tumour consists of islands of transitional epithelium (Walthard nests) in a dense fibrotic stroma, giving a largely solid appearance. The vast majority is benign, but borderline or malignant specimens have been reported. Almost three-quarters occur in women over the age of 40 and about half are incidental findings, being recognized only by the pathologist. Although some can be large, the majority is less than 2 cm in diameter. Some secrete oestrogens and abnormal vaginal bleeding is a common presentation.

Clear cell (mesonephroid) tumours

These arise from serosal cells showing little differentiation, and are only rarely benign. The typical histological appearance is of clear or 'hobnail' cells arranged in mixed patterns.

Benign sex cord stromal tumours

Sex cord stromal tumours represent only 4 per cent of benign ovarian tumours. They occur at any age from prepubertal children to elderly, postmenopausal women. Many secrete hormones and present with the results of inappropriate hormone effects.

Granulosa cell tumours

These are all malignant tumours but are mentioned here because they are generally confined to the ovary when they present and so have a good prognosis. However, they do grow very slowly and recurrences are often seen 10–20 years later. They are largely solid in most cases. Call-Exner bodies are pathognomonic but are seen in less than half of granulosa cell tumours. Some produce oestrogens and most appear to secrete inhibin.

Theca cell tumours

Almost all are benign, solid and unilateral, typically presenting in the sixth decade. Many produce oestrogens in sufficient quantity to have systemic effects such as precocious puberty, postmenopausal bleeding, endometrial hyperplasia and endometrial cancer. They rarely cause ascites or Meig's syndrome.

Fibromas

These unusual tumours are most frequent around 50 years of age. Most are derived from stromal cells and are similar to thecomas. They are hard, mobile and lobulated with a glistening white surface. Less than 10 per cent are bilateral. While ascites occurs with many of the larger fibromas, Meig's syndrome – ascites and pleural effusion in association with a fibroma of the ovary – is seen in only 1 per cent of cases.

Sertoli–Leydig cell tumours

These are usually of low-grade malignancy. Most are found around 30 years of age. They are rare, being less than 0.2 per cent of ovarian tumours. They are often difficult to distinguish from other ovarian tumours because of the variety of cells and architecture seen. Many produce androgens and signs of virilization are seen in three-quarters of patients. Some secrete oestrogens. They are usually small and unilateral.

Age distribution of ovarian tumours

In younger women, the most common benign ovarian neoplasm is the germ cell tumour, and amongst older women, the epithelial cell tumour (Fig. 11.1). The percentage of ovarian neoplasms that are benign also changes with the age of the woman (Fig. 11.2).

Presentation

S Symptoms

Presentation of benign ovarian tumours
- Asymptomatic
- Pain
- Abdominal swelling
- Pressure effects
- Menstrual disturbances
- Hormonal effects
- Abnormal cervical smear

Asymptomatic

Many benign ovarian tumours are found incidentally in the course of investigating another unrelated problem, during a routine examination while performing a cervical smear or at an antenatal clinic. As pelvic ultrasound, and particularly transvaginal scanning, is now used more frequently, physiological cysts are

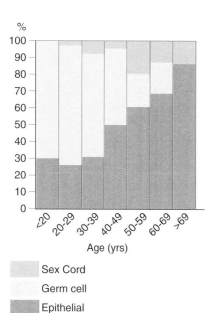

Figure 11.1 Histological distribution (%) of benign ovarian neoplasia treated surgically by age.

detected more often. Where ultrasound was used in trials of screening for ovarian cancer, the majority of tumours detected were benign. About 50 per cent of simple cysts less than 6 cm in diameter will resolve spontaneously if observed over a period of six months. A further 25 per cent regress in the following two years. Use of an oral contraceptive pill may encourage the resolution of physiological cysts.

Pain

Acute pain from an ovarian tumour may result from torsion, rupture, haemorrhage or infection. Torsion usually gives rise to a sharp, constant pain caused by ischaemia of the cyst and areas may become infarcted. Haemorrhage into the cyst may cause pain as the capsule is stretched. Intraperitoneal bleeding mimicking ectopic pregnancy may result from rupture of the tumour. This happens most frequently with a luteal cyst. Chronic lower abdominal pain sometimes results from the pressure of a benign ovarian tumour but is more common if endometriosis or infection is present.

Abdominal swelling

Patients seldom note abdominal swelling until the tumour is very large. A benign mucinous cyst may occasionally fill the entire abdominal cavity. The bloating that women complain of so often is rarely due to an ovarian tumour.

Miscellaneous

Gastrointestinal or urinary symptoms may result from pressure effects. In extreme cases, oedema of the legs, varicose veins and haemorrhoids may result. Sometimes, uterine prolapse is the presenting complaint in a woman with an ovarian cyst.

Occasionally the patient will complain of menstrual disturbances but this may be coincidence rather than due to the tumour. Rarely, sex cord stromal tumours present with oestrogen effects such as precocious puberty, menorrhagia and glandular hyperplasia, breast enlargement or postmenopausal bleeding. Secretion of androgens may cause hirsutism and acne initially, progressing to frank virilism with deepening of the voice or clitoral

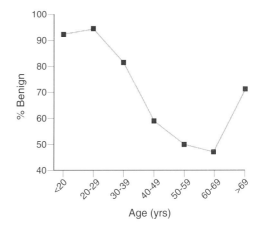

Figure 11.2 Proportion of surgically treated ovarian tumours which are benign falls with increasing age until the eighth decade. (Modified from Koonings *et al.* 1989.)

hypertrophy. Very rarely indeed thyrotoxicosis may result from ectopic secretion of thyroid hormone.

Rarely, a patient with an abnormal cervical smear will be found to have an ovarian tumour, the removal of which is followed by resolution of the cytological abnormality. Surprisingly, these are often benign tumours.

Differential diagnosis

The differential diagnosis of benign ovarian tumours is broad, reflecting the wide range of presenting symptoms.

A full bladder should be considered in the differential diagnosis of any pelvic mass. In premenopausal women, a gravid uterus must always be considered. Fibroids can be impossible to distinguish from ovarian tumours. Rarely, a fimbrial cyst may grow sufficiently to cause anxiety.

Ectopic pregnancy may present as a pelvic mass and lower abdominal pain, especially if there has been chronic intraperitoneal bleeding. Often a ruptured, bleeding corpus luteum will be mistaken for an ectopic gestation. It may be difficult to differentiate between appendicitis and an ovarian cyst. Co-operation between gynaecologist and surgeon is essential to avoid unnecessary surgery on simple ovarian cysts in young women and the effects this may have upon subsequent fertility. Pelvic inflammatory disease may give rise to a mass of adherent bowel, a hydrosalpinx or pyosalpinx.

S Symptoms

Pain
Ectopic pregnancy
Spontaneous abortion
Pelvic inflammatory disease
Appendicitis
Meckel's diverticulum
Diverticulitis

Abdominal swelling
Pregnant uterus
Fibroid uterus
Full bladder
Distended bowel
Ovarian malignancy
Colorectal carcinoma

Pressure effects
Urinary tract infection
Constipation

Hormonal effects
All other causes of menstrual irregularities, precocious puberty and postmenopausal bleeding

If the tumour is ovarian, malignancy must be excluded. In the vast majority of cases this can only be done by a laparotomy. Even then, careful histological examination may be necessary to exclude invasion. Frozen section will only rarely be of value. A rectal tumour or diverticulitis may also cause a pelvic mass. Hodgkin's disease may present as a pelvic mass of enlarged pelvic lymph nodes.

Investigation

The investigations required will depend upon the circumstances of the presentation. The patient presenting with acute symptoms will usually require emergency surgery whereas the asymptomatic patient or the woman with chronic problems may benefit from more detailed preliminary assessment.

Gynaecological history

Details of the presenting symptoms and a full gynaecological history should be obtained with particular reference to the date of the last menstrual period, the regularity of the menstrual cycle, any previous pregnancies, contraception, medication and family history (particularly of ovarian, breast or bowel cancer).

General history and examination

Indigestion or dysphagia might indicate a primary gastric cancer metastasizing to the pelvis. Similarly, a history of altered bowel habit or rectal bleeding would suggest diverticulitis or rectal carcinoma. However, ovarian carcinoma may also present with these features.

If the patient has presented as an acute emergency, look for evidence of hypovolaemia. Hypotension is a relatively late sign of blood loss, as the blood pressure will be maintained for some time by peripheral arteriolar and central venous vasoconstriction. When decompensation occurs, it often does so very rapidly. It is vital to recognize the early signs – tachycardia and cold peripheries.

The breasts should be palpated and the neck, axillae and groins examined for lymphadenopathy. A malignant ovarian tumour may cause a pleural effusion. This is much less commonly found with a benign tumour. Some patients may have ankle oedema. Very occasionally foot drop may be noted as a result of compression of pelvic nerve roots. This would not occur with a benign tumour but suggests a malignancy with lymphatic involvement.

Abdominal examination

The abdomen should be inspected for signs of distension by fluid or by the tumour itself. Dilated veins may be seen on the lower abdominal wall. Gentle palpation will reveal areas of tenderness and peritonism may be elicited by asking the patient to cough or alternately suck in and blow out her abdominal wall. Male hair distribution may suggest a rare androgen-producing tumour.

The best way of detecting a mass that arises from the pelvis is to palpate gently with the radial border of the left hand, starting in the upper abdomen and working caudally. This is the reverse of the process taught to every medical student for feeling the liver edge. Using only the right hand is the commonest reason for failing to detect pelviabdominal masses.

Shifting dullness is probably the easiest way of

demonstrating ascites but it remains a very insensitive technique. It is always worth listening for bowel sounds in any patient with an acute abdomen. Their complete absence in the presence of peritonism is an ominous sign.

Bimanual examination

This is an essential component of the assessment because, even in expert hands, ultrasound examination is not infallible. By palpating the mass between both the vaginal and abdominal hands, its mobility, texture and consistency, the presence of nodules in the Pouch of Douglas and the degree of tenderness can all be determined (Fig. 11.3). While it is impossible to make a firm diagnosis with bimanual examination, a hard, irregular, fixed mass is likely to be invasive.

Ultrasound

- Transabdominal and transvaginal ultrasound can demonstrate the presence of an ovarian mass with reasonable sensitivity and fair specificity and, although it cannot distinguish reliably between benign and malignant tumours, solid ovarian masses are more likely to be malignant than their cystic counterparts.
- The use of colour-flow Doppler may increase the reliability of ultrasound.
- Neither computerized tomographic scanning nor

magnetic resonance imaging has significant advantages over ultrasound in this situation and both are more expensive.

Ultrasound-guided diagnostic ovarian cyst aspiration

This investigation has been introduced gradually into gynaecological practice from the subspecialty of assisted reproduction where ultrasound-guided egg collection is now commonplace This has happened without the benefit of appropriate trials to indicate its potential efficacy.

Unfortunately, this technique has up to a 71 per cent false-negative rate and a 2 per cent false-positive rate for the cytological diagnosis of malignancy. There is a risk of disseminating malignant cells along the needle track or into the peritoneal cavity but the size of that risk is not established.

Overall, ultrasound-guided aspiration of ovarian cysts cannot be recommended as a diagnostic tool.

Radiological investigations

- A chest X-ray is essential to detect metastatic disease in the lungs or a pleural effusion which may be too small to detect clinically. Occasionally an abdominal X-ray may show calcification, suggesting the possibility of a benign teratoma.
- An intravenous urogram is often performed but is seldom useful.
- A barium enema is indicated only if the mass is irregular or fixed, or if there are bowel symptoms.
- A computerized tomography scan is seldom indicated.

Blood test and serum markers

It is always sensible to measure the haemoglobin and an elevated white cell count would suggest infection. Platelet count and clotting screen may be useful in the rare case of a large intra-abdominal bleed. Blood may be cross-matched if necessary.

Serum markers have yet to establish a role in the routine management of most ovarian tumours. However, a raised serum Ca_{125} is strongly suggestive of ovarian carcinoma, especially in postmenopausal

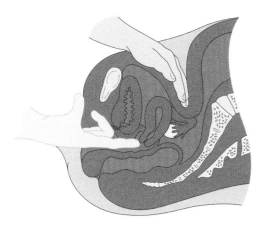

Figure 11.3 Bimanual examination involves palpating the pelvic organs between both hands.

women. Women with extensive endometriosis may also have elevated levels but the concentration is usually not as high as that seen with malignant disease. The beta-human chorionic gonadotrophin concentration might be measured to exclude an ectopic pregnancy but trophoblastic tumours and some germ cell tumours secrete this marker. Oestradiol levels may be elevated in some women with physiological follicular cysts and sex cord stromal tumours. Sertoli–Leydig tumours may cause an increase in androgen concentrations. Raised alpha-fetoprotein levels suggest a yolk sac tumour.

Management

The management will depend upon the severity of the symptoms, the age of the patient and therefore the risk of malignancy and her desire for further children.

The asymptomatic patient

The older woman
Women over 50 years of age are far more likely to have a malignancy and have little to gain from the conservative management of a pelvic mass more than 5 cm in diameter. Physiological cysts are, by definition, unlikely. However, the capacity of the postmenopausal ovary to generate benign cysts is greater than previously thought, occurring in up to 17 per cent of asymptomatic women. Over 50 per cent of small, simple cysts will resolve spontaneously but almost 30 per cent will remain static. Even in this age group, only 29–50 per cent of all ovarian cysts will be malignant (Fig. 11.4).

Therefore, efforts have been made to define criteria that would enable unnecessary surgery to be avoided in this older age group. Evaluation of the cyst is with tumour markers, ultrasound and colour-flow Doppler studies and careful follow up. Simple, unilateral cysts less than 6 cm in diameter with Ca_{125} less than 35 u/mL and normal vascular resistance patterns are likely to be benign and may safely be managed conservatively. In these cases, if there is no change in the cyst at the second ultrasound at three months, follow up with six-monthly ultrasound and Ca_{125} estimation is safe. Most will resolve in three years but some do persist for up to seven years.

The role of laparoscopic surgery in the assessment

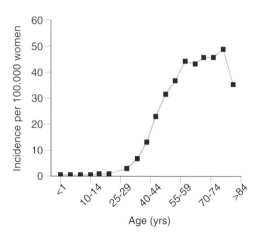

Figure 11.4 The incidence of ovarian cancer in England and Wales (Office of Population and Censuses and Surveys 1985). Note how uncommon ovarian cancer is before the age of 35 years.

and treatment of apparently benign cysts in this age group is controversial. Whilst the small cysts described above may be managed without surgery, there may be a small role for the laparoscopic assessment and treatment of larger (perhaps up to 10 cm), but otherwise apparently, benign cysts. Nonetheless this should only be in the hands of those that are both experienced in laparoscopy and are prepared to perform definitive surgery for an unexpected ovarian carcinoma under the same anaesthetic. Complete and intact removal of the cyst should be achieved. For the more general gynaecologist, laparoscopy may be useful to confirm that the ultrasound lesion is ovarian but the open approach is still recommended if the ovary is to be removed.

Premenopausal women
Young women of less than 35 years are both more likely to wish to have the option of further children and less likely to have a malignant epithelial tumour. However, ovarian cysts more than 10 cm in diameter are unlikely to be physiological or to resolve spontaneously. A normal follicular cyst up to 3 cm in diameter requires no further investigation. A clear unilocular cyst of 3–10 cm identified by ultrasound should be re-examined 12 weeks later for evidence of diminution in size. If the cyst persists, such women may be followed with six-monthly ultrasound and Ca_{125} estimations as described above. The use of a combined oral contraceptive is unlikely to accelerate

Criteria for observation of an asymptomatic ovarian tumour

- Unilateral tumour
- Unilocular cyst without solid elements
- Premenopausal women – tumour 3–10 cm in diameter
- Postmenopausal women – tumour 2–6 cm in diameter
- Normal Ca_{125}
- No free fluid or masses suggesting omental cake or matted bowel loops

the resolution of a functional cyst and hormonal treatment of endometriosis does not usually benefit an endometrioma. If the cyst does enlarge, laparoscopy or laparotomy may be indicated.

The patient with symptoms

If the patient presents with severe, acute pain or signs of intraperitoneal bleeding an emergency laparoscopy or laparotomy will be required. More chronic symptoms of pain or pressure may justify pelvic ultrasound if no mass can be felt, but ultrasound is unlikely to contribute to the investigation of a woman in whom both ovaries can be clearly felt to be of a normal size.

The pregnant patient
An ovarian cyst in a pregnant woman may undergo torsion or may bleed. There is said to be an increased incidence of these complications in pregnancy, although the evidence for this is poor. Very occasionally, a cyst can prevent the presenting fetal part from engaging. A dermoid cyst may rupture or leak slowly, causing peritonitis. However, an ovarian cyst is usually discovered incidentally at the antenatal clinic or on ultrasound, and occasionally at caesarean section.

The pregnant woman with an ovarian cyst is a special case because of the dangers of surgery to the fetus. These have probably been exaggerated in the past and no urgent operation should be postponed solely because of a pregnancy. Thus, if the patient presents with acute pain due to torsion or haemorrhage into an ovarian tumour or if appendicitis is a possibility, the correct course is to undertake a laparotomy regardless of the stage of the pregnancy. The likelihood of labour ensuing is small. However,

the operation should be covered by tocolytic drugs and performed in a centre with intensive neonatal care when possible.

If an asymptomatic cyst is discovered, it is prudent to wait until after 14 weeks' gestation before removing it. This avoids the risk of removing a corpus luteal cyst upon which the pregnancy might still be dependent. In the second and third trimesters, the management of an asymptomatic ovarian cyst may be either conservative or surgical. The risks to the mother and fetus of an elective procedure need to be balanced against the chances of a cyst accident, an unexpected malignancy or spontaneous resolution. Cysts less than 10 cm in diameter, which have a simple appearance on ultrasound, are unlikely to be malignant or to result in a cyst accident, and may therefore be followed ultrasonographically: many will resolve spontaneously. If the cyst is unresolved 6 weeks postpartum, surgery may be undertaken then. The role for cyst aspiration in pregnancy, either diagnostically or therapeutically, is small.

Ovarian cancer is uncommon in pregnancy, occurring in less than 3 per cent of cysts. However, a cyst with features suggestive of malignancy on ultrasound, or one that is growing, should be removed surgically. The tumour marker Ca_{125} is not useful in the pregnant woman, since elevated levels occur frequently as an apparently physiological change. Management may need to include a caesarean hysterectomy, bilateral salpingo-oophorectomy and omentectomy.

The female fetus
Fetal ovarian androgen synthesis commences at 12 weeks', and oestradiol and progesterone at 20 weeks' gestation. Thus, small follicular cysts up to 7 mm in diameter may occur in up to a third of newborn girls. However, larger cysts are rare and, usually, isolated findings. Most are follicular cysts although luteal cysts, cystic teratomata and granulosa cell tumours also occur. They may undergo torsion or haemorrhage, and occasionally necrosis of the pedicle may result in the 'disappearance' of the ovary. Rarely, small bowel compression may cause polyhydramnios, but diaphragmatic splinting and consequent pulmonary hypoplasia does not seem to occur.

Most follicular cysts resolve spontaneously either antenatally or, more commonly, postnatally. Consideration may need to be given to the antenatal aspiration of a very large cyst if it is felt that it may obstruct labour or be ruptured during vaginal delivery, although this is reported rarely. Therefore, delivery by caesarean section is not indicated. Cysts that have not resolved by six months of age should be explored surgically.

The prepubertal girl

Ovarian cysts are uncommon and often benign. Teratomata and follicular cysts are the most common. Theca and granulosa cell tumours may secrete hormones. Presentation may be with abdominal pain or distension, or precocious puberty, either isosexual or heterosexual. Management depends upon relief of symptoms, exclusion of malignancy and conservation of maximum ovarian tissue without jeopardizing fertility.

Treatment

Treatment is mostly surgical, although there may be a few women in whom cyst aspiration is indicated.

Therapeutic ultrasound-guided cyst aspiration

The theoretical advantages of this technique are avoidance of surgery and a reduction in cyst accidents. However, it assumes that the cyst fluid is unable to reaccumulate, and that both physiological (likely to resolve spontaneously) and malignant cysts can be reliably excluded beforehand. Cytological assessment of the aspirated fluid is performed routinely but cannot be relied upon to exclude malignancy (see above).

The role of this technique therefore remains controversial. The best candidate is a young woman with a unilateral, unilocular, anechoic, thin-walled cyst less than 10 cm in diameter. The recurrence rate is 27 per cent if the fluid is clear and 68 per cent if it is bloodstained. A tumour in a young woman that appears to be largely solid on ultrasound is likely to be a germ cell tumour and requires removal. An acutely painful ovary may be due to torsion and surgery is essential.

There may be a small place for cyst aspiration in women in whom surgery is considered to be high risk, either because of co-existing medical problems or because dense pelvic adhesions envelop the ovaries.

Examination under anaesthesia

Prior to any laparoscopy or laparotomy for a suspected ovarian tumour, it is prudent to perform a bimanual examination under anaesthesia to confirm the presence of the mass.

Laparoscopic procedures

Laparoscopy may be of value if there is uncertainty about the nature of the pelvic mass. Thus it may be possible to avoid a laparotomy when there is no pathology. However, it can be difficult to exclude ovarian disease in the presence of marked pelvic inflammatory disease.

The second indication for laparoscopy is if the patient has a cyst suitable for laparoscopic surgery. This decision should be made after a full history and careful bimanual examination, ultrasound assessment and a thorough laparoscopic appraisal of the whole abdominal cavity, particularly the contralateral ovary. The patient should be aware of the possibility, and consented for, a laparotomy in case malignancy is found or unexpected laparoscopic complications encountered.

The advantages are those of laparoscopic surgery in general: less postoperative pain, shorter hospital stay and quicker return to normal activities. It may also result in less adhesion formation than an open procedure, although the evidence is not convincing. However, the consequences of spillage of cyst contents, incomplete excision of the cyst wall and an unexpected histological diagnosis of malignancy are considerable disadvantages. Up to 83 per cent of malignant ovarian tumours found by chance at a laparoscopic operation for a 'cyst' are treated

Indications for laparoscopy

- Uncertainty about the nature of the mass
- Tumour suitable for laparoscopic surgery
  - Age less than 35 years
  - Ultrasound shows no solid component
  - Simple ovarian cyst
  - Endometrioma

inadequately. Dermoid cysts are better removed by laparotomy because of the serious consequences of leakage of the cyst contents.

Laparoscopic surgery is best reserved for young women under 35 years of age in whom the likelihood of malignant disease is small and in whom conservation of ovarian tissue is more important. These operations require considerable expertise in laparoscopic manipulation and should not be attempted without appropriate training.

Laparotomy

A clinical diagnosis may not be possible without a laparotomy and even then histological examination is essential for a confident conclusion. Frozen section is seldom of value in this situation, as a thorough examination of the tumour is required to exclude invasive disease.

If there is any possibility of invasive disease, a longitudinal skin incision should be used to allow adequate exposure in the upper abdomen. If wider exposure is required after making a transverse incision, the ends of the wound can be extended cranially to fashion a flap from the upper edge of the wound. A sample of ascitic fluid or peritoneal washings should be sent for cytological examination at the beginning of the operation. It is essential to explore the whole abdomen thoroughly and to inspect both ovaries.

In a young women less than 35 years of age an ovarian tumour is very unlikely to be malignant. Even if the mass is a primary ovarian malignancy, it is likely to be a germ cell tumour, which is responsive to chemotherapy. Thus, ovarian cystectomy or unilateral oophorectomy are sensible and safe treatments for unilateral ovarian masses in this age group. It is sometimes said that the contralateral ovary should be bisected and a sample sent for histology in case the tumour is malignant. In practice, most gynaecologists are unwilling to biopsy an apparently healthy ovary lest this results in infertility from periovarian adhesions. Even when the lesion is bilateral, every effort should be made to conserve ovarian tissue. This policy is made possible by the effectiveness of modern chemotherapy for germ cell tumours.

Since epithelial cancer is so much more likely in a woman over the age of 44 years with a unilateral ovarian mass, she is probably best advised to have a total abdominal hysterectomy, bilateral salpingo-oophorectomy and infracolic omentectomy. However, there is evidence to suggest that unilateral oophorectomy in selected cases of epithelial carcinoma confined to one ovary may give equally good results as the traditional radical approach. It would seem reasonable to individualize treatment of women of 35–44 years of age where there are greater benefits to the patient from a conservative approach and where the risks may well be less. If conservative surgery is planned, preliminary hysteroscopy and curettage of the uterus are essential to exclude a concomitant endometrial tumour, a thorough laparotomy is especially important and an appropriate plan of action must be decided in advance with the patient should more widespread disease be found.

Key Points

- Asymptomatic, simple ovarian cysts often resolve spontaneously
- Ovarian cysts are very rarely malignant before the age of 35, especially when less than 10 cm in diameter
- Solid ovarian tumours are often malignant – in young women these are usually germ cell or sex cord stromal tumours
- There is only a limited place for aspiration of cysts
- Conservative management is appropriate for most young women:
    - Observation of cystic lesions <10 cm;
    - Laparoscopic treatment should be considered;
    - Unilateral oophorectomy even for solid lesions
- Women over 45 years of age with a unilocular ovarian cyst greater than 6 cm or with any other type of ovarian tumour should usually be advised to have a total abdominal hysterectomy and bilateral salpingo-oophorectomy
- A bimanual examination under anaesthesia should be performed prior to any surgery for ovarian tumours to confirm that a mass is still palpable

References for further reading

Bailey C L, Ueland F R, Land G L, DePriest P D, Gallion H H, Kryscio R J, van Nagell J R Jr. The malignant potential of small cystic ovarian tumours in women over 50 years of age. *Gynecological Oncology* 1998; **69**: 3–7.

Levine D, Gosink B, Wolf SI, Feldesman MR, Pretorius DH. Simple adnexal cysts: the natural history in postmenopausal women. *Radiology* 1992; **184**: 653–9.

Parker WH. Laparoscopic management of the adnexal mass in postmenopausal women. *J Gynaecol Tech* 1995; **1**: 3–6.

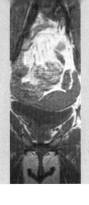

Malignant disease of the uterus and cervix

OVERVIEW

Although cervical screening has reduced the incidence of cervical cancer, overall the incidence is rising in younger women. Surgery remains the mainstay of treatment for early-stage disease whilst radiotherapy is used for more advanced stages. Postmenopausal bleeding is the commonest presenting symptom of endometrial cancer. Although formerly endometrial cancer was thought to carry a good prognosis it is now recognized that the 5-year survival for endometrial carcinoma is similar to that of cervical carcinoma.

Premalignant disease of the cervix

Introduction

Each year there are approximately 2000 deaths in England and Wales from carcinoma of the cervix. Cervical cytological screening is designed to detect over 90 per cent of cytological abnormalities. In theory cervical screening fulfils many of the criteria of a successful screening procedure. The cervical smear test will diagnose the vast majority of cytological abnormalities and the treatment of precancer is simple, safe, nondestructive and usually curative. As a result of women having regular cervical screening the incidence of cervical carcinoma has fallen. The premalignant lesion may persist for many years before an invasive cancer develops and indeed a cancer may never develop.

These premalignant lesions cause no symptoms and are not recognizable with the naked eye.

Epidemiology

Cervical cancer occurs almost exclusively among women who are, or have been, sexually active. The cause is unknown. There is increasing evidence that infection by certain strains of human papilloma virus (HPV) is a factor. Studies have shown that between 10 and 30 per cent of sexually active women have acquired HPV infection of the genital tract by the age of 30 years. The proportion of women infected is higher if the woman or her partner have had several sexual partners. There seems to be an increased risk with the earlier age of onset of intercourse. The genesis of HPV infection is complex: the strains HPV 16 and 18 are particularly implicated in the

Transformation zone

The ectocervix is covered by squamous epithelium, a stratified epithelium very similar to skin, but lacking keratin, the protein that makes skin waterproof. The canal of the cervix however is lined by columnar epithelium, only one cell thick, and the point where these two epithelia meet is called the squamocolumnar junction (SCJ).

The position of the SCJ varies throughout the reproductive life (Fig. 12.1). During infancy it lies just at the external os, but as the cervix increases in volume during puberty and also pregnancy the SCJ is said to roll out onto the ectocervix. The delicate columnar epithelium exposed to the acid environment of the vagina undergoes a process of metaplasia whereby it becomes squamous epithelium.

The transformation zone is that part of the cervix that extends from the widest part of skin that was originally columnar epithelium into the current SCJ. This area is often characterized by Nabothian follicles, which are retention cysts from previous endocervical glands that have been covered by the advancing squamous epithelium.

The area of columnar epithelium seen on the ectocervix appears red because the single cell thickness of columnar epithelium allows the vascular stroma to be seen. This red area has been incorrectly called cervical erosion. To further compound this error, for many years, women with this normal red appearance on their cervix were treated for cervical erosion by cautery under general anaesthetic.

Dysplasia

The process of metaplasia can be disrupted by external influences and can lead to disordered squamous epithelium called dysplastic epithelium.

The human papilloma virus (HPV) is now implicated in this process although HPV infection alone does not appear to be sufficient to cause dysplasia. Dysplastic epithelium lacks the normal maturation of cells as they move from the basal layer to the superficial layer. The nuclei tend to be larger, more variable in size and shape and more actively dividing than healthy squamous epithelium. Dysplasia has been graded as mild, moderate or severe depending on the degree of cytological atypia and also the thickness of the epithelium involved. Mild dysplasia tends to affect only the deepest third of the epithelium from the basal layer upwards with maturation seen more superficial to that. Moderate dysplasia affects two-thirds of the thickness of the epithelium with severe dysplasia showing no maturation throughout the full thickness.

A simpler classification of these abnormalities has been proposed where HPV infection alone and CIN I (cervical intraepithelial neoplasia) are grouped as 'low grade squamous intraepithelial lesions (SIL)' and CIN II and III as 'high grade SIL'. In broad terms CIN I corresponds to mild dysplasia, CIN II to moderate dysplasia and CIN III to severe dysplasia.

---

development of cervical abnormality. Smoking and immune suppression appear to be additional factors which may act as co-agents after initial problems that may stem from HPV infection.

Cytology – cervical smears

Exfoliative cervical cytology was a technique developed by Papanicolaou to collect the cells that had been shed from the skin of the cervix, spread them on a glass slide and stain them using a specially developed technique. Originally cells were washed from the vagina and collected in the posterior fornix. However a more efficient technique of exfoliative cytology involves scraping the cervix to collect cells and cervical mucous directly.

The normal cells shed from healthy squamous

epithelium have extremely small nuclei are flattened and pyknotic. On the other hand, cells from dysplastic epithelium where little maturation has occurred have large nuclei, a large degree of cytological atypia and increased nuclear cytoplasmic ratio.

Whilst cytology does not define where the abnormality is, in skilful hands it has a high degree of sensitivity and specificity and a low cost which makes it suitable for a screening technique.

Colposcopy

The colposcope is a binocular operating microscope with magnification of between five and 20 times. It has been used to examine the cervix in detail to identify dysplastic abnormalities on the ectocervix.

The cervix is first examined for abnormal vessel

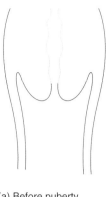

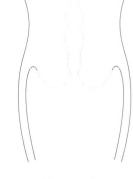

(a) Before puberty

(b) At puberty

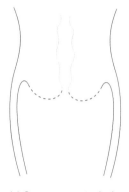

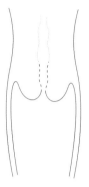

(c) Squamousmetaplasia

(d) Menopausal

 Original squamous epithelium

Original columnar epithelium

Squamous epithelium formed by metaplasia of columnar epithelium

Figure 12.1 The position of the squamocolumnar junction (SCJ) varies in position throughout the reproductive life.

patterns. These are known to be associated with premalignant and malignant lesions of the cervix. To assist in identification of abnormal vessels the cervix may be washed with normal saline and may be viewed through a green filter, which highlights the blood vessels as black lines.

Application of 5 per cent acetic acid to the area highlights dysplastic areas as white, compared with the pink of the squamous epithelium (Fig. 12.2). The acetic acid coagulates protein of cytoplasm and nuclei and since abnormal epithelium is of a high nuclear density this prevents light from passing through the epithelium which thus appears white. Acetowhite epithelium and an abnormal subepithelial capillary pattern may be revealed as mosaicism or punctation.

Occasionally there are very atypical vessels. Mosaic vessels are arranged parallel to the cervix giving a crazy paving appearance whereas punctation is recognized by dilated, elongated vessels arranged in a punctate pattern. Abnormal branching vessels are more suggestive of microinvasive carcinoma (Fig. 12.3). Schiller's test identifies normal squamous epithelium. Normal, mature squamous epithelium contains abundant glycogen that stains dark brown with iodine and the test involves the application of Lugol's solution (iodine and potassium iodide in water) to the ectocervix. The normal squamous epithelium will stain dark brown whereas columnar epithelium, abnormal squamous epithelium and immature normal squamous epithelium will not.

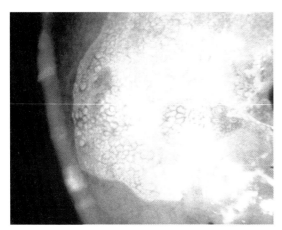

Figure 12.2 This figure shows acetowhite epithelium. (Courtesy of Mr KS Metcalfe.)

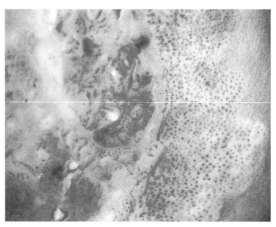

Figure 12.3 Abnormal vascular patterns. (Courtesy of Mr KS Metcalfe.)

Usually a colposcopic-directed biopsy will be taken of the more abnormal areas of the epithelium to confirm the diagnosis. Colposcopy is considered complete if healthy columnar epithelium is identified within the endocervical canal. If the transformation zone extends beyond view then it is incomplete as more abnormal lesions may be seen beyond the field.

Management of the patient with an abnormal cervical smear

Ideally every patient with an abnormal smear should be examined with the colposcope. The practical problem is that the instance of cytological abnormalities appears to be increasing, particularly with the minor grades and resources cannot keep pace with the escalating demand.

Therefore, at present patients with smears suggestive of CIN II or III will undergo colposcopy while those with more minor changes, such as mild dyskaryosis or inflammation, will have a repeat smear. An important point to remember is that a smear will demonstrate dyskaryosis while histological examination is necessary to demonstrate dysplasia.

Natural history of CIN

It has been known for many years that CIN will progress to cervical carcinoma in some instances. The rate of invasion of CIN III lesions is approximately 1.8 per cent per year or 36 per cent over 20 years.

Initially it was believed that CIN III tended to develop from CIN I and II and only CIN III lesions would progress to invasive cancer. Most authors now believe that CIN III lesions probably arise as such. Apparent progression from CIN I to CIN III is explained on the basis of a smaller area of CIN III only becoming apparent with time as the lesions enlarge, hence apparent to be the result of progression.

The risk of invasion of CIN I and II abnormalities has not been clearly defined. While the risk for CIN I appears to be much less than CIN III the difficulty is in defining whether the abnormality in the cervix is truly a pure CIN lesion or whether there are small areas of more significant abnormalities. Certainly cervical malignancies are seen in association with CIN I abnormalities.

Treatment of CIN

CIN has the potential to be an invasive malignancy but does not have malignant properties. Because of this, treatment involves completely removing the abnormal epithelium. This can be done by either an excisional technique or by destroying the abnormal epithelium. It should be remembered that cervical glands can go as far as 5 mm into the stroma of the cervix and that these can be involved with CIN. Treatment, therefore, must be directed to a depth of 5 mm.

Currently, ablative techniques, such as cold coagulation, are used which heats the abnormal epithelium to approximately 100°C and therefore destroys it. Another method is cryotherapy, which involves freezing the abnormal epithelium. This technique is used widely in the United States but its disadvantage is that it does not treat down to the 5 mm depth that is sometimes necessary. Laser vaporization was widely used but is less popular now as it has been superseded by other techniques that are easier. The advantage of ablative therapy is that it is quick, cheap and an easy technique to learn. The principle disadvantage is that no histology is available for review. In all large series of ablative therapy a small number of invasive cancers were overlooked at the time of original diagnosis and were treated in error with ablation. Approximately 1 per cent of patients treated for CIN III will have an unsuspected invasive carcinoma. Using ablative therapy this will not be discovered until the patient is symptomatic or returns for her first check-up.

Excisional techniques include the now popular large loop excision of transformation zone (LLETZ) using a diathermy generator (Fig. 12.4). Other excisional techniques use either a carbon dioxide laser, a diathermy needlepoint or a scalpel with the old-fashioned knife cone biopsy (Fig. 12.5).

LLETZ has become extremely popular because it is quick and easy to perform. However, its major disadvantage is that it is not easy to tailor the excision to the exact area of the abnormality. In consequence, a high rate of incomplete excisions is seen in up to 40 or even 50 per cent of cases. Laser cone biopsy, on the other hand, allows very accurate excision with good visibility but is a more difficult technique to learn and requires slightly longer to perform than LLETZ.

Knife cone biopsy requires a general anaesthetic and has a very high incident of both primary and secondary haemorrhage. Excellent histology can be obtained on a laser or needlepoint cone excision with much lower morbidity.

The follow-up of patients treated for CIN is controversial. In some areas one or two follow-up colposcopies are offered but in others follow-up is entirely by cytology. Women who have undergone treatment for CIN III have approximately a three-fold incidence of invasive carcinoma compared with the background population. Whether this justifies more intensive screening programmes in the long-term has not been clearly defined. Certainly for the first five years women should be offered smears every year and possibly for longer than this.

Malignant disease of the cervix

The development of invasive disease

If CIN is left untreated, after a variable length of time, it may develop the ability to invade through the basement membrane of the epithelium into the stroma beneath. The very earliest signs of invasion can be seen as just a few cells budding through the basement membrane but this may progress to a larger lesion and eventually become a frankly invasive carcinoma. The best estimate of the risk of invasion for high grade CIN is that about 1.8 per cent per year will develop invasive disease.

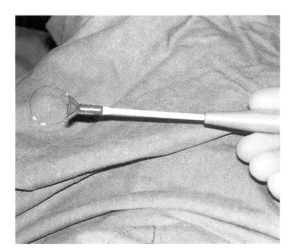

Figure 12.4 A LLETZ loop. (Courtesy of Mr KS Metcalfe.)

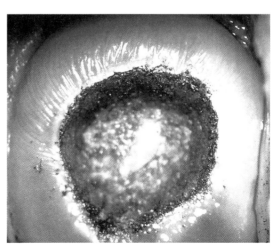

Figure 12.5 The cervix after LLETZ. (Courtesy of Mr KS Metcalfe.)

Microinvasive carcinoma of the cervix

Very early invasive lesions are grouped together in the category of microinvasion. This definition was developed to define a group of patients that could be treated by local therapy alone because the risk of spread to the lymph nodes was lower. By definition, patients with microinvasive cancer are not symptomatic and do not have an obvious lesion on examination of the cervix.

Clinical presentation

The vast majority of patients with cervical cancer will have either intermenstrual bleeding or postmenopausal bleeding at the time of presentation. In addition, patients will often complain of a profuse, offensive vaginal discharge, which may be bloodstained. Other symptoms, such as pain, are uncommon until very late stage.

In all patients with abnormal vaginal bleeding the possibility of either a cervical or uterine carcinoma should be considered and these possibilities should only be discounted after they have been formally excluded. Pain occurs at very late disease.

In addition some patients will present with vaginal bleeding in pregnancy. Every patient with bleeding in pregnancy must have a vaginal examination with inspection of the cervix after the possibility of placenta praevia has been excluded.

On inspection, cancer of the cervix presents as a nodule or small ulcer. It often bleeds on contact. As it advances it becomes a crater-shaped ulcer or often a friable warty looking mass. As the carcinoma progresses, the mobility of the cervix varies and the cervix eventually becomes fixed. Figure 12.6 shows a hysterectomy specimen with cervical carcinoma. Rectal examination will allow a more thorough clinical assessment. Occasionally pyometra occurs, causing uterine enlargement.

Staging

The FIGO classification is the most commonly used staging. This is based on an examination under anaesthetic with an intravenous urogram and cystoscopy, although special imaging techniques and subsequent pathological results are not included. Staging is useful because it affects the choice of treatment.

P | **Understanding the pathophysiology**

Most cervical carcinomas are of the squamous cell type, resembling the epithelium of the ectocervix. In modern series between 85 and 90 per cent of carcinomas are of squamous type. The other principal type is adenocarcinoma with cells resembling the epithelium lining the endocervical canal. Both of these carcinomas tend to arise commonly at the SCJ where the process of metaplasia is shifting the path of differentiation from glandular epithelium of the canal lining to squamous epithelium of the ectocervix. Presumably both the adenocarcinoma and the squamous carcinoma rise from the same precursor cells and, interestingly, the biological behaviour of both common types of carcinoma is very similar (see Fig. 12.1).

Carcinoma of the cervix may spread by direct infiltration and also via the lymphatic vessels. Infiltration occurs or undergrowth may spread downwards into the vaginal wall, forward into the bladder, lateral into the parametrium and paracolpos. Lymphatic spread occurs outwards in the parametrium to the external and internal iliac nodes including those in the obturator fossa and backwards into the uterosacral ligaments and the presacral nodes. From these nodes spread is to the common iliac and para-aortic nodes. Blood spread is unusual.

Table 12.1 – FIGO classification of cervical cancer

Histological stage

Stage 0	CIN 3 (carcinoma *in situ*)
Stage IA	microinvasive carcinoma
Stage IB	invasive carcinoma confined to the cervix
Stage IIA	tumour extending to the upper third of the vagina
Stage IIB	tumour extending to the parametrium but not to the pelvic side wall
Stage IIIA	tumour involving the lower third of the vagina
Stage IIIB	tumour extending to the pelvic side wall (often obstructing a ureter, when seen on IVU)
Stage IVA	tumour involving the bladder or the rectum
Stage IVB	extra pelvic spread, e.g. liver or lung metastasis.

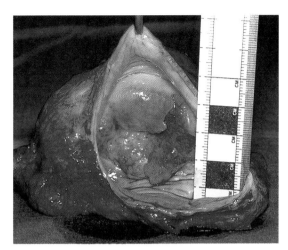

Figure 12.6 A hysterectomy specimen with cervical cancer. (Courtesy of Mr KS Metcalfe.)

The staging is designed to be applicable whether the patient is treated in the Third World countries where high technology imaging is not available or whether the patient is treated by radiotherapy where later pathological findings cannot be included.

Treatment

Preclinical lesions

Patients who have preclinical disease that invades to a depth of less than 3 mm and a width of 7 mm can safely be treated by complete local excision. This is usually in the form of a colposcopically-directed cone biopsy.

Patients with disease invading to a depth of between 3–5 mm have a risk of nodal disease of approximately 5 per cent and accordingly, unless the patient was very keen to be treated conservatively, these patients should be offered radical treatment.

Invasive cervical carcinoma

Treatment for clinical invasive carcinoma is either by surgery, radiotherapy or a combination of the two. If the disease is apparently confined to the cervix, then either surgery or radiotherapy may be offered depending on the skills available in the unit to which the patient is referred. Both forms of treatment are probably equally effective, although for premenopausal women in particular, surgery is thought to offer lower morbidity. Once the disease has spread outside the cervix, radiotherapy is usually the mainstay of treatment.

Surgery

The standard surgical procedure for carcinoma of the cervix is a Wertheim's hysterectomy, which involves removal of the uterus and the paracervical tissues surrounding the cervix and the upper vagina. In addition, the pelvic lymph nodes are carefully dissected as a therapeutic manoeuvre to remove as many of the nodes as possible. The pelvic lymph nodes include the external iliac, internal iliac, common iliac, obturator and presacral nodes.

The dissection of the pelvic nodes is both diagnostic and therapeutic. If a large number of nodes are involved, then it is usual to offer the patient adjuvant radiotherapy. However, we know that if only one or two lymph nodes are involved, the pelvic dissection may well be therapeutic in this situation. During this procedure the ovaries may be conserved, particularly if the patient has squamous pathology, preserving a normal hormonal milieu.

Although the vagina is shortened by 2–3 cm, the remaining vagina is pliable and physical sexual function is preserved. The principal complications seen following this procedure are related to difficulty with complete bladder emptying because of division of the parasympathetic nerve supply to the bladder that runs within the uterosacral ligament.

Careful attention to bladder emptying to prevent urinary retention is important in the immediate postoperative period. On rare occasions patients rarely suffer from lymphoedema.

Radiotherapy

Radical radiotherapy for cervical carcinoma involves the use of a linear accelerator to treat the whole pelvis with external beam therapy to shrink the central carcinoma and also to treat the possible sites of regional metastasis.

Internal sources are then placed in the upper vagina and within the canal of the cervix to provide a very high dose to the central tumour. The external beam therapy is usually given in approximately 25 fractions over a five-week period, followed by two internal treatments in the following week. Most patients tolerate this treatment well, although some damage to the bladder and bowel is inevitable.

Diarrhoea during treatment is usual although this often settles after treatment is finished. A radiation menopause is induced in premenopausal women and inevitably there is some loss of elasticity within the vagina with narrowing. This can be reduced by the use of vaginal dilators and early resumption of intercourse. Recently studies have shown that the addition of chemotherapy during radiotherapy increases the cure rate by approximately 10 per cent and this has now become the standard treatment. Radiotherapy is also used in an adjuvant setting following surgery if more than one or two lymph nodes are positive, if excision margins are close or if the tumour was bulky and had a high chance of recurrence. In advanced cancer of the cervix, radiotherapy may be used in a palliative setting to reduce vaginal bleeding and discharge and to assist in local control of the disease. Chemotherapy may also be used in an adjuvant setting. Response rates are typically 60 per cent and chemotherapy is best used in the neo-adjuvant setting prior to surgery rather than following surgery.

Carcinoma of the cervix and pregnancy

Difficult problems may arise if a woman with cervical carcinoma is also pregnant. In early pregnancy external irradiation may be given; abortion of a dead fetus will follow and then local irradiation with caesium can be given. Later in pregnancy the uterus must be emptied by hysterotomy or Caesarean Section before caesium can be inserted. Many surgeons prefer to treat these cases by Wertheim's hysterectomy, even at the time of Caesarean Section.

Pelvic exenteration

Pelvic exenteration may be considered after radiotherapy in a few selected cases of recurrent disease, where the disease has spread into the bladder or rectum, but where clinical evidence of distant metastases is absent. This is a major operation.

Anterior exenteration consists of removal of the uterus, vagina and bladder, with implantation of the ureters into an artificial bladder made from an ileal loop. If the rectum also has to be removed, total exenteration, the ureters are implanted into an ileal loop and a terminal colostomy is formed. Chemotherapy with combined cytotoxic drugs, including cisplatin, is producing encouraging results and is regarded as preferable in extensive recurrent disease.

Carcinoma of the cervical stump after hysterectomy

The stump of cervix left after subtotal hysterectomy is just as prone to the development of carcinoma as when the uterus is intact. The results of treatment of stump carcinoma are much worse than when the uterus is intact.

Intracavitary radiotherapy is prejudiced because an intrauterine container cannot be used, and vaginal irradiation may not deliver a dose sufficient to destroy the growth without risk of damage to the bladder or rectum. Surgical treatment is prejudiced by the previous operation.

Palliative treatment

Palliative treatment is required for the distressing symptoms that may arise in the advanced stages of the disease. Patients with growths that are too advanced for curative treatment, and also those with recurrent disease, must be kept free from pain and as comfortable as possible. Expert nursing is necessary, especially when incontinence compels frequent changing of pads and sheets.

At first, codeine, pethidine and similar analgesic drugs may be sufficient to control pain; at a later stage opium and its derivatives are required, and the pain may call for progressively larger doses, which may cause nausea and vomiting. A combination containing a phenothiazine may then be effective. Anaesthetists skilled in this field may be able to help with nerve-blocking procedures involving thecal injection of phenol or alcohol. Surgical division of the spinothalamic tract (cordotomy) will also give relief.

Surgical measures will sometimes be required for the unpleasant complication of a vaginal fistula. While a few surgeons will transplant the ureters or perform a colostomy, such procedures may only prolong the act of dying.

The more local operation of colpocleisis may be preferable; this means surgical closure of the lower vagina, so that if there is both a vesicovaginal and rectovaginal fistula the urine and discharge from the growth will be passed through the anus.

P **Understanding the pathophysiology**

The commonest subtype of endometrial carcinoma is usually called endometrioid because it resembles the normal proliferative endometrium although the architecture is much more complicated. Squamous metaplasia can occur within adenocarcinomas and this can result in benign adenocanthoma or malignant change, termed adenosquamous carcinoma. Papillary serous and clear cell carcinomas are particularly aggressive forms of endometrial carcinoma and primary squamous cell carcinoma of the endometrium is extremely rare.

Prognosis

The prognosis of invasive cervical carcinoma varies depending on the method of treatment chosen, the experience of the radiotherapist or surgeon, and on the country.

An illustrative general statement might be that the expectation of five-year survival is:

Stage I	>85%
Stage II	50%
Stage III	25%
Stage IV	5%

In stages IB and IIA there is little difference between the results of surgery and radiotherapy.

When the disease recurs it does so within one year in 50 per cent of patients, within two years in 75 per cent and within five years in 90 per cent.

Malignant disease of the body of the uterus

Introduction

The most common malignant disease affecting the uterus is endometrial carcinoma, which arises from the lining of the uterus. However, sarcomas also arise from the stroma of the endometrium or from the myometrium and these will be discussed later in the chapter.

Table 12.2 – Risk factors in postmenopausal and premenopausal women

Factors known to increase the likelihood of developing the disease are listed below.
1. Obesity
2. Impaired carbohydrate tolerance
3. Nulliparity
4. Late menopause
5. Unopposed oestrogen therapy
6. Functioning ovarian tumours
7. Previous pelvic irradiation
8. Sequential oral contraceptives with dimethisterone
9. Family history of carcinoma of breast, ovary or colon.

Epidemiology

Endometrial cancer can occur in women in their 20s, but the vast majority of cases occur in women over 45 years of age. The median age of presentation is just over 60 years of age. The highest incidence is in white North Americans for reasons that are not clear.

Aetiology

The cause of endometrial carcinoma is unknown although a number of factors that increase the risk of endometrial cancer are listed in Table 12.2. Many of the factors are related to an increase in oestrogen levels. In the postmenopausal period the majority of circulating oestrogen is derived from aromatization of peripheral androgens. This conversion takes place principally in adipose tissue. In addition, postmenopausal women with diabetes have increased oestrogen levels.

Nulliparity and late menopause are both associated with increased risk of endometrial cancer, which may be explained by the prolonged oestrogenic effect on the endometrium.

Women who use oral contraception or progestogens have up to a 50 per cent reduction in the incidence of endometrial cancer and protection lasts for many years after the discontinuation of these treatments. Cigarette smoking has also been associated with the reduced risk of endometrial cancer.

Clinical presentation

As noted above, 75–80 per cent of women with endometrial carcinoma will present with post-menopausal bleeding. However, a postmenopausal discharge, particularly a bloodstained discharge, may well be associated with carcinoma. In the pre-menopausal period, most women with endometrial carcinoma will present with intermenstrual bleeding although one-third of premenopausal women will present with heavy periods only. Figure 12.7 shows a uterus with adenocarcinoma of the endometrium.

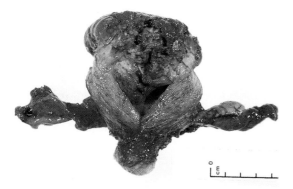

Figure 12.7 Shows a uterus with adenocarcinoma of the endometrium. (Courtesy of Mr KS Metcalfe.)

Diagnosis

Traditionally, postmenopausal bleeding was investigated by a dilatation and curettage. More recently however diagnosis has shifted to the out-patient setting with ultrasound determination of endometrial thickness and out-patient sampling of the endometrium using instruments such as a pipelle sampler. Out-patient hysteroscopy may be undertaken although it is rarely necessary. Ultrasound also allows the ovaries to be imaged, as a number of patients with postmenopausal bleeding will have ovarian pathology.

Staging

The FIGO classification and staging of endometrial carcinoma are shown in Table 12.3.

Table 12.3 – FIGO staging of carcinoma of the corpus uteri

Stage	Description
I	The carcinoma is confined to the corpus
II	The carcinoma has involved the corpus and the cervix but has not extended outside the uterus
III	The carcinoma has extended outside the uterus but not outside the true pelvis
IV	The carcinoma has extended outside the true pelvis or has obviously involved the mucosa of the bladder or rectum. A bullous oedema as such does not permit a case to be allotted to stage IV

Prognosis

Prognosis of the disease is related to stage, which now include grade of disease, myometrial invasion and lymph node involvement. Other factors such as age and body morphology are also important. The higher the age the more likely the patient is to succumb to the disease.

It is now believed that squamous metaplasia does not imply a worse prognosis but the presence of malignant squamous components (adenosquamous carcinoma) is thought to be associated with a poorer outcome. These tumours appear to be increasing in frequency.

Treatment

Stage I
The treatment of choice in patients with endometrial carcinoma is total abdominal hysterectomy and bilateral salpingo-oophorectomy. Radiotherapy is also necessary if invasion of the myometrium has occurred to more than the inner half of the myometrium.

Stage II
In a surgically fit patient at this stage of the disease a radical hysterectomy and bilateral pelvic lym-

phadenectomy with para-aortic node sampling should be performed. If the patient is surgically unfit then radiotherapy may be used.

Stage III

If the node suggests spread of disease then obviously adjuvant radiotherapy is necessary with surgery.

Stages III and IV

Treatment needs to be individualized to the patient but surgery is not usually the first line of treatment. Radiotherapy is performed and then occasionally residual disease may be involved by surgical intervention.

Progestogens

Although there is no randomized study to suggest that progestogens are beneficial there appears to be some belief that these are helpful in preventing recurrence after treatment of early stage disease.

Carcinoma of the endometrium has traditionally been the poor relation of gynaecological malignancies with the majority of cases being treated outside major cancer centres. Such an approach stems from the belief that the cancer carries a good prognosis. However, the five-year survival figures approximate to those of cancer of the cervix.

Sarcoma and mixed mesodermal tumours of the uterus

Leiomyosarcoma

Leiomyosarcoma may arise in the uterine muscle. Very rarely, such a tumour may arise by transformation of a previously benign fibromyoma; this occurs in less than 0.2 per cent of fibromyomata. Sarcoma also occasionally arises in the stroma of the endometrium – endometrial stromal sarcoma.

Tumours of this group grow more rapidly and are softer than fibromyomata. They may increase in size after the menopause, when fibromyomata remain unchanged or shrink. On naked-eye inspection the tumour may be seen to have invaded the uterine wall or the capsule of the fibromyoma, and the cut surface often shows small haemorrhages and areas of degen-

erative softening. Microscopically, they consist of spindle-shaped or rounded cells, many of them pleomorphic, with little stroma and primitive blood vessels. Histological diagnosis of malignancy depends on the number of mitoses per high-power field (HPF). Patients with more than ten mitoses per HPF are regarded as having malignant disease. Distant metastasis via the bloodstream and direct spread to adjacent structures often occur.

These tumours occur in adults, who usually complain of uterine bleeding. Rapid growth of the tumour, with increasing pain, may give rise to suspicion of its nature, but in many cases the diagnosis is made only after the tumour has been removed. In rare cases a sarcoma may be slow growing, and its nature discovered only when it recurs after operation.

Mixed mesodermal tumours

This covers tumours that contain heterologous mesenchymal elements. In adults they may occur when a large fleshy mass protrudes from the uterine wall into the uterine cavity. Histological examination shows that it contains some elements resembling sarcoma and others resembling carcinoma, together with bizarre components such as cartilage and striped muscle. Metastasis via the bloodstream is common, as is local recurrence after removal. The patient complains of bleeding from the uterus, and sometimes of pain. Tumours of this type occasionally follow uterine irradiation. The prognosis is poor.

Sarcoma botryoides (embryonal rhabdomyosarcoma) is a variety of the same type of tumour that is seen in infants and young children. There is a blood-stained watery discharge and the vagina is found to contain grape-like masses of soft growth, usually arising from the cervix. Among the myxomatous cells of the tumour primitive striped muscle cells (rhabdomyoblasts) can be demonstrated. Local recurrence often follows removal and distant metastases occur.

Treatment

If the diagnosis is suspected in adults before operation, total hysterectomy and bilateral salpingo-oophorectomy is performed, followed by external radiotherapy.

In many cases the diagnosis is made only after hysterectomy has been performed for supposed fibromyomata; a decision whether to proceed to additional radiotherapy must then be taken, depending on the extent and nature of the disease. The prognosis is poor, except for leiomyosarcoma arising in a fibromyoma.

In children, as with many other forms of malignant disease, the prognosis with conventional treatment has been very poor. The modern use of a combination of external irradiation and chemotherapy has altered the outlook and allowed a less radical surgical approach to be taken. Exenteration is now rarely indicated in the treatment of these tumours.

Key Points

- Cervical cancer occurs almost exclusively amongst women who are or have been sexually active
- The cause of cervical cancer is unknown
- The advent of regular cervical screening and colposcopy has reduced the incidence of invasive cervical cancer. However, overall, the incidence of cancer is rising in younger women under the age of 45
- Squamous cell carcinoma is the most common type and has a similar prognosis to adenocarcinoma
- Metastatic spread is mainly lymphatic but overall half of women with cervical cancer die within 5 years
- Treatment is dependent on surgical staging
- Surgery is most often performed in the young woman patient with Stage I disease
- Radiotherapy is used for the older and less fit patients regardless of size of the tumour and for women in the bulky stage Ib and IIa tumours or for more advanced disease
- The overall 5-year survival for carcinoma of the uterus is 65%. Most risk factors for development of this cancer share common basis – excessive unopposed oestrogen stimulation of the endometrium
- Post-menopausal bleeding is the most common presenting symptom in 80% of women
- Total abdominal hysterectomy and bilateral salpingo oophorectomy is the treatment of choice for Stage I disease
- More recently lymphadenectomy for enhancing staging has been recommended
- The value of adjuvant progestogen therapy is not established

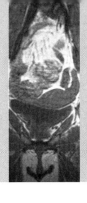

Chapter 13

Malignant disease of the ovary

OVERVIEW

Carcinoma of the ovary is most common in the wealthy nations of the World. There are just under 6000 cases each year in the UK. Whilst the incidence of ovarian cancer is similar to that of cancer of the endometrium and of the cervix, more women die from ovarian cancer than from carcinoma of the cervix and body of the uterus combined.

CANCER OF THE OVARY

Introduction

Most ovarian tumours are of epithelial origin. These are rare before the age of 35 years, but the incidence increases with age to a peak in the 50–70 year old age group (Fig. 13.1). Most epithelial tumours are not discovered until they have spread widely. Surgery and chemotherapy, mainly with carboplatin or cisplatin and taxol, form the mainstay of treatment for epithelial tumours. The results are poor. Less than 25 per cent of women with ovarian cancer are alive after five years.

Only 3 per cent of ovarian cancers are seen in women younger than 35 years and most of these are non-epithelial cancers such as germ cell tumours. In contrast to epithelial tumours, germ cell tumours can be treated very successfully with conservative surgery and modern, multidrug chemotherapy. Fertility can often be conserved.

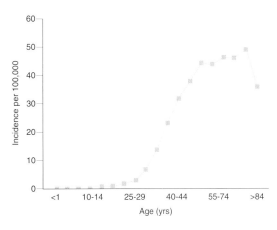

Figure 13.1 The incidence of ovarian cancer in England and Wales (Offices of Population Censuses and Surveys 1985).

Aetiology

'Incessant ovulation' theory

Epithelial tumours are most frequently associated with nulliparity, an early menarche, a late age at menopause and a long estimated number of years of ovulation. Oral contraceptive use reduces the risk four-fold. However, even without oral contraceptives, increasing age at first birth reduces the risk of ovarian cancer. This and other anomalies cast doubt upon the 'incessant ovulation' theory.

Infertility treatment

Infertility, especially when it is unexplained, is associated with both ovarian and endometrial cancer. However, case controlled studies have suggested that there might possibly be a link between ovarian cancer and prolonged attempts at induction of ovulation.

Genetic factors

Familial ovarian cancer

There is a family history in between 5 and 10 per cent of women with epithelial ovarian cancers – usually serous adenocarcinomas. A woman with one affected close relative has a lifetime risk of 2.5 per cent, twice the risk in the general population. With two affected close relatives, the lifetime risk increases to 30–40 per cent. A particular feature of familial cancers is the relatively early age at which they occur.

Most of these families also have cases of breast or colorectal cancer in the family. The defective gene in the breast/ovary families is most commonly the tumour suppressor gene BRCA1 (81 per cent). BRCA2 is defective in about 14 per cent. Families with colorectal cancer have defects in the DNA repair genes but this is seldom found in association with familial ovarian cancer. A woman who has inherited a defective BRCA1 gene in a well-documented family has a 60 per cent risk of breast cancer by 50 years of age and an 80 per cent lifetime risk. However, the risk of ovarian cancer is much lower, being nearer 40 per cent.

Management of women with a family history of ovarian cancer

Genetic testing for BRCA1 is now possible but is impracticable and unreliable as mutations are found far less often than would be expected, even in women with a strong family history. There are considerable problems in interpreting the results in women with only one or two affected relatives. There may be a spectrum of mutations with very different levels of risk. Even a negative test result may not provide the expected reassurance.

Once identified with the help of a clinical geneticist, women with a high risk of ovarian and breast cancer are difficult to advise. The main risk is breast cancer but prophylactic, bilateral mastectomy is a drastic step for any woman to take. None of the available screening tests for ovarian cancer is effective and false positive results can result in unnecessary surgery. Annual ovarian ultrasonography with colour-flow Doppler studies and serum Ca_{125} estimation every 6–12 months are recommended but it is uncertain how much protection this offers. Prophylactic bilateral oophorectomy, usually combined with hysterectomy is recommended for clearly defined high-risk women after completion of their family at about 45 years of age. This does not remove the risk entirely as carcinoma of the peritoneum has occurred after this procedure.

P | **Understanding the pathophysiology**

Familial ovarian cancer
- Familial ovarian cancer is rare (5–10 per cent)
- Suggestive history
- At least two first-degree relatives with ovarian, breast or colorectal carcinoma
- Cases usually diagnosed before 50 years of age
- Defective genes include BRCA1 and BRCA2
- Risk of ovarian cancer (40 per cent) in these families is less than risk of breast cancer (80 per cent)
- Genetic testing remains impracticable and unreliable

Simplified histological classification of ovarian tumours

I   Common epithelial tumours (benign, borderline or malignant)
    A. Serous tumour
    B. Mucinous tumour
    C. Endometrioid tumour
    D. Clear cell (mesonephroid) tumour
    E. Brenner tumour
    F. Undifferentiated carcinomas

II   Sex cord stromal tumours
    A. Granulosa stroma cell tumour
    B. Androblastoma: Sertoli–Leydig cell tumour
    C. Gynandroblastoma

III   Germ cell tumours
    A. Dysgerminoma
    B. Endodermal sinus tumour (yolk sac tumour)
    C. Embryonal cell tumour
    D. Choriocarcinoma
    E. Teratoma
    F. Mixed tumours

IV   Metastatic tumours

Classification of ovarian tumours

Ovarian tumours can be solid or cystic. They may be benign or malignant and in addition there are those which, while having some of the features of malignancy, lack any evidence of stromal invasion. These are called borderline tumours.

Primary ovarian tumours are divided into epithelial type (implying an origin from surface epithelium); sex cord gonadal type (also known as sex cord stromal type, or sex cord mesenchymal type, and originating from sex cord mesenchymal elements), and germ cell type.

Pathology of epithelial tumours

Well-differentiated epithelial carcinomas tend to be more often associated with early stage disease, but the degree of differentiation does correlate with survival, except in the most advanced stages. Diploid tumours tend to be associated with earlier stage disease and a better prognosis. Cell type is not of itself prognostically significant. Comparing patients stage for stage and grade for grade, there is no difference in survival between different epithelial types. However, mucinous and endometrioid lesions are likely to be associated with earlier stage and lower grade than serous cystadenocarcinomas.

Serous carcinoma

Most serous carcinomas have both solid and cystic elements but some may be mainly cystic. They often affect both ovaries. Well-differentiated tumours have a papillary pattern with stromal invasion. Psammoma bodies (calcospherules) are often present. At the other end of the spectrum is the anaplastic tumour composed of sheets of undifferentiated neoplastic cells in masses within a fibrous stroma. Occasional glandular structures may be present to enable a diagnosis of adenocarcinoma to be made. All gradations between these two are seen, sometimes in the same tumour.

Mucinous carcinoma

Malignant mucinous tumours account for 10 per cent of the malignant tumours of the ovary. They are usually multilocular, thin-walled cysts with a smooth external surface containing mucinous fluid. Mucinous tumours are amongst the largest tumours of the ovary and may reach enormous dimensions. A cyst diameter of 25 cm is quite common.

Endometrioid carcinoma

These are ovarian tumours that resemble endometrial carcinomas. There is little to characterize an ovarian tumour as being of endometrioid type by naked eye examination. Most are cystic, often unilocular, and contain turbid brown fluid. Five to 10 per cent are seen in continuity with recognizable endometriosis. Ovarian adenoacanthoma, with benign-appearing squamous elements, account for almost 50 per cent of some series of endometrioid tumours.

It is important to note that 15 per cent of endometrioid carcinoma of the ovary are associated with endometrial carcinoma in the body of the uterus. In most cases these are two separate primary tumours.

Clear cell carcinoma (mesonephroid)

These are the least common of the malignant epithelial tumours of the ovary, accounting for 5 to 10 per cent of ovarian carcinomas. The appearance from which the tumours derive their name is the clear cell pattern but, in addition, some areas show a tubulo-cystic pattern with the characteristic 'hob-nail' appearance of the lining epithelium.

As there is a very strong association between clear cell tumours of the ovary and ovarian endometriosis, and because clear cell and endometrioid tumours frequently co-exist, it has been suggested that the clear cell tumour may be a variant of endometrioid tumour.

Borderline epithelial tumours

Ten per cent of all epithelial tumours of the ovary are of borderline malignancy. These show varying degrees of nuclear atypia and an increase in mitotic activity, multilayering of neoplastic cells and formation of cellular buds, but no invasion of the stroma. Most borderline tumours remain confined to the ovaries and this may account for their much better prognosis. Peritoneal lesions are present in some cases and, although a few are true metastases, many do not progress and some even regress after removal of the primary tumour. The histological diagnosis of borderline malignancy can be difficult, particularly in mucinous tumours. Most borderline tumours are serous or mucinous in type.

Natural history

Some two-thirds of patients with ovarian cancer present with disease that has spread beyond the pelvis. This is probably due to the insidious nature of the signs and symptoms of carcinoma of the ovary but may sometimes be due to a rapidly growing tumour. Due to the non-specific nature of most of these symptoms, a diagnosis of ovarian cancer is seldom considered until the disease is in an advanced stage.

Metastatic spread

The pelvic peritoneum and other pelvic organs become involved by direct spread. The peritoneal fluid, flowing to lymphatic channels on the under-surface of the diaphragm, carries malignant cells to the omentum, the peritoneal surfaces of the small and large bowel and the liver and the parietal peritoneal surface throughout the abdominal cavity and on the surface of the diaphragm. Metastases on the undersurface of the diaphragm may be found in up to 44 per cent of what otherwise seems to be stage I–II disease (Table 13.1).

Lymphatic spread commonly involves the pelvic and the para-aortic nodes. Spread may also occur to nodes in the neck or inguinal region. Haematogenous spread usually occurs late in the course of the disease. The main areas involved are the liver and lung, although metastases to bone and brain are sometimes seen.

Clinical staging

Clinical staging is an important prognostic indicator (see Table 13.2). Peritoneal deposits on the surface of the liver do not make the patient stage IV, the parenchyma must be involved. Similarly, the presence of a pleural effusion is insufficient to put the patient in stage IV status unless malignant cells are found on cytological examination of the pleural fluid.

Table 13.1 – Pelvic and para-aortic node metastases

	Nodes involved	
	Pelvic nodes	Para-aortic nodes
Stage I–II	30%	19%
Stage III–IV	67%	65%

Table 13.2 – FIGO staging for primary ovarian carcinoma

Stage		FIGO definition (simplified)
I		Growth limited to ovaries
	Ia	Growth limited to one ovary
		no ascites; no tumour on external surfaces; capsule intact
	Ib	Growth limited to both ovaries
		no ascites; no tumour on external surfaces; capsule intact
	Ic	Tumour either Stage Ia or Ib but tumour on surface of one or both ovaries; or with ascites present containing malignant cells
II		Growth involving one or both ovaries with pelvic extension
III		Growth involving one or both ovaries with peritoneal implants outside the pelvis or positive retroperitoneal or inguinal nodes. Superficial liver metastases equals Stage III.
IV		Growth involving one or both ovaries with distant metastases. If pleural effusion is present there must be positive cytology to allot a case to Stage IV. Parenchymal liver metastasis equals Stage IV.

Diagnosis

Abdominal pain or discomfort is the commonest presenting complaint and distension (Fig. 13.2) or feeling a lump the next most frequent. Patients may complain of indigestion, urinary frequency, weight loss or, rarely, abnormal menses or postmenopausal bleeding. A hard abdominal mass arising from the pelvis is highly suggestive, especially in the presence of ascites. A fixed, hard, irregular pelvic mass is usually felt best by combined vaginal and rectal examination. The neck and groin should also be examined for enlarged nodes.

Haematological investigations include a full blood count, urea, electrolytes and liver function tests. A chest X-ray is essential. It is sometimes advisable to carry out a barium enema or colonoscopy to differentiate between an ovarian and a colonic tumour and to assess bowel involvement from the ovarian tumour itself. An IVP (intravenous urogram) is occasionally useful. Ultrasonography may help to confirm the presence of a pelvic mass and detect ascites before it is clinically apparent. In conjunction with Ca_{125} estimation it may be used to calculate a 'risk of malignancy score'. In most women, the diagnosis is far from certain before the laparotomy and the operation is undertaken on the basis that there is a large mass that needs to be removed regardless of its nature.

Markers for epithelial tumours

Ca_{125} is the only marker in common clinical use. It can also be raised in benign conditions such as endometriosis. Ca_{125} is useful for monitoring women receiving chemotherapy to assess response. A persistent rise in Ca_{125} may precede clinical

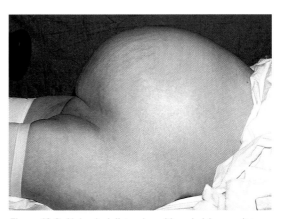

Figure 13.2 Abdominal distension with underlying ovarian mass and ascites. (Courtesy of K Metcalfe.)

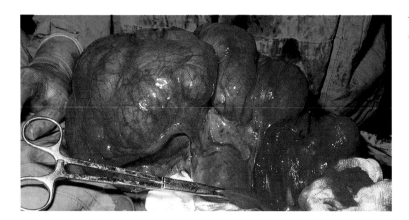

13.3 Resected ovarian carcinoma. (Courtesy of K Metcalfe.)

evidence of recurrent disease, in some cases, by several months. However, the values can be normal even in the presence of small tumour deposits.

Screening

Because carcinoma of the ovary tends to be asymptomatic in the early stages and most patients present with advanced disease, much effort has been made to define a tumour marker that could be used for screening purposes. So far, none has become available which is truly specific and which is suitable for the early detection of epithelial tumours. Ultrasound is not suitable as a primary screening tool because it is too expensive and has a high false-positive rate. The most promising approach is a combination of Ca_{125} with ultrasound for those women with persistently raised values.

In our present state of knowledge and with the available technology, screening the general population is neither useful nor safe. Patients should be enrolled in trials to assess new screening techniques but should not be led to believe that these have proven value.

Surgery

Surgery is the mainstay of both the diagnosis and the treatment of ovarian cancer. A vertical incision is required for an adequate exploration of the upper abdomen. A sample of ascitic fluid or peritoneal washings with normal saline should be taken for cytology. The pelvis and upper abdomen are explored carefully to identify metastatic disease.

The therapeutic objective of surgery for ovarian cancer is the removal of all tumour. While this is achieved in the majority of stage I and stage II cases, it is usually impossible in more advanced disease. Because of the diffuse spread of tumour throughout the peritoneal cavity and the retroperitoneal nodes, microscopic deposits will persist in almost all cases even when all macroscopic tumour appears to have been excised. Thus, while surgery alone may be curative in many Stage I cases, additional therapy is essential for most of the remainder. Fig. 13.3 shows an ovarian tumour at surgery.

Surgery for epithelial ovarian cancer

Primary surgery – to determine diagnosis and remove tumour
- Total abdominal hysterectomy
- Bilateral salpingo-oophorectomy
- Infracolic omentectomy

Conservative primary surgery
- Young, nulliparous women with Stage Ia disease
- No evidence of synchronous endometrial cancer
- Unilateral salpingo-oophorectomy

Interval debulking surgery
- Women with bulky disease after primary surgery
- Must respond after 2–4 courses of chemotherapy
- Chemotherapy resumed after surgery

Second-look surgery
- At the end of chemotherapy
- No place in current management

Borderline tumours
- Ovarian cystectomy or oophorectomy adequate in young women
- Hysterectomy and bilateral salpingo-oophorectomy in older women

The resection of all visible tumour usually requires a total hysterectomy, bilateral salpingo-oophorectomy and infracolic omentectomy. However, in a young, nulliparous woman with a unilateral tumour and no ascites, unilateral salpingo-oophorectomy may be justifiable after careful exploration to exclude metastatic disease, and curettage of the uterine cavity to exclude a synchronous endometrial tumour. If the tumour is subsequently found to be poorly differentiated or if the washings are positive, a second operation to clear the pelvis will be necessary.

Borderline disease usually presents as a Stage Ia tumour confined to one ovary. It is often not recognized as malignant. If an ovarian cystectomy has been performed in a young woman and it seems likely that the disease has been removed completely, there is probably little to be gained from further surgery. In cases of doubt, a second laparotomy should be performed to explore the abdomen thoroughly and to remove the rest of the affected ovary. Older women who have no wish to have children, have little to gain from conservative surgery and it is probably still prudent to recommend bilateral oophorectomy and hysterectomy.

When bulky disease remains after initial surgery, a second laparotomy may be performed on those women who respond after two to four courses of chemotherapy. The chemotherapy is then resumed as soon as possible after the second operation. This is called 'interval debulking'. A large European study of this approach suggests that the median survival in this poor prognosis group may be increased by six months and that the survival at three years may be improved from 10 to 20 per cent.

Second-look surgery is defined as a planned laparotomy at the end of chemotherapy. The objectives are, firstly, to determine the response to previous therapy in order to document accurately its efficacy and to plan subsequent management and, secondly, to excise any residual disease. While there is no doubt that second-look surgery gives the most accurate indication of the disease status, the evidence suggests that neither the surgical resection of residual tumour nor the opportunity to change the treatment have any effect on the patient's survival. Second-look procedures therefore have no place outside clinical trials at the present time.

Selecting patients with postoperative treatment

Women with stage 1a or Ib disease and well- or moderately-differentiated tumours may not require further treatment. The benefit of adjuvant therapy for women with stage Ic disease remains uncertain but many oncologists will advise chemotherapy. All other patients with invasive ovarian carcinoma require adjuvant therapy. There is no evidence that adjuvant therapy affects the outcome in women with borderline tumours.

Radiotherapy

Radiotherapy is now almost never used in the routine management of ovarian carcinoma. A potential exception is radio-immunotherapy in which radioactive Ytrium is linked to a monoclonal antibody which recognizes an antigen found on most ovarian cancers. This is given intraperitoneally. It remains an experimental treatment.

Chemotherapy

Chemotherapy for epithelial ovarian cancer:
* Stages II–IV – possibly stage Ic;
* Carboplatin or cisplatin and taxol.

Chemotherapy is given both to prolong clinical remission and survival, and for palliation in advanced and recurrent disease. It is commenced as soon as possible after surgery and is usually given for five or six cycles at three- to four-weekly intervals.

The platinum drugs, cisplatin and its analogue carboplatin, are heavy metal compounds that cause cross-linkage of DNA strands in a similar fashion to alkylating agents. These are considered to be the most effective drugs in general use in the management of ovarian carcinoma, and are the most widely used cytotoxic drugs either alone or in combination.

Cisplatin is a very toxic drug. Until the advent of the 5HT antagonists (ganesetron and ondansetron), severe nausea and vomiting, sometimes lasting several days, was a serious problem. Permanent renal damage will occur unless cisplatin is given with adequate hydration with intravenous fluids. Peripheral neuropathy and hearing loss are reported with increasing cumulative doses. Electrolyte disturbances, such as hypomagnesaemia, are seen occasionally. Unlike most chemotherapeutic agents, marrow toxicity is not usually a problem, with the exception of anaemia.

Carboplatin is as effective as cisplatin in the treatment of ovarian cancer. It causes less nausea and vomiting than cisplatin and has no significant renal toxicity. Neurotoxicity is rare and hearing loss is subclinical. The lack of renal toxicity means that there is no need to give carboplatin with intravenous hydration. The dose is calculated in relation to the glomerular filtration rate, using the area under the curve (AUC) formula.

Paclitaxel (taxol) is now considered to be part of the standard treatment for ovarian cancer given in combination with cisplatin or carboplatin. It is usually given as a four-hour infusion after a premedication regime of dexamethasone 20 mg, diphenhydramine 50 mg and ranitidine or cimetidine to prevent hypersensitivity reactions. Paclitaxel is derived from the bark of the Pacific yew tree (*taxus brevifolia*) and has a mechanism of action which is unique among cytotoxic drugs.

Sensory neuropathy and neutropenia are more common with higher doses and infusions for 24 hours result in a higher incidence of grade 4 neutropenia. Other forms of toxicity, such as myalgia and arthralgia, are dose dependent but never severe. Nausea and vomiting is very mild but loss of body hair is usually total, irrespective of dose and schedule. Bradycardia and hypotension usually do not cause symptoms.

Results – epithelial tumours

Borderline epithelial tumours

Women with borderline ovarian epithelial tumours confined to the ovaries have a good long-term prognosis, with very few women dying from their disease. Even with extra-ovarian spread, the 15-year survival for serous borderline epithelial tumours is around 90 per cent. For stage III mucinous tumours the 15-year survival rate is only 44 per cent.

Invasive epithelial ovarian cancer

Survival for epithelial ovarian cancer is dependent mainly on stage, size of residual tumour at the end of initial surgery and grade of tumour. The five-year survival rate ranges from 60 to 70 per cent for women with stage I disease to 10 per cent for stages III–IV. Since the majority of patients present with advanced disease, the overall five-year survival in the UK is only 23 per cent.

While women with Stage I tumours with grade 1 or 2 histology have a five-year survival rate of over 90 per cent, those with poorly differentiated tumours do much worse. In more advanced tumours, the amount of residual tumour at the end of initial surgery is significant in terms of prognosis.

The survival figures for cancer of the ovary have changed little over the last 20 years and remain poor for women with advanced disease despite more radical surgery and improvements in chemotherapy. Most studies do show some improvement in median survival in patients with minimal residual disease following surgery and who respond to postsurgical treatment. However this benefit has not been sufficiently long lasting to affect five-year survival rates. There is no doubt that even if long-term survival has not been improved, modern cytotoxic therapy has improved the quality of life for many patients with advanced ovarian cancer in spite of the side effects.

Non-epithelial tumours

Non-epithelial tumours constitute approximately 10 per cent of all ovarian cancers. Because of their rarity and their sensitivity to intensive chemotherapy, it is especially appropriate to refer these patients for specialist care.

Sex cord stromal tumours

Granulosa and theca cell tumours
The most common sex cord stromal tumours are the granulosa and theca cell tumours. They often produce steroid hormones, in particular oestrogens, which can cause postmenopausal bleeding in older women and sexual precocity in prepubertal girls. Granulosa cell tumours usually secrete inhibin. This can be used to monitor the effects of treatment.

Theca cell tumours are usually benign. Granulosa cell tumours occur at all ages, but are found predominantly in postmenopausal women. The staging system for these tumours is the same as for epithelial tumours. Most present as stage I. Bilateral tumours are present in only 5 per cent of cases.

Pathology

Granulosa cell tumours are normally solid but cystic spaces may develop when they become large. Some are predominantly cystic. Like most tumours of the sex cord stromal tumour group, the cut surface is often yellow because of neutral lipid related to sex steroid hormone production. Areas of haemorrhage are also common.

Treatment

The surgical treatment is the same as for epithelial tumours. Unilateral oophorectomy is indicated only in young women with stage Ia disease. The effect of adjunctive therapy is difficult to assess as granulosa cell tumours can recur up to 20 years after the initial diagnosis. Radiotherapy has been largely replaced by chemotherapy in advanced or recurrent cases. In cases of late recurrence, further surgery should be considered before any other therapy is given. The five-year survival is around 80 per cent overall but recurrence is associated with a high mortality.

Sertoli–Leydig cell tumours

Half of these rare neoplasia produce male hormones which can cause virilization. Rarely oestrogens are secreted. The prognosis for the majority with local-

ized disease is good and treatment is the same as for granulosa cell tumours.

Germ cell tumours

Dysgerminomas

Dysgerminomas account for 2–5 per cent of all primary malignant ovarian tumours. Nearly all occur in young women less than 30 years old. They spread mainly by lymphatics. All cases need a chest X-ray and a computerized tomography (CT) scan. Serum alpha-fetoprotein (AFP) and ßhCG must be assayed to exclude the ominous presence of elements of choriocarcinoma, endodermal sinus tumour or teratoma. Occasionally some cases of pure dysgerminoma have raised levels of ßhCG. Pure dysgerminomas have a good prognosis as they are normally stage I tumours (75 per cent), most being stage Ia.

Pathology

Dysgerminomas are solid tumours that have a smooth or nodular, bosselated external surface. They are soft or rubbery in consistency, depending upon the proportion of fibrous tissue contained in them. They may reach a considerable size; the mean diameter is 15 cm. Approximately 10 per cent are bilateral; they are alone among malignant germ cell tumours in having a significant incidence of bilaterality. Elements of immature teratoma, yolk sac tumour or choriocarcinoma are found in about 10 per cent of dysgerminomas. Very thorough sampling of all dysgerminomas must be undertaken by the histopathologist to exclude the presence of these more malignant germ cell elements as this indicates a worse prognosis.

Other germ cell tumours

Yolk sac (endodermal sinus) tumours

Yolk sac (endodermal sinus) tumours are the second most common malignant germ cell tumour of the ovary, making up 10–15 per cent over all and reaching a higher proportion in children. It may present as an acute abdomen due to rupture of the tumour following necrosis and haemorrhage. The tumour is usually well-encapsulated and solid. Areas of necrosis and haemorrhage are often seen, as are small cystic spaces. Its consistency varies from soft to firm and rubbery and its cut surface is slippery and mucoid. It

---

Non-epithelial tumours

Sex cord stromal
- Granulosa cell tumour
- Theca cell tumour
- Sertoli–Leydig tumour

Germ cell
- Dysgerminoma
- Yolk sac (endodermal sinus) tumour
- Teratoma

Treatment of non-epithelial tumours

Sex cord stromal tumours
- Mainly treated by surgery – hysterectomy and bilateral salpingo-oophorectomy
- Unilateral salpingo-oophorectomy only in young women with Stage Ia disease
- Chemotherapy (when required) same regimens as used for epithelial tumours

Germ cell tumours
- Mainly conservative surgery because the patients are usually young
- Combination chemotherapy is highly effective when required

---

often secretes AFP, which can be used to monitor treatment.

Teratomas

Mature teratomas are benign, the most common being the cystic teratoma or dermoid cyst found at all ages but particularly in the third and fourth decades. Not all solid teratomas are immature type.

Immature teratomas are composed of a wide variety of tissues and comprise about 1 per cent of all ovarian teratomas. They are unilateral in almost all cases and appear as solid masses that have smooth and bosselated surfaces. The cut surface shows mainly solid tissue, although small cystic spaces are visible. Blood levels of ßhCG and AFP should be estimated even when the tumour appears to be a straightforward immature teratoma.

Results of treatment of epithelial tumours

- Borderline tumours
- Excellent long-term prognosis in most cases
- Most of those who die have pseudomyxoma peritonei
- Invasive tumours – 5-year survival rates
- 90 per cent for stage Ia & b well- or moderately differentiated tumours
- 10 per cent for stage III
- 23 per cent overall

Treatment

A malignant germ cell tumour should be suspected prior to surgery if a young woman has what appears to be a predominantly solid tumour on ultrasound examination. Such patients should be referred to a gynaecological oncologist.

Early disease is treated by surgery. In young women with Stage Ia disease, unilateral oophorectomy may suffice but in older patients hysterectomy and bilateral salpingo-oophorectomy is recommended. Women are suitable for conservative surgery if they have a unilateral encapsulated tumour, no ascites, no evidence of abnormal lymph nodes at surgery and a negative CT scan of the para-aortic nodes.

Stage I malignant teratomas and dysgerminomas may be followed up closely without further treatment. For the remainder, chemotherapy has replaced radiotherapy, particularly in the young age groups in which this tumour is most common, as most patients will wish fertility to be preserved. Short courses of cisplatin chemotherapy given in combination with bleomycin and etoposide (BEP) is curative in the 90 per cent of patients without adverse features. More intensive regimens are used for patients with adverse features.

CANCER OF THE FALLOPIAN TUBE

Primary carcinoma of the fallopian tube is extremely rare comprising only 0.3 per cent of gynaecological malignancies. However, only early fallopian tube carcinomas can be distinguished with certainty from ovarian disease. A study of screening for ovarian cancer detected three cases of early fallopian tube carcinoma and 19 ovarian tumours, a relative prevalence 25 times greater than expected. This suggests that fallopian tube carcinoma may be more common than is realized.

Primary carcinoma is usually unilateral. The mean age at diagnosis is 56 years. Many of the patients are nulliparous (45 per cent) and infertility is reported in up to 71 per cent of these women. Tumour spread is identical to that of ovarian cancer and metastases to pelvic and para-aortic nodes are common. Most tumours involving the fallopian tube are metastatic from ovarian cancer but secondary spread from the breast and gastrointestinal tract can also occur.

Pathology

Carcinoma of the fallopian tube usually distends the lumen with tumour. The tumour may protrude through the fimbrial end and the tube may be retort-shaped, resembling a hydrosalpinx. It is usually very similar to the serous adenocarcinoma of the ovary histologically. There may be evidence of *in situ* disease in the tubal epithelium.

Staging

The FIGO clinical staging is similar to that used for ovarian cancer. Probably because of the difficulty in distinguishing between advanced ovarian and advanced fallopian tube carcinoma, 74 per cent of fallopian tube carcinomas are diagnosed at stage I–IIa, the remaining 26 per cent are stage IIb–IV.

Clinical presentation and management

Most cases of cancer of the fallopian tube are diagnosed at laparotomy. The diagnosis is seldom considered preoperatively. The usual presenting symptom is postmenopausal bleeding and the diagnosis should be considered, particularly if the patient also complains of a watery discharge and lower abdominal pain. Unexplained postmenopausal bleeding or abnormal cervical cytology without obvious cause demands a careful bimanual examination and pelvic ultrasound. Laparoscopy may be required in doubtful cases.

The management of cancer of the fallopian tube is the same as for cancer of the ovary with surgery to remove gross tumour. This will almost always involve a total abdominal hysterectomy and bilateral salpingo-oophorectomy. Postoperative chemotherapy will be required with platinum analogues for all but the earliest cases. The treatment of carcinoma metastasized to the fallopian tube is determined by the management of the primary tumour.

Results

The overall five-year survival rate is around 35 per cent. The prognosis is improved if the tumour is detected early. The five-year survival for Stage Ia cases is in the region of 70 per cent but in Stages Ib–IIIc survival falls to 25–30 per cent. Chemotherapy with platinum agents improves the survival.

Key Points

- Epithelial ovarian cancer is usually advanced at presentation and, except when the disease is confined to the ovaries and is well- or moderately well-differentiated, it has a poor prognosis
- Oral contraceptive use protects against the development of ovarian cancer
- Inheritance plays a significant role in approximately 5 per cent of epithelial ovarian cancers. The BRCA1 gene is associated with 80 per cent of families with both breast and ovarian cancer. The risk of ovarian cancer in these families is less than the risk of breast cancer. BRCA1 does not appear to be responsible for many sporadic cases of ovarian cancers
- Population screening for ovarian cancer is not yet justified with the techniques evaluated so far
- Standard treatment of epithelial carcinoma is surgery followed by a platinum agent in combination with paclitaxel. This approach allows many women to lead a relatively symptom-free life for periods of up to three to four years
- A young woman with a solid ovarian tumour should be referred to a gynaecological oncologist as she may have a curable germ cell tumour. If the diagnosis is made postoperatively she should always be referred to a specialist team
- Primary carcinoma of the fallopian tube is treated like ovarian carcinoma

References for further reading

Eng C, Stratton M, Ponder B, Murday V, Easton D, Sacks N, Watson M, Eeles R. Familial cancer syndromes. *Lancet* 1994; **343**: 709–13.

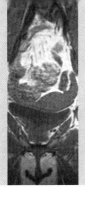

Conditions affecting the vulva and vagina

OVERVIEW

Although carcinoma of the vulva and vagina are rare there are a number of benign conditions that commonly present in this area. Vulval itching is a particularly prevalent condition and in addition to local epithelial disorders, including vulval intraepithelial neoplasia, other generalized skin disease must be excluded. Tumours in the vagina are uncommon but vaginal discharge and atrophy are common presenting symptoms.

THE VULVA

Benign disease

During the ageing process the labia majora lose their fat and elastic tissue content and become smaller and the vaginal introitus is exposed. In the elderly woman only a narrow cleft indicates presence of the introitus. The vulval epithelium becomes thin. These changes may lead to vulval irritation although, of course, irritation may occur at any age.

Pruritus vulvae

It must be remembered that the skin covering the vulva may be involved in any generalized dermatological disorder but its special anatomical situation makes it liable to a number of inflammatory conditions that are confined to the genital area. Infections are common after the menopause and these are covered in Chapter 16. Constant vaginal discharge or urinary incontinence may lead to irritation, scratching and damage to macerated skin.

Whatever the cause of the vulval itching it is usually mediated by the release of histamines, which lead to scratching which aggravates the itch. Over a period of time the itch–scratch cycle may initiate a variety of histological changes in the vulval skin.

Non-neoplastic epithelial disorders

There is a lot of confusion over the classification; the latest classification is shown in Table 14.1.

Table 14.1 – Classification of non-neoplastic epithelial disorders

Non-neoplastic disorders
Lichen sclerosus
Squamous cell hyperplasia (formerly hyperplastic dystrophy)
Other dermatoses

Vulval intraepithelial neoplasia (VIN)
Squamous VIN
  VIN I Mild dysplasia
  VIN II Moderate dysplasia
  VIN III Severe dysplasia or carcinoma *in situ*
Non-squamous VIN
  Paget's disease

Lichen sclerosus

This is the commonest condition found in elderly women complaining of vulval itching but may also be seen in children and younger women. The cause is not known but it is associated with autoimmune disorders. The skin may be reddish or of normal colour and the skin looks thin with a crinkled surface and white shiny plaques. The contours of the vulva slowly disappear and labial adhesions form. If the patient has been scratching the area the skin will become thickened (lichenified). It is uncertain if lichen sclerosus leads to vulval cancer; vulval intraepithelial neoplasia (VIN) and lichen sclerosus can co-exist in the same patient. Approximately 4 per cent of women with lichen sclerosus develop invasive cancer.

Squamous cell hyperplasia

The skin is usually reddened with exaggerated skin folds. In certain areas after rubbing lichenification can be seen. The term squamous cell hyperplasia is applied to those women who have histological evidence of this without a clinical evidence for the cause.

Other dermatoses

These problems are often seen by dermatologists but knowledge of this area is important. The most common general diseases causing itching of the vulva are diabetes, uraemia and liver failure. In diabetes the vulva, as well as being itchy, is swollen and dark red in colour.

Allergic dermatitis

The skin is usually red and swollen and may later become thickened. Secondary infection may occur. The commonest irritants are perfumed soap, synthetic materials and washing powders although there are many other contacts, allergens or irritants.

General skin diseases

Psoriasis, intertrigo, lichen planus and scabies may affect the vulva. In lichen planus the lesions on the vulva are characteristically a purple-white papule with a shiny surface and regular outline. There is a variant of this condition that is erosive and can lead to pain and bleeding as well as itching. In this latter condition there is a slight risk of malignancy.

Vaginal infections

Although these are covered elsewhere (Chapter 16) these are the most common cause of vulval itching, particularly in younger women. Candidiasis and trichomoniasis are the commonest causes. Human papilloma virus is not thought to cause pruritis vulvae.

Investigation of pruritis vulvae

History

The history is important and it must be remembered that psychological problems may predispose to this condition and must be enquired about. In addition, the patient's general health should be assessed and questions asked about sexual relationships. The history must also include any treatments that may have been applied which may affect the appearance both clinically and histologically.

The area should be carefully inspected and if there are any white plaques (leukoplakia) or suspicious areas, then a biopsy should be considered for histological diagnosis. If there is discharge then vaginal swabs should be taken to exclude infection.

Treatment

Any aetiological factor detected should be treated. Perfumed sprays and synthetic under garments should be avoided. Topical corticosteroids are usually prescribed. A high potency steroid cream such as Dermovate should be applied for four to six weeks. This normally resolves the condition. If biopsies show vulval dysplasia then surgical therapy should be considered and this will be discussed later in this chapter.

Vulva atrophy in younger women

Vulva atrophy can occur in younger women and this is a cause of considerable distress because it prevents intercourse or makes it uncomfortable. The conditions mentioned previously should be investigated but treatment is usually very difficult.

Chronic vulval pain (vulvodynia)

Vulvodynia is a term applied to a feeling of vulval burning. In addition there may be stinging, irritation, rawness and sometimes pain in the whole vestibule. Often there is no itching.

Treatment is usually unsatisfactory. Low dose antidepressants and psychotherapy may be tried once other causes have been excluded. The aetiology is unclear.

Vulval ulcers

The causes of benign vulval ulcers are listed in Table 14.2.

Benign tumours

Cystic lesions

Epidermoid and sebaceous cysts can be difficult to differentiate. Management involves excision of the

---

Table 14.2 – Vulval ulcers

The causes of benign vulval ulcers are:
Aphthous ulcers
Herpes genitalis
Primary syphilis
Crohn's disease
Behçet's disease
Lipschutz ulcers
Lymphogranuloma venereum
Chancroid
Donovanosis
Tuberculosis

---

cyst. Cysts may also arise from the duct of the Bartholin's gland that lies in subcutaneous tissue below the lower third of the labium majorum. When a duct becomes blocked a tense retention cyst forms. The patient usually presents only after infection has supervened and a painful abscess has formed.

Incision and a marsupialization of the abscess and antibiotic therapy give excellent results. The pus from the abscess should be sent for culture in media suitable for the detection of gonococcal infection.

Non-epithelial tumours

Lipomas and fibromas are the commonest benign tumours of the vulva that arise from non-epithelial tissues.

Epithelial tumours

Squamous papillomata and skin tags are common and benign. Secondary syphilis may present as a maculopapular rash which can affect the vulva (see Chapter 16).

Condyloma acuminata are small papules that are sometimes sessile and often polypoid. These are due to infection by the human papilloma virus and may be seen over the whole perineal region. Treatment usually involves out-patient application of trichloroacetic acid. Podophyllin is less effective and more toxic but may also be used. Occasionally electrodiathermy is required to remove these warts.

Malignant disease

Vulval intraepithelial neoplasia

Vulval intraepithelial neoplasia (VIN) is seen more commonly now but this is probably due to a greater awareness of the problem. Both squamous and adenocarcinoma *in situ* (Paget's disease) occur on the vulva, the latter is very rare. There are three grades of VIN just as those for CIN, from mild to severe dysplasia. However VIN does not have the same malignant potential.

Pruritus vulvae may be present but usually the patients are asymptomatic and the condition is often found after treatment for pre-invasive or invasive disease in other sites of the lower genital tract. The lesions are often raised above the surrounding skin and have a rough surface; the colour is variable. If 5 per cent acetic acid is applied the areas of VIN turn white and mosaicism or punctation may be visible. Biopsies will confirm a diagnosis. Usually therapy (e.g. surgical excision) is not recommended as VIN occurs in the younger population and this is an important consideration. Observation with regular biopsies may be necessary. If symptoms are persistent then surgery using either laser vaporization or a skinning vulvectomy may be necessary.

Carcinoma of the vulva

Vulval carcinoma accounts for approximately 5 per cent of genital tract cancers in the UK. It is most commonly seen in older women with a median age of over sixty years. Little is known about the aetiology of vulval cancer. Most invasive cancers (85 per cent) are squamous, some 5 per cent are melanomas and the remainder are made up of carcinoma of Bartholin's gland, other adenocarcinomas and basal cell carcinomas. In a third of cases of Paget's disease there is an adenocarcinoma in underlying apocrine glands.

Melanomas and Paget's disease carry an especially poor prognosis.

Symptoms and signs

A patient may present with a hard nodule or ulcer with vulval itching, bleeding, soreness or irritation. Later there may be a purulent discharge.

A lump or ulcer may be visible and usually has a sloughing base and raised edges. Fifty per cent of cases start on one labium majus, 25 per cent on a labium minus. If the cancer is large then lymph node involvement will occur and this is usually seen in approximately half of the cases when they first present. Nodal involvement is usually in the inguinal regions on the side of the observed lesion. However, bilateral lymphadenopathy may be seen because the lymph supply crosses the midline in the anterior part of the vulva. Figure 14.1 shows a very advanced vulval carcinoma.

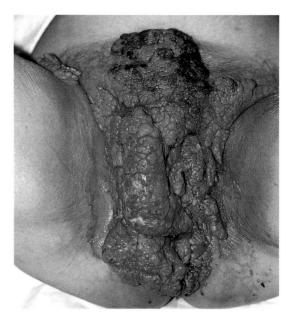

Figure 14.1 A very advanced vulval carcinoma. (Courtesy of K Metcalfe.)

Treatment

Treatment is tailored to the individual. In cases of microinvasion, a wide local excision may be all that is required. In other cases radical removal of the affected vulva with wide margins and complete removal of the groin nodes is necessary. The most common complication of surgery is wound breakdown.

Although radiotherapy is not used as a primary treatment for vulval cancer it is used for the management of women with positive groin nodes and can reduce their size.

Prognosis

The prognosis depends on the stage at which the growth is first treated and is very much worse if the glands are involved. The size of the lesion affects the outcome; lesions less than 2 cm in diameter have twice as good a prognosis as larger tumours. If there is no nodal invasion and the tumour is less than 1 cm in size then there is 90 per cent five-year survival. Unfortunately if nodal involvement has occurred then the five-year survival rate is only 20 per cent. The FIGO staging of vulval cancer is shown in Table 14.3.

Table 14.3 – The FIGO staging of vulval cancer

Stage I   Confined to vulva and/or perineum, 2 cm or less maximum diameter. Groin nodes not palpable.

Stage II   Confined to vulva and/or perineum, more than 2 cm maximum diameter. Groin nodes not palpable.

Stage III   Extends beyond the vulva-vagina, lower urethra or anus; or unilateral regional lymph node metastasis.

Stage IVa   Involves the mucosa of rectum or bladder; upper urethra; or pelvic bone; and/or bilateral regional lymph node metastases.

Stage IVb   Any distant metastasis including pelvic lymph node.

THE VAGINA

Benign disease

Vaginal discharge

It can be difficult to assess the significance of vaginal discharge as often the patient is just seeking reassurance. The best guide is to ask whether the amount or character of the discharge has altered from the patient's usual pattern.

Physiological discharge

Changes in the activity of the vaginal epithelium and in the vaginal secretions that occur at different times during a woman's life have a profound influence on the defence against vaginal infection. A normal vaginal secretion consists of transudate containing desquamated vaginal epithelial cells, mucous secreted by the cervical glands and to some extent secretion from the endometrial glands. There is a cyclical variation of the amount of secretion; it is heavier in the premenstrual period and also at ovulation there is an increase in secretion of clear cervical mucous. There are no glands in the vagina and the transudate passes through the stratified epithelium.

The epithelium contains glycogen, which is converted to lactic acid by Doderlein's bacilli that are normally present in the vagina. The vaginal fluid is acidic and prevents multiplication of pathogenic organisms.

Vaginitis is one of the most common gynaecological complaints and about 90 per cent of women suffer from infection of the vagina caused by *Candida*, bacterial vaginosis or *Trichomonas*. The causes of infective vaginitis and discharge are discussed in Chapter 16.

Speculum examination will show a healthy looking vagina with a small amount of discharge; an area of ectopy may be visible on the cervix. Bacterial vaginosis can be diagnosed by microscopic examination of a slide which will show characteristic 'clue cells'. Swabs will grow other organisms.

Vaginal discharge in children

Vaginal discharge in the young child is often due to infection secondary to atrophic vaginitis. A foreign body is sometimes found or occasionally threadworms are involved. Rarely a vaginal tumour is responsible. The vagina and anus should be inspected for signs of trauma, atrophy should be noted and, if possible, swabs taken.

In cases of doubt, general anaesthetic is usually necessary to allow adequate inspection of the vagina without frightening the child. Any foreign bodies should be removed and appropriate antibiotics initiated. Advice on hygiene may be necessary.

Miscellaneous causes

A number of other problems may present as vaginal discharge. A foreign body, e.g. a tampon, will cause a purulent bloodstained discharge. A bloody discharge may result from tumours in the vagina, cervix, uterus or fallopian tubes. Very rarely a fistula may be found and this may involve the bladder or rectum. In a young child an important cause of recurrent vaginal discharge may be an ectopic ureter.

Atrophic vaginitis

Symptoms of vaginal atrophy occur in many women after the menopause. Vaginal dryness, dyspareunia, superimposed infection and bleeding are common problems. Often symptoms of the lower urinary tract, e.g. dysuria, frequency and urgency, may co-exist. Examination will show pale, thin vaginal epithelium often with petechial haemorrhage. In extreme cases the vulva becomes atrophic, the labia shrink and the introitus contracts. Appropriate hormone replacement therapy will reverse these symptoms.

Benign tumours

Tumours in the vagina are uncommon, the commonest are Condyloma acuminata (warts). Endometrial deposits may be seen in the vagina. A simple mesonephric (Gartner's duct) or paramesonephric cyst may be seen, especially high up near the fornices. Adenosis (multiple mucus-containing vaginal cysts) is a rare condition that even more rarely gives rise to symptoms. A variety of abnormalities is reported in daughters of women who took Diethylstilboestrol during their pregnancy but none have been corroborated.

Vaginal intraepithelial neoplasia (VAIN)

The terminology and pathology of vaginal intraepithelial neoplasia (VAIN) is analogous to that of CIN. VAIN is seldom seen alone and is usually a vaginal extension of CIN. Diagnosis is made colposcopically. The usual treatment involves laser vaporization. If there are recurrent symptoms such as bleeding, carcinoma may be difficult to exclude and more radical surgery such as excision will be required.

Carcinoma of the vagina

Primary squamous cell carcinoma of the vagina is rare but carcinoma of the cervix very commonly spreads to the vaginal vault and in cases of endometrial carcinoma isolated vaginal metastases may occur usually in the lower third of the anterior wall. Endometrial cancer may also recur in the vaginal vault and the pelvic connective tissue after removal of the uterus. The aetiology of vaginal cancer is poorly understood. Although 92 per cent of carcinomas are squamous, clear cell adenocarcinomas, melanomas, rhabdomyosarcomas and endodermal sinus tumours are also seen. The commonest site for primary cancer is the upper vagina on the posterior wall. This usually occurs postmenopausally and occasionally follows chronic ulceration, which accompanies complete uterovaginal prolapse. Symptoms usually include vaginal discharge with bleeding and occasionally postcoital bleeding. If this advances then a fistula may develop either in the rectum or the bladder.

Invasive vaginal cancer is usually treated with radiotherapy. A stage I lesion in the upper vagina can usually be treated by radical hysterectomy with radical vaginectomy and pelvic lymphadenectomy. Exenteration is required for more advanced lesions.

The FIGO staging of vaginal cancer is shown in Table 14.4.

The five-year survival FIGO for stage I disease ranges between 60 and 90 per cent but advanced disease carries a poor prognosis.

Table 14.4 – Modified FIGO staging of vaginal cancer

Stage	Definition
Stage 0	Intraepithelial neoplasia
Stage I	Invasive carcinoma confined to vaginal mucosa
Stage IIa	Subvaginal infiltration not extending to parametrium
Stage IIb	Parametrial infiltration not extending to pelvic wall
Stage III	Extends to pelvic wall
Stage IVa	Involves mucosa of bladder or rectum
Stage IVb	Spreads beyond the pelvis

Key Points

- Vulval itching is very common especially in post-menopausal women and may be due to atrophy but the commonest cause is lichen sclerosus
- One must not forget that other dermatoses can also affect this region
- Treatment may be necessary but a biopsy should be taken if there are suspicious areas
- In most cases a strong steroid cream is helpful
- Carcinoma of the vulva is relatively rare and only counts for 5 per cent of genital tract cancer in the UK
- This usually presents with a hard nodule or ulcer but may present with bleeding. Treatment is usually surgical
- Vaginal discharge may be physiological
- Infective causes are candida, bacterial vaginosis or Trichomonas
- Carcinoma of the vagina is extremely rare
- Radiotherapy is the commonest treatment but surgery may be relevant for early-stage cancers

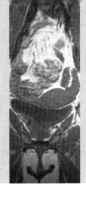

Imaging in gynaecology

OVERVIEW

Transvaginal sonography has transformed the practice of gynaecology. It is used routinely to investigate pelvic pain, abnormal vaginal bleeding, in the differential diagnosis of pelvic masses and in the investigation of early pregnancy complications. It also has an essential role in the investigation of the infertile couple and monitoring of fertility treatment. Other imaging modalities, such as CT scanning and MRI are complementary techniques which may provide extra information in certain conditions especially in assessing the spread of cervical and uterine carcinoma.

Introduction

The principal imaging technique in gynaecology is diagnostic ultrasound. This is because it is inexpensive and can be performed in the clinic or by the bedside as part of the gynaecological examination. Traditionally, a gynaecological scan was performed with a transabdominal transducer, with the patient's distended bladder acting as a window to the pelvic organs. The majority of scans are now performed with a high frequency transvaginal probe which, because of its proximity to the pelvic organs, provides superior images. Furthermore, the avoidance of having to fill the bladder makes this also the preferred route of investigation amongst patients. Most young gynaecologists are now trained in transvaginal scanning and the pelvic scan may in the future become a standard part of the out-patient gynaecological assessment. Already, most hospitals will have a gynae-

cological emergency scanning unit where a team of doctors, nurses and sonographers will provide a rapid diagnostic service which will include a transvaginal scan and blood biochemistry for women with acute pelvic pain and bleeding in early pregnancy.

Other imaging modalities used in gynaecology include radiography, computerized tomography (CT) and magnetic resonance imaging (MRI) all of which can give, in certain circumstances, additional information to that provided by the ultrasound scan.

DIAGNOSTIC ULTRASOUND

The technique employs high frequency (3–7.5 mHz) low-intensity pulsed sound waves, which are transmitted through the abdomen or pelvis by an ultrasound transducer. A typical transvaginal transducer is shown in Figure 15.1. The array of elements at the

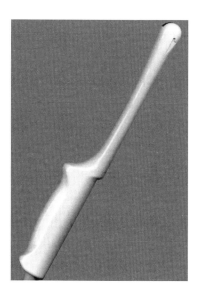

Figure 15.1 Transvaginal ultrasound transducer.

tip is triggered in sequence and updated 20 times per second (frame rate). Reflected signals from surfaces or discontinuities within organs are displayed as a 2-dimensional echo map and the frequent updates provide 'real time' information so that, for example, the embryonic fetal heart rate can be accurately recorded. Doppler ultrasound information can also be provided by the same transducer. Doppler ultrasound makes use of the phenomenon of the Doppler frequency shift where the reflected wave will be at a different frequency from the transmitted one if it interacts with moving structures such as red cells flowing along a blood vessel. The Doppler shifted signals can be displayed as a colour map of blood vessels superimposed on top of the grey scale image. Quantitative information about the actual velocity or resis-

tance to flow can be obtained from a graphic display of the Doppler signals throughout the cardiac cycle called the flow velocity wave form. Colour Doppler is especially useful in gynaecology for it can illustrate the process of normal and abnormal angiogenesis (i.e. the generation of new blood vessels). Normal angiogenesis around the follicle increases up to the time of ovulation, during the formation of the corpus luteum and in the endometrium during the late follicular and luteal phase of the menstrual cycle. Abnormal angiogenesis is associated with certain pathological conditions, in particular cancer. For example, ovarian carcinoma is typified by high blood velocities and a chaotic arrangement of blood vessels.

Normal pelvic appearance

Uterus

On transvaginal sonography the uterus and cervix can be visualized and measured in longitudinal and transverse planes. The uterine muscle is of uniform 'grainy' texture around a central endometrial strip. The endometrium changes in morphology and thickens throughout the cycle. It is initially thin (<3 mm) but in mid-cycle has three distinct lines (triple layer) which indicate good receptivity (Fig. 15.2). In the luteal phase it becomes thick and white, indicating a change to the secretory phase (Fig. 15.3). Blood flow in the main uterine arteries also changes during the cycle with increased flow (low

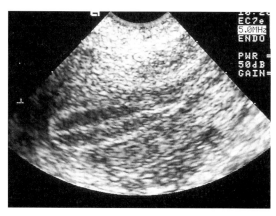

Figure 15.2 Mid-cycle endometrium with typical triple line appearance.

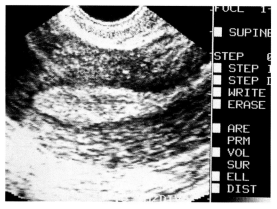

Figure 15.3 Echogenic endometrium typical of secretory phase.

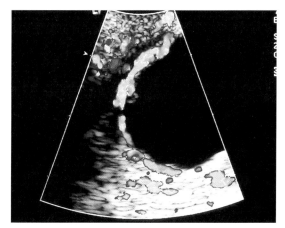

Figure 15.4 Pre-ovulatory follicle with intense vascularity in the theca layer.

vein. During the reproductive years the growth of the follicles (each of which contains an oocyte) can be charted. Early in the cycle several follicles of about 5 mm can be identified in each ovary but after day 8 a dominant follicle can be seen in one of the ovaries and its growth can be tracked. Prior to ovulation the follicular diameter is about 20 mm and after follicular rupture an irregular solid cystic structure, the corpus luteum can be seen. Colour Doppler can be used to show the increased vascularity around the growing follicle which is greatest just before ovulation (Fig. 15.4). This becomes even more intense during the formation of the vascular corpus luteum (Fig. 15.5).

Pathological appearances

Uterus

pulsatility) found in the luteal phase probably to improve the process of implantation. After the menopause the uterus becomes smaller and the endometrium thin and should always be <5 mm.

Fallopian tubes

Normal fallopian tubes cannot be seen by ultrasound as distinct from the surrounding bowel. The fimbrial ends of the tubes can only be seen if there is free fluid in the pouch of Douglas.

Ovaries

The ovaries are identified as lozenge-shaped structures lateral to the uterus, usually related to the internal iliac

Fibroids are easily identified as discrete circular structures arising in the myometrium. Sometimes they are so large that they are best assessed by a transabdominal scan. The position (i.e subserous, intramural, submucus, cervical) and size of the fibroid can be documented. Adenomyosis causes a diffuse thickening of the myometrium with spots of hypo- and hyperechogenicity. Endometrial polyps will cause local thickening of the endometrium. Sometimes the diagnosis of an endometrial lesion can be elucidated by instilling saline through the cervix by means of a catheter. Saline sonohysterography can determine, for example, if a thickened endometrium is due to hyperplasia or a polyp (Fig. 15.6).

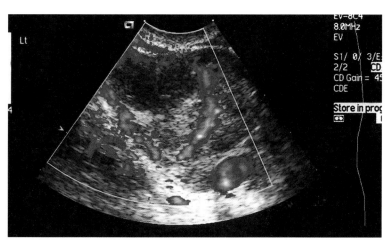

Figure 15.5 Normal ovary in luteal phase with vascular corpus luteum.

Fallopian tubes

Chronic tubal damage frequently results in a hydrosalpinx, which on ultrasound is seen as an elongated (retort-shaped) cystic structure adjacent to the uterus. Acute salpingitis will not be detected unless a pyosalpinx develops although the transvaginal scan will elicit tenderness indicative of peritonitis.

Ovaries

Polycystic ovaries can exist as an isolated phenomenon or as part of polycystic ovarian syndrome. They are usually larger than normal ovaries and have a necklace of small follicles (about 5 mm) round a dense central stroma. Colour Doppler usually demonstrates intense vascularity in this stroma.

Ovarian cysts are easily identified by ultrasound. It is important to determine whether they are:

1. functional;
2. neoplastic.

Functional cysts are usually simple in appearance (smooth internal wall and clear contents) but occasionally they will have lace-like contents indicating blood clots. They usually disappear over a period of 2–4 weeks.

Neoplastic cysts can also have a simple appearance but more often are complex with locules or internal papillae. Dermoid cysts have a typical appearance of a mixture of tissues of different echogenicity, while endometriotic cysts have typical 'ground glass' contents of unclotted blood. The more complex a cyst, the more locules and the larger the internal papillae

the more likely is the cyst to be malignant. Other malignant features are bilaterality, fixity and associated pelvic fluid. Intense vascularity on colour Doppler with high velocity signals is another feature suggesting malignancy (Fig. 15.7).

Clinical applications

Menstrual disorders

If the symptom is menorrhagia, ultrasound will reveal whether there are abnormalities of the endometrium (hyperplasia, polyps) myometrium (fibroids, adenomyosis) or ovaries (functional cysts) to explain the symptoms. Postmenopausal bleeding should always be investigated by transvaginal scan. A thick endometrium (≥ 5 mm) with endometrial blood flow is suggestive of endometrial cancer. Oligomenorrhoea is frequently associated with polycystic ovaries, which have a classical ultrasound appearance. Intrauterine adhesions typical of Asherman's syndrome will only be revealed if saline sonohysterography is used.

Pelvic pain

Ultrasound will demonstrate certain causes of pelvic pain both acute (ectopic pregnancy, haemorrhagic or torted cyst) and chronic (ovarian endometriosis, pyosalpinx). Lesser degrees of peritoneal endometriosis or salpingitis cannot be diagnosed by ultrasound. Generally speaking, if the tubes are not

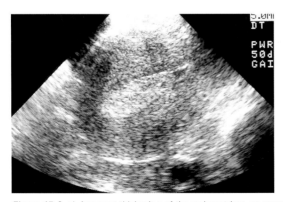
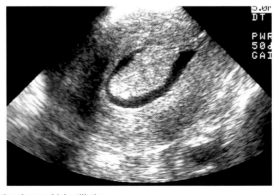

Figure 15.6 a) Apparent thickening of the endometrium on conventional scan. b) Instillation of saline through the cervix (saline sonohysterography) reveals an endometrial polyp.

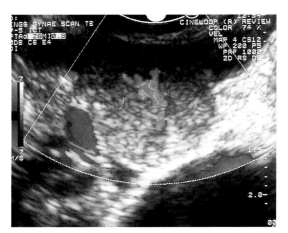

Figure 15.7 Early ovarian cancer showing abnormal angio-genesis.

visible and the ovaries and uterus are seen to move freely on abdominal palpation, it is unlikely there is significant pathology to explain the pain.

Lower abdominal mass

The differential diagnosis of a lower abdominal mass (e.g. uterine fibroids, ovarian cysts, pelvic kidney, hydrosalpinx) can usually be successfully made by transvaginal sonography. Rarely a pedunculated fibroid can be confused with a solid ovarian tumour, but a skilled sonographer will reveal on ultrasound and colour Doppler the connecting stalk and blood vessels in the case of a pedunculated fibroid.

Monitoring of infertility treatment

Transvaginal sonography has now become an essential part of infertility investigation and management.

Initial assessment
An initial (pivotal) ultrasound scan will provide essential information on the normality of the uterus and ovaries. Uterine fibroids adenomyosis, hydrosalpinges, polycystic ovaries or ovarian cysts may require treatment. Sometimes assessment of tubal patency with a contrast agent (HyCoSy) is performed at this examination.

Follicle tracking
This is used in the following circumstances:
i.   To diagnose ovulation in women with irregular cycles or polycystic ovaries and to time intrauterine insemination.
ii. To determine the number of follicles and the timing of hCG administration during superovulation therapy. In general hCG is withheld if more than two follicles are above 17 mm in diameter in order to avoid high multiple gestation.
iii. To determine if the ovaries are poorly responsive (<6 mature follicles) or hyper-responsive (>20 mature follicles) during IVF superovulation therapy. In the former case the stimulation regime may have to be altered while in the latter case hCG administration may be withheld in order to avoid ovarian hyperstimulation syndrome.

Management of IVF cycles
Transvaginal sonography is an essential part of IVF management. In addition to follicle tracking it is used to guide the needle for oocyte aspiration, which is usually done under sedation.

Early pregnancy scanning

Normal early pregnancy

The normal early gestation sac can be first seen in the endometrium on transvaginal sonography five weeks after the last menstrual period (three weeks after conception). The embryo and fetal heart pulsations are first seen at six weeks. From then until 14 weeks the growth of the embryo is measured from its crown–rump length (CRL).

Some key chronological landmarks in early human development seen on transvaginal sonography are given below:

5 weeks: early gestational sac (mean diameter 10 mm)
5 ½ weeks: yolk sac visible within the gestation sac
6 weeks: small embryo (CRL 3 mm) seen adjacent to yolk sac. Fetal heart pulsation seen (Fig. 15.8)
6½ weeks: embryo CRL 6 mm, heart rate 125 beats per minute (bpm)
7 weeks: embryo CRL 10mm, heart rate 150 bpm

8 weeks: embryo CRL 16mm, heart rate 175 bpm, fetal body movements now seen

Early pregnancy problems

Bleeding and pain in early pregnancy can be due to early miscarriage or ectopic pregnancy. The two important investigations required when these symptoms occur are:

1. quantitative βhCG;
2. transvaginal ultrasound scan.

Interpretation of the findings based on these tests requires skill and experience. In brief:

- If the βhCG is >1000 IU then a gestational sac should be seen in the uterus. If no gestational sac can be seen then ectopic pregnancy should be suspected. Other ultrasound features of ectopic pregnancy are:
  - i   A gestation sac visible outside the uterus (Fig. 15.9)
  - ii An adnexal mass suspicious of haematocoele
  - iii Free fluid (blood) in the pelvis
- If there is a gestation sac with a diameter of >20 mm then an embryo should be seen inside. If no embryo is seen than a blighted ovum should be suspected (Fig. 15.10).
- If there is an embryo in the sac of >10 mm then fetal heart pulsations should be seen. If no pulsations are visible then a missed miscarriage should be suspected (Fig. 15.11).

If an ectopic pregnancy is suspected, then laparoscopy should be immediately arranged. A suspected blighted ovum or early missed miscarriage does not require the same urgent management; in fact a delay of one week will confirm that the embryo is not viable and in some cases enable spontaneous miscarriage to take place without the need for surgical evacuation.

OTHER IMAGING MODALITIES

Standard radiography

This is rarely used to image the pelvic organs. In the past it was employed to determine if there was calcification in ovarian cysts (such as occurs in dermoids or cystadenomas), but this is now more effectively done by ultrasound. A standard method of evaluating Fallopian tubal patency is to inject radiopaque dye through the cervix and image the filling of the tubes and peritoneal spill under fluoroscope control (X-ray hysterosalpingography or HSG).

CT scanning

This provides superior soft tissue imaging compared to standard radiography. In CT scanning, the attenuation of a finely columnated beam of radiation by

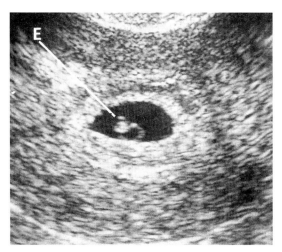

Figure 15.8 6 week embryo (E) with yolk sac. Fetal heart pulsations are visible at this stage.

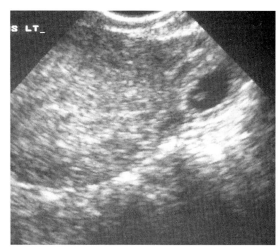

Figure 15.9 Ectopic pregnancy showing gestation sac and embryo outside the uterus.

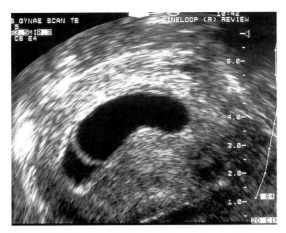

Figure 15.10 Large gestation sac with no embryo visible, confirming the diagnosis of blighted ovum.

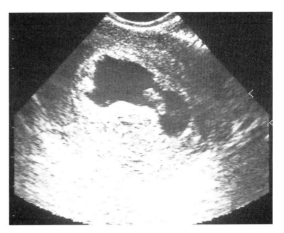

Figure 15.11 Irregular gestation sac with small embryo. Absence of fetal heart pulsations confirms the diagnosis of missed miscarriage.

different tissues is measured, the final images being computer constructed using a filtered back projection technique. Reconstruction is limited to the transaxial or transverse planes. CT scans provide better information than ultrasound on the parametrial spread of cervical cancer and in particular lymph node metastasis. Following radiation treatment, CT scanning is not useful in distinguishing between fibrosis and tumour recurrence.

MRI

This technique does not use ionizing radiation and produces impressive imaging of soft tissues. It also has the advantage of providing sectional images in any plane. The technique utilizes the effect of powerful magnetic forces on spinning hydrogen protons, which when knocked off their axes by pulsed radio waves produce radio frequency signals as they return to their basal state. These signals reflect the clinical composition of the tissue (i.e. the amount and distribution of hydrogen protons) and thus the images provide significant improvement over ultrasound in tissue characterization. MRI has the disadvantage when compared with ultrasound of being many times more expensive and requires the patient to be isolated in a scanning chamber. The images are also more likely to be affected by movement artefact, although the female pelvis is suitable for MRI examination because of the minimal effect of respiratory motion on the pelvic organs. MRI is probably more effective in assessing parametrial spread of cervical cancer than

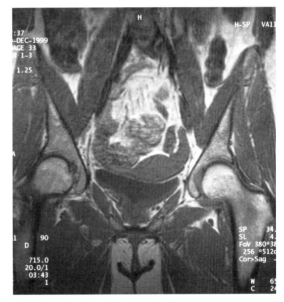

Figure 15.12. MRI of pelvis showing uterus and dilated fallopian tubes. Courtesy of K Dewberry.

CT scanning, but is less useful in detecting lymph node spread. MRI has also been shown to be superior to ultrasound in detecting the depth of myometrial invasion in cancer of the endometrium, thereby improving the staging of this disease. MRI is probably no better than ultrasound in staging ovarian cancer, although it may be better in detecting recurrences.

MRI is able to visualize the pelvic floor more effectively than ultrasound (Fig. 15.12) and has been reported to be superior to ultrasound in detecting small deposits of peritoneal endometriosis.

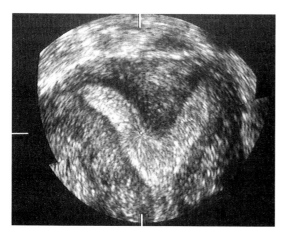

Figure 15.13 3-D scan of uterus showing septum dividing the endometrial cavity.

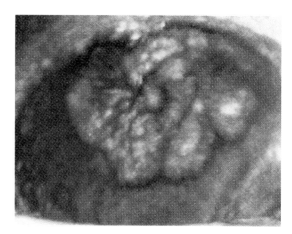

Figure 15.14 3-D surface rendered view of ovarian cyst showing papilliferous projection.

New developments

Screening for ovarian cancer

Several studies have demonstrated that routine examination of the ovaries in postmenopausal women will permit the detection of ovarian cancer at an early treatable stage (stage I) with a consequent improvement in five-year survival. In this regard ultrasound may be more effective than single or serial serum Ca_{125} screening. The extent to which routine transvaginal scanning or serum Ca_{125} measurement will improve mortality from ovarian cancer is at present being investigated in a prospective trial funded by the Medical Research Council. The convenience of serum screening backed up by ultrasound in positive cases may turn out to be the best option when looking for sporadic ovarian cancer in a non-selected population of women over 50 years of age. However, in women with a strong family history of ovarian cancer, or who carry the BRCA1 gene, then six-monthly ultrasound scans would appear to provide the greatest chance of detecting ovarian cancer at stage 1.

3-D ultrasound imaging

3-D transvaginal transducers are now available, which capture a block (or volume) of echoes instead of the thin slices provided by 2-D transducers. This capture only takes 5 to 10 seconds and the digitally stored volume of echoes can be analysed in different ways to increase the range of diagnostic options. For example, the volume can be resliced in any plain and coronal views of the uterus can now be obtained for the first time. This will improve the diagnosis of congenital uterine abnormalities and an example of subseptate uterus is illustrated in Figure 15.13. Surface rendering of the volume can be performed especially if there are fluid interfaces and realistic views of ovarian cysts can be obtained with this technique (Fig. 15.14).

Key Points

- Transvaginal ultrasound is the principal imaging technique in gynaecology
- This technique can identify pathology of the uterus, endometrium, fallopian tubes and ovaries
- It is particularly useful in:
  - i. the diagnosis of functional ovarian disorders such as polycystic ovaries and in the monitoring of fertility treatment
  - ii. the differential diagnosis of lower abdominal masses; it can identify features suggestive of malignancy, but not with absolute certainty
- The transvaginal scan is a necessary investigation for women with pain and bleeding in early pregnancy and can demonstrate features diagnostic of early miscarriage and ectopic pregnancy. Together with the quantitative βhCG, it is the key investigation in the Early Pregnancy Diagnostic Unit (EPU), which is a walk-in service now offered by most hospitals
- CT scanning and MRI are ancillary imaging investigations in gynaecology, which are mainly used to assess the spread of cervical and endometrial carcinoma. X-ray fluoroscopy is used in the evaluation of tubal patency (HSG)

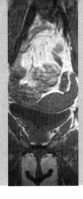

Infections in gynaecology

OVERVIEW

Most women experience an infection of the urogenital tract at some time. The most common symptomatic infections are vulvovaginal candidiasis (thrush) and urinary tract infections. The sexually transmissible bacterial infections, *Chlamydia* and gonorrhoea, can be carried asymptomatically for months or even years. Viral infections such as human papilloma virus and herpes simplex virus may persist for life. Upper genital tract infection is a threat to a woman's future fertility. The long-term sequelae of damage to the fallopian tubes include ectopic pregnancy and tubular factor infertility.

Worldwide, HIV infection is predominantly acquired sexually and in some parts of the world as many as 25–30 per cent of pregnant women are now infected. Clinicians need to be aware of the way that HIV alters the manifestations of, and host susceptibility to, other infections.

Principles of management of sexually transmissible infections

Many gynaecological infections are sexually transmissible. Others, such as *Candida* and urinary tract infection, are frequently triggered by sexual intercourse although the organism is colonizing the woman beforehand. It takes practice to be comfortable taking a sexual history from a patient. If the clinician is embarrassed, this is quickly transmitted to the patient. It is also difficult to take a sexual history if the patient's friends or relatives are present, or in a ward or cubicle in which there is inadequate privacy and sound-proofing. It is sometimes necessary therefore, to postpone seeking a detailed history until the right atmosphere can be provided. In order to assess the risk of an individual having acquired a sexually transmitted disease, it is necessary to find out:

- when sexual intercourse last took place;
- whether this was oral, vaginal or anal;
- what contraception was used;
- when the woman last had a different sexual partner;
- a travel history and knowledge about the origin of partners which may indicate a risk of a tropical infection seldom seen in the UK;
- previous pregnancies, menstruation.

Enquire about intravenous drug use in the patient and her partners. Do not assume that a woman is heterosexual until you have ascertained the sex of her partners.

If one sexually transmissible infection is present then there may be others. Ideally, therefore, a full screen should be performed for *Chlamydia*, gonorrhoea, vaginal infections and serological tests for syphilis, hepatitis B, HIV and hepatitis C if indicated. If facilities are not available for such a screen, the patient should be referred to a genitourinary medicine (GUM) clinic.

To break the chain of infection and prevent reinfection, it is essential that the patient avoids intercourse until she is sure that her partner(s) has been screened and received appropriate treatment. Follow-up evaluation and tests of cure are essential for individuals infected with *Neisseria gonorrhoeae* and are advisable for other infections.

Lower genital tract infections

At birth, the neonate has been exposed to high levels of oestrogen and progesterone from her mother and the vagina is lined with stratified squamous epithelium. Sometimes a baby girl has a withdrawal bleed, analogous to a period, as the effect of maternal oestrogen wanes. It is possible for *Trichomonas vaginalis* to be transmitted at birth but the infection usually clears spontaneously.

In young females the vagina is lined with a simple cuboidal epithelium. The pH is neutral and it is colonized by organisms similar to skin commensals. Under the influence of oestrogen at puberty, stratified squamous epithelium develops and lactobacilli become the predominant organisms. A drop in the pH accompanies this change to a level of approximately 3.5 to 4.5. Following the menopause, atrophic changes occur with a return to bacterial flora similar

to that of the skin. The pH again rises to 7.0.

Vaginal discharge can originate from anywhere in the upper or lower genital tract (Table 16.1). Discharge arising from the vagina itself can be physiological or due to bacterial vaginosis, candidiasis or *Trichomonas* infection (Fig. 16.1 a–d). Its presence can be very alarming for a woman, particularly if she is concerned that she might have caught a serious sexually transmitted infection.

Physiological discharge

Normal vaginal discharge is white, becoming yellowish on contact with air, due to oxidation. It consists of desquamated epithelial cells from the vagina and cervix, mucus originating mainly from the cervical glands, bacteria and fluid which is formed as a transudate from the vaginal wall. More than 95 per cent of the bacteria present are lactobacilli. The acidic pH is maintained by the lactobacilli and through the production of lactic acid by the vaginal epithelium metabolizing glycogen. Physiological discharge increases due to increased mucus production from the cervix in mid-cycle. It also increases in pregnancy and sometimes when women begin using a combined oral contraceptive pill.

Vaginal candidiasis

Over three-quarters of women have at least one episode of vaginal candidiasis. A few women get frequent recurrences. The organism is carried in the gut, under the nails, in the vagina and on the skin. The yeast *Candida albicans* is implicated in more

---

Table 16.1 – Differential diagnosis of vaginal discharge

Symptoms and signs	Candidiasis	Bacterial vaginosis	Trichomoniasis	Cervicitis
Itching or soreness	++	–	+++	–
Smell	May be 'yeasty'	Offensive, fishy	May be offensive	–
Colour	White	White or yellow	Yellow or green	Clear or coloured
Consistency	Curdy	Thin, homogeneous	Thin, homogeneous	Mucoid
pH	<4.5	4.5–7.0	4.5–7.0	<4.5
Confirmed by	Microscopy and culture	Microscopy	Microscopy and culture	Microscopy, tests for *Chlamydia* and gonorrhoea

Factors predisposing to vaginal candidiasis

- Immunosuppression
- HIV
  Immunosuppressive therapy, e.g. steroids
- Diabetes mellitus
- Vaginal douching, bubble bath, shower gel, tight clothing, tights
- Increased oestrogen
  Pregnancy
  High dose combined oral contraceptive pill
- Underlying dermatosis, e.g. eczema
- Broad-spectrum antibiotic therapy

than 80 per cent of cases. *C. glabrata*, *C. krusei* and *C. tropicalis* account for most of the rest. Sexual acquisition is rarely important although the physical trauma of intercourse may be sufficient to trigger an attack in a predisposed individual.

The classical presentation is with itching and soreness of the vagina and vulva with a curdy, white discharge, which may smell yeasty, but in some cases there may be itching and redness with a thin watery discharge. The pH of vaginal fluid is usually normal, between 3.5 and 4.5. Microscopy and culture of the vaginal fluid can confirm a diagnosis (Fig. 16.1b). Asymptomatic women from whom *Candida* is grown on culture do not require treatment.

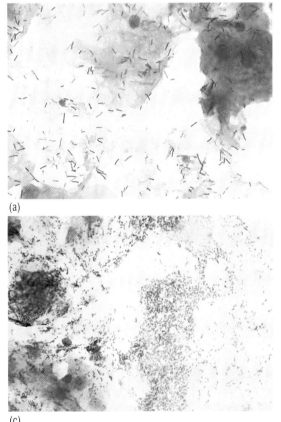

(a)

(c)

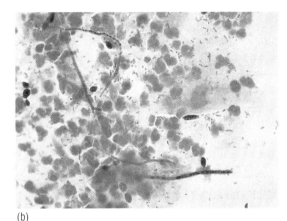

(b)

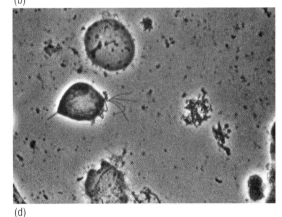

(d)

Figure 16.1 Vaginal and cervical flora. All are 1000x magnified.
a) Normal. Lactobacilli, seen as large Gram-positive rods, predominate. Squamous epithelial cells are Gram-negative with a large amount of cytoplasm.
b) Candidiasis. There are speckled Gram-positive spores and long pseudohyphae visible. There are numerous polymorphs present and the bacterial flora is abnormal, resembling bacterial vaginosis.
c) Bacterial vaginosis - there is an overgrowth of anaerobic organisms including *Gardnerella vaginalis* (small Gram-variable

cocci), and a decrease in the numbers of lactobacilli. A 'clue cell' is seen. This is an epithelial cell covered with small bacteria so that the edge of the cell is obscured.
d) Trichomoniasis - an unstained 'wet mount' of vaginal fluid from a woman with *Trichomonas vaginalis* infection. There is a cone-shaped flagellated organism in the centre, with a terminal spike and 4 flagellae visible. In practice the organism is identified under the microscope by movement, with amoeboid motion and its flagellae waving.

Recurrent *Candida*, or *Candida* not responding to treatment, is relatively uncommon. If this appears to be the case, it is important to consider other diagnoses, particularly herpes simplex, which causes localized ulceration and soreness, and dermatological conditions such as eczema and lichen sclerosus et atrophicus.

As a general rule it is better to use a topical treatment rather than systemic. This minimizes the risk of systemic side effects. Vaginal creams and pessaries can be prescribed at a variety of doses and duration of treatment. For uncomplicated *Candida*, a single dose treatment, such as clotrimazole 500 mg, is adequate. Some women have a preference for oral therapy, particularly if treatment is required at the time of menstruation. A single 150 mg tablet of fluconazole is usually effective but its activity is limited to *C. albicans* strains. Longer courses of treatment are needed when there are predisposing factors that cannot be eliminated, such as steroid therapy. If recurrences occur frequently it is worth performing a full blood count to check for anaemia and checking thyroid function, but usually these are normal. Many clinicians prescribe treatment to be taken once or twice a month for a few months.

Bacterial vaginosis

Bacterial vaginosis (BV) is the commonest cause of abnormal vaginal discharge in women of childbearing age. Studies in antenatal clinics and gynaecology clinics show a prevalence of approximately 12 per cent in the UK. It is commoner in women of Afro-Caribbean origin and in those who have an intrauterine contraceptive device (IUCD). Higher prevalence is generally reported in women undergoing elective termination of pregnancy. It is probably commoner in women with sexually transmitted infections, but has been reported in virgins, and it may be particularly common in lesbian women. The condition often arises spontaneously around the time of menstruation and may resolve spontaneously in mid-cycle.

When BV develops, the predominantly anaerobic organisms that are usually present in the vagina at low concentration increase in concentration up to a thousand-fold. This is accompanied by a rise in vaginal pH to between 4.5 and 7.0 and ultimately the lactobacilli may disappear. The organisms most commonly associated with BV are *Gardnerella vaginalis*, *Bacteroides* (*Prevotella*) *spp.*, *Mobiluncus spp.* and *Mycoplasma hominis*. At present we do not know what triggers these dramatic changes in the vaginal ecology.

The principle symptom of BV is an offensive fishy smelling discharge; it is characteristically thin, homogeneous and adherent to the walls of the vagina and may be white or yellow. The smell is particularly noticeable around the time of menstruation or following intercourse, however, semen itself can give off a weak fishy smell.

The diagnosis is commonly made in clinical practice using the composite (Amsel) criteria:
- vaginal pH >4.5;
- release of a fishy smell on addition of alkali (10 per cent potassium hydroxide);
- a characteristic discharge on examination;
- presence of 'clue cells' on microscopy.

'Clue cells' are vaginal epithelial cells so heavily coated with bacteria that the border is obscured. BV can also be diagnosed from a Gram-stained vaginal smear. Large numbers of Gram-positive and Gram-negative cocci are seen, with reduced or absent large Gram-positive bacilli (lactobacilli). Culture of a high vaginal swab yields mixed anaerobes and a high concentration of *Gardnerella vaginalis*. However, *G. vaginalis* can be grown from cultures taken from up to 50 per cent of women with normal vaginal flora. Its presence is not, therefore, diagnostic of BV.

The simplest and cheapest treatment for BV is metronidazole 400 mg twice a day for five days, or 2 g as a single dose. Topical preparations are available in the form of metronidazole gel 0.75 per cent or clindamycin cream 2 per cent. Initial cure rates are over 80 per cent but up to 30 per cent of women relapse within one month of treatment.

It is now established that women with BV are at a greater risk of second trimester miscarriage and preterm delivery during pregnancy, which may result in perinatal mortality or cerebral palsy. Women with a prior history of second trimester loss or idiopathic preterm birth should be screened for BV and treated with metronidazole early in the second trimester. It has also been demonstrated that treating women with BV with metronidazole prior to termination of pregnancy reduces the subsequent incidence of endometritis and pelvic inflammatory disease. Women with BV are also at increased risk of infections after surgery.

In some women the vaginal flora is in a dynamic state, with BV developing and remitting spontaneously. Symptomatic women with recurrent BV can become frustrated as the condition responds rapidly to treatment with antibiotics but may also relapse rapidly. Regular treatment once or twice a month as prescribed for women with recurrent candidiasis is sometimes helpful.

Trichomoniasis

This sexually transmissible infection can be carried asymptomatically for several months before causing symptoms. The incidence has been falling in the UK over the last 10 to 15 years. In men it is often carried asymptomatically but may present as non-gonococcal urethritis (NGU). In women it causes a vulvovaginitis that can be severe, accompanied by a purulent, sometimes offensive vaginal discharge. In many cases BV develops as well.

Examination shows a yellow or green vaginal discharge with inflammation sometimes extending out onto the vulva and adjacent skin. Punctate haemorrhages can occur on the cervix, giving the appearance of a 'strawberry cervix'.

The diagnosis is confirmed by culture, preferably in a specific medium such as Fineberg–Whittington. Microscopy of vaginal secretions mixed with saline has a 60 per cent sensitivity for detecting the organism. Numerous polymorphonuclear cells are seen and the motile organism is identified from its shape and four moving flagellae.

Treatment is with metronidazole, either 2 g as a single dose or 400 mg twice a day for five days. The woman should be advised to send her sexual partner(s) for treatment before resuming intercourse together.

Trichomoniasis has occasionally been identified in the upper genital tract of women with pelvic inflammatory disease but is probably not an important cause of genital tract pathology. It can be isolated from the bladder. Occasionally persistent trichomoniasis is seen. This may be due to poor compliance with medication, poor absorption or a resistant organism. Review the history to rule out re-infection from an untreated partner. The usual approach is to use higher doses of metronidazole, initially 400 mg three times a day, increasing to 1 g per rectum or intravenously twice a day. Neurological toxicity may be encountered with high doses. Unfortunately, alternative treatments are limited, but include

arsphenamine pessaries and clotrimazole, which has an inhibitory effect on *Trichomonas vaginalis*.

Vaginal discharge in children

Vaginal infections are common in childhood and mostly not related to sexual abuse. Streptococcal infections are the commonest cause. *Shigella spp.* can cause a haemorrhagic chronic vaginitis, often with no history of diarrhoea. Recurrent vaginal infections should lead to suspicion of a foreign body. An examination under anaesthesia may be necessary to exclude or remove the cause.

Pinworms (*Enterobius vermicularis*) are common and migrate from the anus at night causing intense irritation and inevitable scratching by the child. The clue to the diagnosis is the nocturnal pattern. A selotape test can be performed to look for eggs if the worms have not been witnessed at night.

If sexual abuse occurs leading to infection with *Chlamydia* or gonorrhoea, a generalized vaginitis occurs. Adequate testing can therefore be performed from vaginal swabs, negating the need to observe the cervix with the aid of a speculum.

Other conditions affecting the vagina

Other causes of discharge include atrophic vaginitis, toxic shock syndrome, Bartholin's abscess and infestations.

Atrophic vaginitis is common in postmenopausal women. Over the five years following cessation of menstruation, the vaginal epithelium atrophies and the lactobacilli are once again replaced by typical skin commensal organisms. This can lead to superficial dyspareunia and vaginal soreness. The treatment of choice is oestrogen replacement with either topical dienoestrol cream or systemic therapy.

Occasionally a true bacterial vaginitis is encountered due to a Streptococcus or other organism. It responds to appropriate antibiotic therapy. Toxic shock syndrome is a rare condition associated with retention of tampons or foreign bodies in the vagina. An overgrowth of *Staphylococci* producing a toxin causes systemic shock with fever, diarrhoea, vomiting and an erythematous rash. There is a 10 per cent mortality rate. More frequently a foreign body or retained tampon merely causes an offensive discharge.

Bartholin's abscess

Bartholin's glands are situated on either side of the vagina opening into the vestibule. Cysts can develop if the opening becomes blocked. These present as painless swellings. If they become infected a Bartholin's abscess develops. Examination reveals a hot, tender abscess adjacent to the lower part of the vagina. Surgical treatment is required. This is usually done by marsupialization. Culture may yield a variety of organisms including *Neisseria gonorrhoeae*, *Streptococci*, *Staphylococci*, mixed anaerobic organisms or *Escherichia coli*.

Infestations

Pubic lice and scabies are transmitted by close bodily contact. Pubic lice (*Phthirus pubis*) attach their eggs to the base of pubic hair. Their claws only attach to thick body hair, so they can also colonize the axillae and eyelashes. Infected individuals may report small itchy papules, or notice debris from the lice in their underwear. Lice are treated by application of topical agents such as malathion, carbaryl or permethrin. Treatment should be repeated after seven days, and be supplied for partners to use simultaneously.

Scabies (*Sarcoptes scabiei*) causes an intensely itchy papular rash. If acquired during intercourse it may be initially confined to the genital area. It responds to applications of malathion or permethrin, however, symptoms may take up to six weeks to resolve completely.

🔧 Key Points

Vaginal infections
- Vaginal candidiasis is an opportunistic infection, not an STD
- Women with asymptomatic candidal colonisation do not require treatment
- Bacterial vaginosis is a common, relapsing condition, with half of those affected being asymptomatic
- Bacterial vaginosis is associated with preterm birth, and upper genital tract infection following TOP, gynaecological surgery and Caesarean section
- *Trichomonas vaginalis* is sexually transmitted. Partners must be treated to prevent reinfection

Upper genital tract infections

Pelvic inflammatory disease (PID) is a broad term used to cover upper genital tract infection, i.e. endometritis, parametritis, salpingitis and oophoritis. These infections usually spread from the vagina or cervix through the uterine cavity. Lymphatic spread may occur, either parametrially or along the surface of the uterus. Although rare, salpingitis has occurred in women who have been sterilized. Infection can also spread from the bowel or can be bloodborne. Many different organisms have been cultured from women with PID, but 80 per cent of cases are triggered by a sexually transmissible infection; either *Chlamydia* or gonorrhoea. *Mycoplasma genitalium* is probably sexually transmitted and has been implicated in PID in women and NGU in men. It is difficult to detect, requiring special culture medium or a polymerase chain reaction (PCR) test. Endogenous anaerobes, such *Bacteroides spp.*, or *Mycoplasma hominis*, often come in as secondary invaders and are responsible for subsequent tubal abscess formation.

PID is an important condition because it results in tubal damage leading to ectopic pregnancy and tubal factor infertility. As many as 20 per cent of women may be left with chronic pelvic pain. The symptoms and signs may be mild and subtle with many women unaware of the significance of mild pelvic pain and possible future fertility. On the other hand, many women are now aware of these complications and seek reassurance about their future fertility when they receive a diagnosis of PID.

Chlamydia trachomatis

Chlamydia trachomatis is the commonest bacterial sexually transmitted infection in industrialized countries. As many as 10 per cent of women of childbearing age are infected in inner cities in the UK. Women under 25 years of age have the highest prevalence. Many infections are asymptomatic: approximately 50 per cent in men and 80 per cent in women. In men it is the most important cause of NGU. In women it causes cervicitis and PID. Genital strains can colonize the throat and cause conjunctivitis. It can infect the rectum, although only *Lymphogranuloma venereum* (LGV) strains cause a severe proctitis.

Chlamydia trachomatis is a small bacterium that is an obligate intracellular pathogen. Serovars A–C cause trachoma, infecting the conjunctiva. Serovars D–K cause genital infections. Specific LGV serovars (L1–L3) cause LGV. The infectious particle is the elementary body that infects columnar epithelial cells in the genital tract. They gain entry to the cells by binding to specific surface receptors. Once inside the cell, inclusion bodies form, which contain the metabolically active reticulate bodies. These divide by binary fission. After a 48-hour life cycle reticulate bodies condense into elementary bodies which are released from the cell surface. Heavily infected cells die but it is the inflammatory response to infection that contributes most to damaging the epithelial surface.

Humoral immunity may protect from re-infection, but antibodies are serovar-specific and the protection is short-lived. Cell-mediated immunity, with activation of cytotoxic T cells and production of interferon-γ is more important for controlling established infection.

Chlamydial infection is diagnosed by specific tests. Initially cell culture techniques were used. ELISA (enzyme-linked immunosorbant assay) tests are now used more commonly, but their sensitivity is limited. It is essential that samples are collected from the endocervix and areas of cervical ectropion so that columnar epithelial cells are harvested. Tests that detect DNA, such as the PCR and the ligase chain reaction (LCR) are much more sensitive. They can be applied to urine samples or vaginal swabs and have detection rates superior to ELISA tests on cervical swabs. This means that non-invasive screening for *Chlamydia* is now possible. Unfortunately higher cost has limited the availability of such tests in the UK. A direct fluorescent antibody (DFA) test can be performed on cervical smears rolled onto a specific collecting slide and fixed in alcohol. ELISA tests cannot be used reliably on rectal or conjunctival swabs, when DFA is more appropriate.

In Scandinavian countries, nationwide screening programmes have reduced the incidence of chlamydial infection, with concomitant reductions in the incidence of PID and ectopic pregnancy. It is likely that a national screening programme will be set up in the UK in the next few years.

Serological tests are not performed routinely in the diagnosis of chlamydial infections. Micro-immuno-fluorescence can be used to detect serum antibodies, which are not present in all infected individuals. The highest antibody titres are found in women with PID or disseminated infection. They are present in 60 per cent of women with tubal factor infertility.

The following treatments are effective for uncomplicated chlamydial infection:
- Doxycycline 100 mg twice a day for seven days;
- Erythromycin 500 mg twice a day for 14 days.
Used in pregnancy;
- Azithromycin 1 g as a single dose;
- Ofloxacin 400 mg daily for seven days.

It is essential that sex partners are screened fully for sexually transmitted infections and prescribed treatment for *Chlamydia*, before sexual intercourse is resumed.

Gonorrhoea

The incidence of gonorrhoea has declined in developed countries in the last two decades. The prevalence is less than 1 per cent in women of childbearing age. Chronic asymptomatic infection is common: 50 per cent of women have no symptoms or signs of infection. Approximately 90 per cent of men, however, are symptomatic. In men, gonorrhoea causes a severe urethritis, with green urethral discharge and dysuria. In women, the spectrum of disease is similar to *Chlamydia*. It may be carried in the throat or cause an exudative tonsillitis. It can cause conjunctivitis in adults. It causes proctitis in women and homosexual men, who may present with purulent discharge, bleeding and rectal pain.

Neisseria gonorrhoeae is a Gram-negative diplococcus. It colonizes columnar or cuboidal epithelium. In chronic infection there is a complex interaction with the host immune system. The expression of antigenic surface proteins changes over time in the face of an effective antibody response. Protective immunity does not appear to develop. Reliable serological tests for gonorrhoea have not been developed. Where antibiotic use is not controlled adequately resistant strains emerge rapidly. Chromosomal mutations conferring reduced sensitivity to penicillin emerge slowly in an incremental way. High-level resistance to penicillin is mediated by a plasmid. The first one described encoded a penicillinase enzyme (PPNG [Penicillinase Producing *Neisseria gonorrhoea*] strains). Chromosomal mutations conferring resistance to quinolone antibiotics have emerged in developing countries in the last decade.

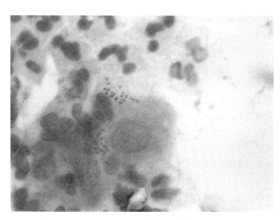

Figure 16.2 Vaginal and cervical flora. 1000x magnified. A Gram-stained smear of cervical secretions showing polymorphs and Gram-negative intracellular diplococci. This appearance is highly suggestive of gonorrhoea.

In GUM clinics, the diagnosis is made presumptively by observing typical Gram-negative intracellular diplococci on Gram-stained smears of urethral, cervical and rectal swabs (Fig. 16.2). It is a fastidious organism, requiring a CO_2 concentration of 7 per cent specific media such as blood agar and antibiotics to inhibit the growth of other organisms. It may fail to grow on culture, particularly if transport to the laboratory is delayed. DNA-based detection tests are available for screening, but culture remains essential to allow antibiotic sensitivity testing.

The following treatments are effective for sensitive strains of gonorrhoea infection:

- Amoxycillin 3 g with probenecid 2 g as a single dose;
- Ciprofloxacin 500 mg as a single dose;
- Spectinomycin 2 g as a single dose (intramuscularly);
- Azithromycin 1 g as a single dose;
- Ceftriaxone 250 mg as a single dose (intramuscularly).

The choice of treatment is dictated by local sensitivity patterns, a history of recent travel and cost. It is essential that sex partners are screened fully for sexually transmitted infections and prescribed treatment for gonorrhoea before sexual intercourse is resumed. More than 50 per cent of women infected with gonorrhoea have a concomitant chlamydial infection. Chlamydial treatment is prescribed routinely, therefore, for all women with gonorrhoea, and their partners.

Because of the possibility of antibiotic resistance and occasional treatment failures, women should have two sets of cultures performed following treatment, as tests of cure. This should include rectal swabs, as infection can spread there from vaginal secretions.

Cervicitis

Mucopurulent cervicitis is a clinical diagnosis based on detecting purulent mucus at the cervical os and is often accompanied by contact bleeding (Fig. 16.3). It can be confused with a benign ectropion but the latter does not usually bleed heavily unless swabbed very vigorously. Women with cervicitis may present with postcoital bleeding or complain of a purulent vaginal discharge. Many, however, are asymptomatic. Cervicitis is often caused by a sexually transmissible agent, with the male partner having NGU. Tests for *Chlamydia* and gonorrhoea should be performed. If ulceration is present, test for herpes simplex.

The treatment is the same as for *Chlamydia*. Chronic cervicitis produces scarring. Nabothian follicles are mucus-containing cysts up to 1 cm in diameter, which are often present following chronic cervicitis.

Pelvic inflammatory disease

As infection ascends into the uterus, endometritis develops. Plasma cells are seen on endometrial biopsy, and germinal centres may develop with chronic chlamydial infection. It may be associated with intermenstrual bleeding.

The first stage of salpingitis involves mucosal inflammation with swelling, redness and deciliation. Polymorphonuclear cells invade the submucosa, followed by mononuclear cells and plasma cells. Inflammatory exudate fills the lumen of the tube, and adhesions develop between mucosal folds. Inflammation extends to the serosal surface and pus exudes from the fimbriae to the ovaries and adnexae. At laparoscopy the tubes are swollen and red in mild cases. In more severe cases the tubes are fixed to adjacent structures by fibrin exudate and adhesions. With pelvic peritonitis all the organs are congested with multiple adhesions producing an inflammatory mass. The omentum usually confines the infection to the pelvis. The infection causes considerable tissue destruction. Tubal or tubo-ovarian abscesses may develop.

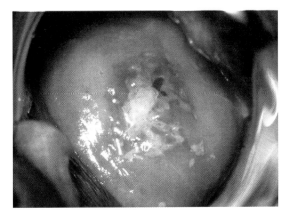

Figure 16.3 Cervicitis. The cervix is inflamed with erythema and contact bleeding from the columnar epithelium. This can be associated with gonorrhoea, *Chlamydia* or non-specific infections.

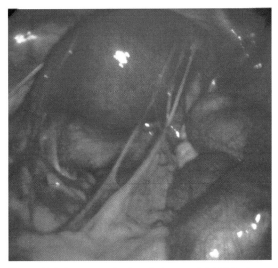

Figure 16.4 Laparoscopic view of uterus and right fallopian tube. The tube is dilated (hydrosalpinx or pyosalpinx) and there are bands of adhesions running from the uterine fundus to the omentum. The part of the left fallopian tube that is visible is also dilated.

Key Points

Pelvic Inflammatory Disease (PID)

- Most episodes of PID are associated with traditional STD pathogens: chlamydia and gonorrhoea
- Secondary invasion with anaerobes is common, so that combinations of antibiotics are required to cover the spectrum of likely pathogens
- Partner notification is an important part of management
- PID is associated with tubal damage leading to ectopic pregnancy and tubal-factor infertility
- Most chlamydial amd gonococcal infections are asymptomatic: 'safer sex' and screening are the best means of prevention

Subsequent scarring may lead to the fimbriae being drawn into the ends of the fallopian tubes, adhering and sealing the ends of the tubes. The uterus and tubes may be pulled back into the pelvis by adhesions, becoming fixed and retroverted. A hydrosalpinx is caused by accumulation of fluid within the tube, which expands and swells. If infected, a pyosalpinx results. Pelvic adhesions organize, matting together the pelvic organs. Some recovery of the ciliated epithelium within the tubes usually occurs.

Clinical features

As infection extends into the uterus, fallopian tubes and ovaries causing pelvic pain and deep dyspareunia. Intermenstrual bleeding may be caused by endometritis. It is not uncommon for women to have an associated urinary tract infection. An abnormal urine dipstick test should not distract one from the diagnosis of pelvic inflammatory disease (PID). The diagnosis of PID is based on the following.

- A history of pelvic pain and deep dyspareunia.
- On examination: cervical motion tenderness (often called cervical excitation) with or without uterine and adnexal tenderness.
- Lower genital tract infection: BV, trichomoniasis or cervicitis.
- In more severe cases: pyrexia, a raised neutrophil count and a raised erythrocyte sedimentation rate (ESR).
- An adnexal mass may be present in 20 per cent of women, usually those who are most systemically unwell.

At best the clinical diagnosis is 70–80 per cent accurate. Laparoscopy is regarded as the 'gold standard' for diagnosis (Fig. 16.4). In early salpingitis, however, the inflammation may not be visible from the serosal surface of the tubes. The important differential diagnoses are shown in Table 16.2. The most important diagnosis to exclude acutely is ectopic pregnancy. If there is any doubt about the possibility of pregnancy a urine pregnancy test should be performed. If early pregnancy is established, an ultrasound scan to look for evidence of an intrauterine pregnancy is essential.

Table 16.2 – Findings at laparoscopy in women undergoing laparoscopy for suspected PID

Diagnosis at laparoscopy	Percentage of women
Salpingitis/PID	65
Normal findings	22
Appendicitis	3
Endometriosis	2
Bleeding corpus luteum	2
Ectopic pregnancy	2
Miscellaneous	4

When PID is suspected, endocervical swabs should be taken for detection of *Chlamydia trachomatis* and *Neisseria gonorrhoeae*. A high vaginal swab should be taken for detection of *Trichomonas* and BV. Laparoscopy should be performed if the clinical diagnosis is uncertain, drainage of an abscess might be required, or if there is no improvement after 24–48 hours of intravenous antibiotic treatment in a systemically unwell woman.

Ambulant patients with mild symptoms can be treated as out-patients. The antibiotic regime should cover both *Chlamydia* and gonorrhoea, as well as an anaerobic organism. It is usual to prescribe Doxycycline 100 mg twice a day for 14 days with five days of metronidazole 400 mg twice a day. If gonorrhoea is suspected, prescribe Ciprofloxacin 500 mg as a single dose in addition. An alternative is to use Ofloxacin 400 mg daily for two weeks with five days of metronidazole 400 mg twice a day. Patients who are systemically unwell, or in whom a tubal abscess is suspected, should be admitted for intravenous antibiotic treatment and may require laparoscopy to definitely establish the diagnosis. Intravenous cephalosporin and metronidazole can be used initially but it is essential that a two-week course of Doxycycline is prescribed to eradicate any possible chlamydial infection.

It is essential that sexual partners are screened for *Chlamydia* and gonorrhoea and prescribed appropriate antibiotic treatment before intercourse is resumed (Fig. 16.5).

Other complications of Chlamydia *and* gonorrhoea

Intra-abdominal spread of *Chlamydia* or gonorrhoea can cause peri-appendicitis or perihepatitis. The latter is termed the Fitz-Hugh Curtis syndrome. Women, and rarely men, present with right hypochondrial pain and tenderness and pyrexia. They are frequently misdiagnosed as having cholecystitis. Careful examination usually elicits signs of salpingitis. At laparoscopy, fine 'violin string' adhesions are seen between the liver capsule and visceral peritoneum. It is cured by a three-week course of appropriate antibiotics.

Disseminated infection with *Chlamydia* may cause Reiter's syndrome or sexually acquired reactive arthritis (SARA). This probably occurs in less than 1 per cent of cases. There is usually an asymmetrical oligoarthritis, affecting large joints of the lower limb. In Reiter's syndrome, the arthritis is accompanied by uveitis and a rash that, if florid, may be similar to psoriasis. It is associated with the presence of human locus antigen (HLA) B27 haplotype, and there is overlap with other seronegative spondarthritides.

Disseminated infection with gonorrhoea occurs rarely, but presents as a septic oligoarthritis, usually affecting the small joints of the hand or wrist, with a scanty papular rash. It is rare but occurs more often in women than men.

Pregnancy and vertical transmission

See Obstetrics by Ten Teachers, Chapter 15.

Other causes of endometritis

Tuberculosis

Mycobacterium tuberculosis can spread through the genital tract via the blood or lymphatics. There is nearly always tuberculosis elsewhere, usually pulmonary. Granulomata develop in the tubes and subse-

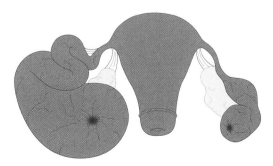

Figure 16.5 Large hydrosalpinx of left tube with a smaller hydrosalpinx on the right side.

quently the other genital organs. Infection may remain subclinical, presenting ultimately with amenorrhoea, infertility, or in a similar fashion to PID, with chronic, low-grade pelvic pain. The endometrium is involved in up to 80 per cent of cases and the ovaries in 20–30 per cent. Abnormal uterine bleeding is a presenting symptom in 10–40 per cent of patients.

Examination is normal in many women but an adnexal mass or fixing of the pelvic organs may be detected. Diagnosis can be confirmed by obtaining endometrial tissue from biopsy or dilatation and curettage. The detection rate is greatest towards the end of the menstrual cycle. Even so, endometrial biopsy does not have 100 per cent sensitivity.

Because the presentation may be subtle, a high index of suspicion is essential. A Mantoux or Heaf test should be reactive in a woman with active tuberculosis unless she is immunosuppressed. A chest X-ray should be performed to look for evidence of pulmonary tuberculosis. After chronic infection, bilateral tubal calcification may be seen on abdominal X-rays.

Actinomycosis

This infection is almost exclusively seen in women with an intrauterine contraceptive device (IUCD). It can be detected on cervical cytology and if there are no clinical features to suggest PID careful monitoring is required. If there is any history of pelvic pain the IUCD should be removed and antibiotic treatment with penicillin initiated. If undetected, actinomycosis can progress to widespread pelvic involvement with an inflammatory mass and fixing of the pelvic organs.

Genital ulcer disease

The diagnosis of genital ulcers can be a considerable challenge for the clinician. In the UK, herpes simplex infection is by far the commonest cause. It is essential, however, to take an adequate sexual and travel history, as there are many other sexually transmissible causes of genital ulcers that are common in tropical countries.

Herpes simplex virus

Most women experience considerable psychological distress upon receiving a diagnosis of genital herpes.

Classification of genital ulcers
Infective
Herpes simplex virus
Primary syphilis
Lymphogranuloma venereum
Chancroid
Donovanosis
HIV
Non-infective
Aphthous ulcers
Trauma
Skin disease, e.g. lichen sclerosis et atrophicus
Behçet's syndrome
Other multisystem disorder, e.g. sarcoidosis
Dermatitis artefacta

They feel contaminated by acquiring an incurable sexually transmitted disease that will inevitably be transmitted to future partners, making future relationships difficult to start. Many are also aware that it can be transmitted to neonates with disastrous consequences. Sensitive discussion and counselling is essential. This may require several follow-up consultations.

Microbiology and diagnosis

Traditionally, herpes simplex virus type I (HSV-I) causes oral lesions (cold sores) and type II (HSV-II) causes genital herpes. Currently cold sores caused by HSV-I infection are becoming less common in the UK. They are commoner in lower socio-economic groups. Fewer adults are infected orally before they become sexually active, and more are therefore susceptible to the virus. Accordingly, 50 per cent of genital lesions are now caused by HSV-I. At present, approximately 20 per cent of GUM clinic attendees have antibodies to HSV-II and 50–60 per cent have antibodies to HSV-I. Less than half those with antibodies to HSV-II are aware that they have herpes, or even report genital ulcers when questioned. Infection is frequently subclinical so that an individual presents many years after acquisition with what is apparently a newly acquired infection. Individuals with one type of HSV infection can develop symptomatic infection from the other type, although there is some partial immunity.

The diagnosis is made by collecting serum from a vesicle with a small gauge needle and syringe or by

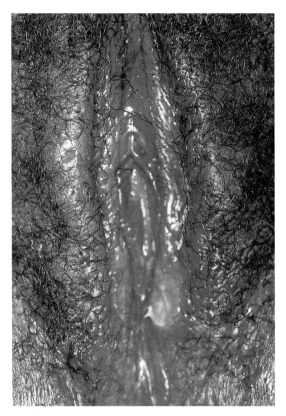

Figure 16.6 Genital herpes. Several ulcers are seen on the vulva. Widespread lesions are seen in primary herpes and in recurrent herpes affecting pregnant or immunosuppressed women.

applying a cotton-tipped swab to ulcers. The virus is demonstrated by electron microscopy or culture in a tissue monolayer. Monoclonal antibodies are used to type the virus once cultured. Serological tests are commercially available, but cannot yet reliably distinguish between antibodies to HSV-I and HSV-II. Demonstration of anti-HSV antibody cannot therefore distinguish genital from orolabial herpes.

Primary herpes

Primary herpes presents up to three weeks after acquisition. There is usually widespread involvement of the vulva and the vagina and cervix can also be affected (Fig. 16.6). Primary pharyngeal or rectal infections are seen following orogenital contact or anal intercourse.

Painful vesicles develop which coalesce into multiple ulcers. Peri-urethral involvement may cause severe pain and urinary retention can result. This may also be partly due to involvement of the sacral nerves. If seen very early, primary herpes may only affect a

small part of the vulva appearing to be a recurrent episode. It is sensible therefore to routinely prescribe a course of antiviral medication for five days for all patients presenting with the first attack, even if the clinical suspicion is of a secondary episode. Diagnosis should always be confirmed by culture, or electron microscopy of a swab taken from the lesion. In primary herpes, partners should be advised to attend although often the infecting lesion has healed.

Treatment includes analgesics and bathing in salt water. Lignocaine gel can be applied to particularly sore areas. Antiviral treatment stops viral replication. Healing occurs over the following week. Aciclovir 200 mg five times a day for five days is the cheapest and most established treatment. Famciclovir and Valaciclovir have greater bio-availablility, but are considerably more expensive.

Recurrent herpes

Following a primary infection, herpes colonizes the neurones in the dorsal root ganglia, establishing a latent infection. Productive infection occurs intermittently when virus particles are produced and track down the axons to the skin. Vesicles and ulcers then occur, usually in the same area. Sometimes distant anatomical sites are affected, if supplied by the same dermatomal nerve root. The spectrum of severity varies.

- Asymptomatic shedding of virus.
- Apparently trivial ulcers, resembling small abrasions on the vulva.
- Localized clusters of vesicles and ulcers over an area of 1–2 cm diameter.
- Widespread or chronic ulceration, resembling a primary infection can be seen in pregnant women.
- If a woman is immunosuppressed, large atypical chronic ulcers may develop. A herpetic ulcer persisting for more than one month is AIDS-defining in an individual with HIV infection.

A diagnosis of herpes can often be made by swabbing small ulcers in women who may present with an unrelated condition, or who think they have recurrent thrush. It is important to advise such patients that herpes is likely, even if the initial swab is negative. The woman should return for a further culture as soon as any similar lesions occur, so that the diagnosis can be confirmed.

Patients with an established history of genital herpes may present with a recurrent episode requesting treatment. Antiviral agents are usually ineffective in treating an established attack, which will resolve just as quickly without specific treatment. It is usual to advise patients to keep the area clean by washing with salt water and to avoid sexual intercourse until fully healed.

A small proportion of individuals with genital herpes develop frequent recurrences (more than six to eight attacks a year) or are considerably incapacitated during attacks. It is then appropriate to prescribe long-term suppression with acyclovir 400 mg twice a day. This considerably reduces the frequency of attacks although they can still occur and the infection can still be transmitted to partners. Many individuals experience a prodrome before the onset of vesicles and ulceration. This is usually a tingling sensation, but may include neuralgic symptoms, with pain in the thigh or perineum. An alternative strategy for these patients is episodic treatment. Prescribe a five-day treatment pack to keep at home. The patient can then initiate treatment when prodromal symptoms arise. This may abort a developing attack of symptomatic herpes.

If individuals with a history of herpes take swabs every day, herpes can be detected on occasions, usually for several consecutive days even though there are no symptoms. Such asymptomatic shedding can transmit infection to a sexual partner. It is important therefore that people with herpes use condoms to reduce the likelihood of transmitting infection. If both partners have a history of genital herpes this is probably not necessary.

Complications
There may be considerable psychological distress associated with a diagnosis of herpes. Counselling may help an individual to come to terms with the diagnosis. Occasionally referral to a psychologist or psychiatrist is indicated. Self-help organizations such as The Herpes Association provide useful support.

Neurological involvement during primary herpes infection is uncommon. It may present as aseptic meningitis, transverse myelitis or autonomic neuropathy. Resolution usually takes one to two months. Although HSV-II is more frequently implicated in aseptic meningitis, HSV-I more often causes encephalitis in adults.

Herpes keratitis is a serious condition that can produce corneal scarring and blindness, particularly if treated inappropriately with steroids in the absence of antiviral agents. Both HSV-I and HSV-II can infect the eye, and direct inoculation from an infected site is the route of spread. The presence of a branching 'dendritic' ulcer visible with fluorescein drops is diagnostic. Recurrent episodes may occur.

Pregnancy and vertical transmission
See *Obstetrics by Ten Teachers*, Chapter 15.

Non-herpes genital ulcers

The differential diagnosis of genital ulcers is wide-ranging from a variety of infections. Malignancy, particularly squamous cell carcinoma may arise on a background of lichen sclerosis et atrophicus or vulval intraepithelial neoplasia. Multisystem disorders, such as Behçet's syndrome, systemic lupus erythematosis and sarcoidosis, may be associated with genital ulceration. It is advisable to arrange for a biopsy if there is any doubt about the diagnosis.

Simple aphthous ulcers can occur on the genital mucosa in the same way as in the mouth. HIV infection may present with genital ulceration, particularly persistent atypical herpetic ulcers. The presentation of other infections is modified by immunosuppression.

Infective genital ulcers
These are more common in tropical countries but can be imported into the UK. At present, the incidence of syphilis is rising in European countries. The correct microbiological diagnosis can be difficult and referral to an appropriate specialist may be appropriate.

Syphilis

Syphilis is a systemic sexually transmissible infection caused by *Treponema pallidum*. *In vitro*, *T. pallidum venereum* causing venereal syphilis cannot be distinguished from *T. pertenue* which causes yaws, *T. pallidum endemicum*, which causes endemic syphilis and *T. carateum*, which causes pinta. These three tropical treponematoses are not sexually transmitted but pass between children and household contacts. A description of them is beyond the scope of this chapter. Clinicians in the UK must be aware that they occur in sub-Saharan Africa, the Caribbean and most of the humid tropics (yaws), in desert regions (endemic syphilis), and isolated parts of Central and South America (pinta). Following such an infection

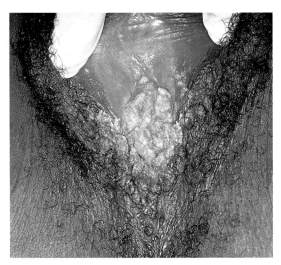

Figure 16.7 Primary syphilitic chancre. A painless rubbery ulcer is seen on the vulva. In many women the chancre is sited on the cervix, in which case the infection may pass asymptomatically.

the serological tests for syphilis may remain positive for life, causing diagnostic confusion. The tropical treponematoses have become less common following mass treatment campaigns in the 1950s and 1960s, but they still occur.

The first manifestation of venereal syphilis is a painless ulcer (chancre) at the site of inoculation. These can be multiple. The regional lymph nodes become enlarged. In women, the commonest site for a chancre is on the cervix. It may therefore pass unnoticed. A chancre usually arises three to six weeks after infection (Fig. 16.7), is painless and will resolve spontaneously without treatment after a few weeks. Chancres usually have a rubbery consistency and are accompanied by inguinal lymphadenopathy.

Secondary syphilis can arise as the chancre disappears or up to six months later. This is manifested by a systemic eruption, most often a non-itchy maculopapular rash. It is symmetrical and involves the palms of the hands and soles of the feet. More florid lesions resembling warts, condylomata lata, are seen in intertriginous areas, particularly perianally. Mucous pathos and linear (snail track) ulcers are seen on the mucosal surfaces. There may be generalized lymphadenopathy. Other manifestations include alopecia, arthritis and meningitis. A sensorineural deafness can occur early in the infection, due to destruction of the hair cells in the inner ear.

The diagnosis of primary syphilis is made by demonstrating the organism by dark field

microscopy. The lesion is cleaned and mildly abraded so that clear serum exudes from the base. This is then collected and mixed with a drop of saline on a microscope slide. The slide is viewed under high power (3800×) using dark field illumination. *T. pallidum* can be seen as tightly wound spiral organisms, which move and bend in a characteristic fashion. Inexperienced observers can be misled by other spirochaetes that may be present on mucosal surfaces, but are less tightly coiled.

Serological tests for syphilis should be requested including a fluorescent treponemal antibody (FTA) test. This is the most sensitive and specific test for syphilis, but is time-consuming to perform, requiring skilled interpretation. Most laboratories routinely perform a specific treponemal test such as the *Treponema pallidum* haemagglutination assay (TPHA) or *Treponema pallidum* particle agglutination (TPPA). A reaginic or non-specific test such as the venereal disease reference laboratory (VDRL) test or rapid plasma reagin (RPR) tests are used in addition. These are diluted down serially to give a titre such as 1 in 64, at the threshold of reaction of the test. In early primary syphilis, however, the serological tests may all be negative. Chancres on the cervix may be misdiagnosed as cervical carcinomas. If there is any doubt biopsies must be taken. An extensive infiltrate of lymphocytes and plasma cells is seen histologically. Specialized stains, such as silver, reveal the presence of spirochaetes.

In secondary syphilis the serological tests are positive with a VDRL titre of usually 1 in 32 or greater. Dark ground examination can be performed from mucosal lesions or condyloma lata. Following treatment of primary or secondary syphilis the titre of VDRL should fall two-fold every three months, becoming negative within two years.

Following resolution of secondary syphilis a period of latency occurs. There are no outward manifestations of infection, which is only detected on serological testing. There is a potential for lesions of secondary syphilis to relapse for up to two years, during which infection can be transmitted to a sexual partner. This is called early latent syphilis.

Primary and secondary syphilis are not life threatening. The importance of the diagnosis rests on the risk of late tertiary syphilis. Neurosyphilis can be manifest within five years of infection in the form of meningovascular syphilis presenting with a stroke. This may subsequently progress to tabes dorsalis, or

Table 16.3 – Treatment for bacterial genital ulcers

Antibacterial agent	Primary syphilis	*Lymphogranuloma venereum*	Chancroid	Donovanosis
Azithromycin	Active, but not fully evaluated	Active, but not fully evaluated	1 Gram Stat	
Ceftriaxone	Active, but not fully evaluated		250 mg Stat IM	
Ciprofloxacin	Not active	Not reliable	500 mg twice/day for 3 days	750 mg twice/day for 21 days minimum
Cotrimoxazole	Not active		May be used, but resistance is common in some areas	960 mg twice/day for 21 days minimum
Doxycycline	100 mg twice/day for 14 days	100 mg twice/day for 21 days		100 mg twice/day for 21 days minimum
Erythromycin	500 mg four times/ day for 14 days	500 mg four times/ day for 21 days	500 mg four times/day for 7 days	500 mg four times/day for 21 days minimum
Penicillin	Procaine penicillin 1.2 MU/day for 12 days			

general paresis of the insane. Approximately 10 per cent of men and 5 per cent of women develop neurosyphilis if not treated in the early stages. Approximately 20 per cent will develop cardiovascular syphilis manifesting as thoracic aortic aneurysm or aortic regurgitation, which can present many years later.

Syphilis is also important because of the risk of vertical transmission. At its most severe this will cause intrauterine death or a severely affected neonate. Neonates at risk should be fully evaluated, including a lumbar puncture, and receive intravenous penicillin. Less severe infection may present during late childhood with the stigmata of congenital syphilis including eighth nerve deafness, interstitial keratitis and abnormal teeth. The risk of congenital infection is greatest, as high as 70 per cent, with primary and secondary syphilis but can occur even five to ten years later. The effects of late congenital syphilis are not prevented unless the mother is treated before 20 weeks' gestation.

Treatment

T. pallidum replicates slowly, with an estimated doubling time of 20 hours. Sustained treponemicidal levels of antibiotic are needed for a minimum of 12 days in early syphilis. The treatment of choice is penicillin. A variety of regimens are used (Table 16.3).

- Procaine penicillin 1.2 MU daily by intramuscular injection for 12 days.
- Benzathine penicillin 2.4 MU by intramuscular injection, repeated after seven days.
- Doxycycline 100 mg two times a day for 14 days.
- Erythromycin 500 mg four times a day for 14 days.

In the UK, administration of procaine penicillin 1.2 MU daily is prescribed commonly. If the infection has been present for more than one year, treatment is extended to 21 days for penicillin regimens and 28 days for oral regimens. Only intravenous penicillin or high doses of procaine penicillin (2.4 MU daily) combined with probenecid (500 mg four times/day) produce acceptable levels of penicillin in the cerebrospinal fluid (CSF) to treat neurosyphilis. In pregnancy the absorption of erythromycin is unreliable. Consider intravenous treatment for penicillin-allergic pregnant women, or desensitization to penicillin.

Partner notification is essential. The sexual history should be reviewed. In some cases partners from a few years previously should be contacted when possible. Children may need to be tested, and siblings if congenital infection is possible. This may be arranged most easily with the help of a GUM clinic.

Tropical genital ulcer disease

Sexually transmitted infections causing genital ulcer disease present considerable diagnostic difficulty. In some cases more than one infecting agent may be present. Most of the aetiological agents cannot be cultured in standard microbiological media. Histological examination of tissue is sometimes the only means of confirming the diagnosis. In many tropical countries where resources are poor, a syndromic approach is taken to treatment of genital ulcers. Recommended treatments are shown in Table 16.3.

Lymphogranuloma venereum

Lymphogranuloma venereum (LGV) is caused by specific serovars (L1–L3) of *Chlamydia trachomatis*. It is found in the Far East, sub-Saharan Africa and South America. In the early stages there is often a small superficial ulcer that can slowly increase in size, but often goes unnoticed. More obvious are the enlarged nodes, which become compressed by the inguinal ligament leading to the 'groove sign'. The nodes can become matted together and discharge pus, forming a bubo. In women, a severe proctocolitis can progress to fistulae and strictures. The diagnosis can be confirmed serologically by a complement fixation test.

Chancroid

Chancroid is an infection caused by *Haemophilus ducreyii*. The geographical distribution is similar to that of LGV. It starts with small shallow ulcers which are usually multiple and painful. The edges are irregular and there is localized lymphadenopathy. The sores may persist for several months and the glands can suppurate through the skin. The organism can only be grown on specialized culture medium and ideally the medium should be inoculated directly from the patient. Even so it may be difficult to obtain a positive culture. There is a characteristic appearance on biopsy when Ducreyii's bacillus may be seen.

Granuloma inguinale (Donovanosis)

Granuloma inguinale is an infection caused by *Klebsiella granulomatis* (previously known as *Calymmatobacterium granulomatis*). It is endemic in India, Papua New Guinea and southern Africa. It is usually a slowly progressive infection starting with discrete papules on the skin or vulva which can enlarge to

form 'beefy red' painful ulcers. These spread slowly around the genitalia and perineum. As they heal, fibrosis can develop which may lead to lymphoedema and elephantiasis. Diagnosis is best confirmed by biopsy or a crush preparation in which Donovan bodies are visible.

Other viral infections

Human papilloma virus

More than 70 different types of human papilloma virus (HPV) have been described. Although strains causing hand warts occasionally spread to the genital area, certain genital strains preferentially infect the genital mucosa. These are thought to be sexually transmitted. Infection is often established asymptomatically and may be carried for years, probably lifelong. In one study genital warts developed in nearly two-thirds of contacts of patients with visible genital warts within three months of starting the relationship. There is less information on the role of asymptomatic shedding of wart virus in those with subclinical lesions. The virus can infect the skin of the vulva and perineum, the vagina, cervix and rectum (Fig. 16.8). Possibly orogenital contact leads to warts developing in the mouth or lips. Warts are frequently multiple and slowly increase in size. They can spread directly to the perianal skin without anal intercourse being practised. The same strains can affect the larynx of a neonate (rarely) but do not usually spread to normal skin.

The majority of genital warts are caused by HPV types 6 and 11; viruses which have little oncogenic potential. HPV types 16 and 18 may cause flat warts

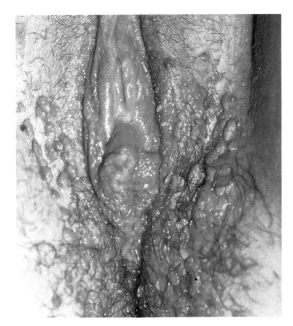

Figure 16.8 Genital warts. Multiple warts are seen over the lower vulva.

and have been linked with the development of cervical carcinoma. The majority of squamous cell carcinomas of the cervix contain DNA sequences from oncogenic HPV strains. It is thought that viral proteins, called E6 and E7, bind to p53 and pRB proteins produced by anti-oncogenes. This leads to dysregulation of the cell cycle and cell proliferation. Carcinomas that lack HPV sequences usually have other mutations which affect P53 gene expression. Several other events need to occur at the molecular level to initiate a cancer cell. Most women infected with HPV 16 or 18 do not develop cancer. Smoking is an important risk factor that should be discouraged.

Visible genital warts are usually treated with physical methods such as cryotherapy. Application of Podophyllin once or twice a week for up to six weeks will produce cure in 50–60 per cent of women. A purified extract of Podophyllotoxin has the advantage of self-application at home: twice a day for three days. Healing may be followed by ulceration, so patients should be instructed on its use with care. Petroleum jelly can be applied to adjacent normal skin to protect it. Surgical treatment is used for intractable cases, employing lasers, electrocautery or scissor excision.

Many women have heard of a link between genital warts and cervical cancer. It is important to explain that most visible genital warts are not caused by oncogenic strains of virus and that the risk of cervical cancer is not greatly increased. If cervical cytology has not been performed within three years, it should be done, but there is no need to advocate yearly smears or any other enhanced surveillance. Women with warts on the cervix should, however, be referred for expert colposcopic assessment. Recent sexual partners should be examined for evidence of genital warts and also other infections. Traditionally, patients with warts have been advised to use barrier methods of contraception during treatment and for the subsequent three months. Not enough is known about the risks of transmission of asymptomatic wart virus carriage to allow evidence-based recommendations to be made. Discuss the role of condoms in the general context of protecting against both acquisition and transmission of sexually transmitted infections with new partners.

Whatever treatment is used, the warts will recur until the immune response controls growth of the wart virus. This can take several weeks or even months in some patients who may become frustrated by such persistence. Patients who are immunosuppressed, such as those with HIV infection or underlying malignancies, are particularly difficult to treat. Immune-based therapies with interferon or topical application of Imiquimod, a cream that stimulates local cytokine release, may be helpful for such patients. A new class of antiviral drugs based on nucleotide analogues is active against HPV and may become useful for its treatment.

Molluscum contagiosum

This pox virus produces painless pearly lesions with a dimple, up to 5 mm in diameter. They are common

🔍 Key Points

Genital warts

- Most genital warts are caused by sexually transmitted strains of human papilloma virus (HPV)
- Long-lasting resolution of visible warts requires a good cell-mediated immune response
- Infections persist for many years, and relapse can occur at any time
- Several types of HPV, particularly 16 and 18, are associated with cervical cancer. Attention should be paid to reversible risk factors such as smoking

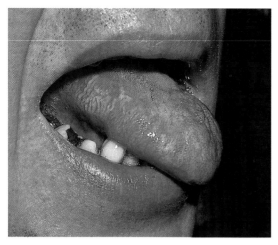

Figure 16.9 Hairy oral leukoplakia (HOL). Filliform white ridges are seen on the lateral border of the tongue. This is almost pathognomic of HIV infection, but may be seen in immunosuppression due to other causes. It can appear early in the course of the disease and is not AIDS defining.

Common Manifestations of AIDS	
Pulmonary	*Pneumocystis carinii* pneumonia
	Tuberculosis – pulmonary or extra-pulmonary
Neurological	Cerebral Toxoplasmosis
	Cryptococcal meningitis
	AIDS dementia
Gastrointestinal	Diarrhoea and wasting syndrome which may be due to infection with *Cryptosporidium*, Microsporidium, Isospora
	Oesophageal candidiasis
Ophthalmic	Cytomegalovirus retinitis
Malignancy	Kaposi's sarcoma (Fig. 16.10a–c)
	Non-Hodgkin's lymphoma
Systemic	*Mycobacterium avium* intracellulare complex (MAC) infection

in childhood and clear after a few months. Adults may acquire infection during sexual intercourse, and they can be mistaken for genital warts. They resolve with cryotherapy or following curettage and application of phenol. The fluid from the vesicles is infectious, and patients should be warned not to pick at them. In immunosuppressed individuals widespread, large, confluent lesions may develop. These are currently almost untreatable, as resolution requires an immune response. Nucleotide analogue drugs show *in vitro* activity against the virus, offering the prospect of antiviral treatment.

HIV infection

Acquired immunodeficiency syndrome (AIDS) was first described in San Francisco in 1983. It is caused by infection with human immunodeficiency virus (HIV). More than 20 million individuals are now infected worldwide and in countries with a high prevalence it is the leading cause of death in young adults. It is a particularly devastating disease because of the stigma of sexual transmission and the risk of vertical transmission to children. Even if a child is not infected, the death of one or both parents threatens their development and survival in many parts of the world. The prevalence is greatest in sub-Saharan Africa where in several cities as many as a third of pregnant women are

infected. A resurgence in tuberculosis has occurred hand-in-hand with the AIDS epidemic.

The onset of immunodeficiency can be manifest in any organ system so that a high index of suspicion is required to recognize the way in which other disease processes are altered. This section will focus on the gynaecological aspects of HIV infection.

Natural history and principles of treatment of HIV infection

Twenty per cent of those infected with HIV experience an acute seroconversion illness a few weeks after acquisition. Clinical features include fever, generalized lymphadenopathy, a macular erythematous rash, pharyngitis and conjunctivitis. A steady decline in immune function over the first few years may be manifest by non-life-threatening opportunistic conditions such as recurrent oral and vaginal candidiasis, single dermatome herpes zoster (shingles), frequent and prolonged episodes of oral or genital herpes or persistent warts. Furry white patches on the sides of the tongue, termed hairy oral leukoplakia (HOL) (Fig. 16.9) may come and go and are pathognomic of immunodeficiency. Persistent generalized lymphadenopathy may be present. Skin problems include seborrhoeic dermatitis, folliculitis, dry skin, tinea pedis and a high frequency of allergic reactions.

Without antiretroviral treatment the median time to the development of AIDS is ten years. Essentially AIDS is defined by the onset of life-threatening opportunistic infections, or malignancies associated with immunodeficiency. The commonest presentations are listed in the box above. There are two strategies used in treatment. Combinations of antiretroviral drugs are prescribed. These may include two or more nucleoside analogue reverse transcriptase inhibitors, such as zidovudine or didinasine, a non-nucleoside reverse transcriptase inhibitor, such as nevirapine, and one or more protease inhibitors such as nelfinavir. If successful the immune system improves after a few months. These drugs, particularly some of the protease inhibitors, have many potential interactions with other drugs through effects on the cytochrome P-450 enzymes. This includes increasing the rate of breakdown of synthetic oestrogens in oral contraceptive pills.

If immunodeficiency has already occurred, treatment and prevention of opportunistic infections is needed. This may include cotrimoxazole to prevent *Pneumocystis carinii* pneumonia (PCP) and, in severely immunosuppresed individuals with CD4 counts, 0.5/L, azithromycin to prevent disseminated *Mycobacterium avium intracellulare* complex (MAC) infection, and ganciclovir to prevent cytomegalovirus (CMV) infection. Regular administration of antifungal agents may be necessary to control oral and vaginal candidiasis.

Virology

HIV is a retrovirus, with its genetic code in a single strand of RNA. Reverse transcriptase is carried within the core to enable proviral DNA to be produced in an infected cell. The outer membrane protein, gp-120, binds to CD4 receptors which are present on T-helper lymphocytes, macrophages, dendritic cells and microglia. Co-receptors, such as the CCR-5 chemokine receptor, are also used to enhance viral entry. Approximately 1 per cent of Caucasians has a homozygous mutation in the receptor, which is associated with resistance to acquiring infection. Another viral protein, p24, surrounds the RNA and enzymes present within the core of the virus which enters the cytoplasm of an infected cell. Once proviral DNA has been integrated into the host genome viral peptides are transcribed. These are cleaved by specific viral protease enzymes before the daughter virus particles are assembled.

Current antiretroviral drugs target reverse transcriptase or viral proteases. The aim of therapy is to reduce the level of virus in the plasma to zero with a combination of antiretroviral agents. If total suppression of viral replication is not achieved, resistant strains of virus will inevitably arise within the patient over the course of a few months. This is because reverse transcription is inherently inaccurate, leading to a high rate of mutation. With each cycle of replication of virus, which takes 48 hours, single point mutations arise, which will confer reduced sensitivity to antiviral agents. If therapy is effective the CD4 lymphocyte count rises progressively, and at least partial immune restoration occurs. Unfortunately HIV infects long-lived memory cells from which the virus can rapidly reseed the body on cessation of therapy. Eradication, and thus cure, is unlikely even after several years of treatment.

Diagnosis

HIV infection is diagnosed by finding antibodies to gp-120. During seroconversion p24 antigen is detectable in the serum before antibodies are produced. We monitor the disease by measuring the level of CD4 lymphocytes in peripheral blood. A normal level is >0.5/L. There is a 10 per cent risk of AIDS developing within one year when the CD4 lymphocyte count drops to 0.2/L. This is the level at which primary prophylaxis against PCP is recommended. Using PCR technology we can also measure the concentration of viral RNA in the plasma. A high level, >100,000 particles/mL, predicts rapid disease development.

As the consequences of receiving a diagnosis of HIV are serious, a test should only be performed with informed consent from the patient. They may wish to discuss it with a partner, for whom the test may have major implications. If you suspect an individual has HIV look for HOL, generalized lymphadenopathy and skin rashes. There is often lymphopenia or thrombocytopenia on a full blood count. Polyclonal IgG production produces a raised total protein level. Kaposi's sarcoma (Fig. 16.10a–c) may be evident with multiple red or purple tumours anywhere on the body.

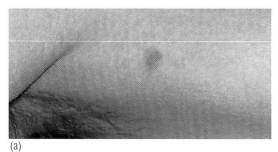

(a)

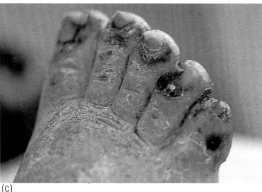

(c)

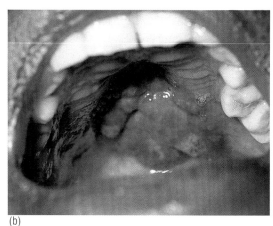

(b)

Figure 16.10 Kaposi's sarcoma.
a) Early lesion is red/purple and palpable.
b) Advanced Kaposi's sarcoma with extensive involvement of the palate. This is usually accompanied by visceral involvement elsewhere, e.g. gut and lung.
c) Advanced Kaposi's sarcoma of the foot producing lymphoedema of the leg and gangrene of the toes. This was a pre-terminal event.

Transmission

In most developing countries HIV is principally spread through vaginal intercourse, with approximately equal numbers of men and women infected. In developed countries the majority of infections have been acquired through homosexual sex or intravenous drug use, although the incidence of heterosexual transmission is increasing. Genital infections are risk factors for HIV transmission and acquisition, including genital ulcer disease, *Chlamydia* and gonorrhoea. BV may also be a risk factor and is very common in some African countries, with a prevalence of 50 per cent or greater. Good control of sexually transmitted infections should reduce the incidence of HIV infection.

Vertical transmission

See *Obstetrics by Ten Teachers*.

Gynaecological manifestations of HIV

HPV infection flourishes in immunosuppressed individuals. Genital warts often persist despite aggressive surgical treatment. Chronic HPV infection can result in the development of cervical carcinoma, vulval intraepithelial neoplasia and Bowen's disease. Because of this most physicians perform cervical cytology annually in women with HIV infection. Persistent atypical warty lesions of the skin or vulva should be biopsied.

Other infections can also be more persistent in HIV infected individuals. There is limited evidence that PID requires longer courses of antibiotics in women with HIV. Careful follow-up is certainly indicated. Postpartum endometritis is common in this group of women, and herpes simplex has been implicated occasionally. Eruptions of secondary genital herpes may become widespread, severe and persist for weeks if not diagnosed and treated. It often presents as deep, painful ulceration (Fig. 16.11).

Although all HIV infected women are urged to use condoms to prevent them transmitting the infection to others, they should also be advised to use a more reliable form of contraception if they do not wish to become pregnant. Medication prescribed for HIV may interact with the metabolism of synthetic oestrogens.

If an HIV infected woman plans to become pregnant discuss the means of reducing the risk of vertical transmission. Discuss also the consequences for

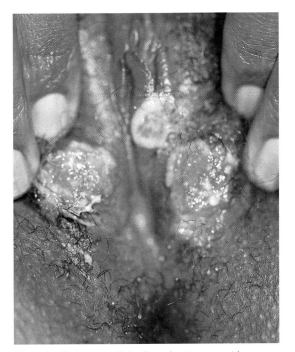

Figure 16.11 Large multiple ulcers due to recurrent herpes simplex in a woman with HIV infec0tion. An ulcer that persists for more than one month is clinically AIDS defining.

the child of possibly losing their mother in childhood. If the partner is HIV-negative, assist the couple to perform artificial insemination by providing information and syringes or pipettes. At present the provision of infertility treatments to HIV infected women is controversial, but has been offered by some gynaecologists.

Key Points

HIV infection

- The incidence of HIV is increasing rapidly worldwide
- A high index of suspicion is needed, as risk factors are not always apparent in affected individuals, some of whom might remain well for 15–20 years without specific treatment
- Treatment with combination anti-retroviral therapy can improve life expectancy and reduce hospital admissions, but it is expensive, complex to manage and there is considerable drug-associated toxicity
- Some of the antiretroviral drugs have major pharmacokinetic interactions, including effects on the combined oral contraceptive pill, some antihistamines and anti-tuberculous medication

CASE HISTORY

A 25-year-old single woman presented with a history of increased non-offensive vaginal discharge, postcoital bleeding, right hypochondrial pain and feeling generally unwell. She had been in a new relationship for one month, having separated from her previous boyfriend three months earlier. On enquiry she reported mild deep dyspareunia. She was taking the oral contraceptive pill and had one previous pregnancy which had been terminated at eight weeks, two years before.

On examination there was a mucoid vaginal discharge and green mucus emerging from the internal os. There was a small ectropion which bled profusely after swabbing. On bimanual examination, the uterus was anteverted and mobile. There was cervical motion tenderness and bilateral adnexal tenderness. There was right hypochondrial tenderness.

The diagnosis of pelvic inflammatory disease with presumptive perihepatitis was made and she was prescribed Doxycycline 100 mg twice a day for three weeks with Metronidazole 400 mg twice a day for five days. A test for *Chlamydia trachomatis* was positive and at review after one week and three weeks her symptoms had resolved.

Both her new and her previous boyfriend tested positive for *Chlamydia trachomatis* when screened in the GUM clinic. She presented one year later with right-sided pelvic pain and amenorrhoea of six weeks. An ectopic pregnancy was confirmed.

Comment

- Both *Chlamydia* and gonorrhoea can be carried for months or years before symptoms develop.
- Postcoital and intermenstrual bleeding are common symptoms of cervicitis and endometritis. Their presence should instigate a search for infection in young sexually active women.
- As many as 20 per cent of women with pelvic inflammatory disease have signs of perihepatitis on laparoscopy. Sometimes right hypochondrial pain overshadows the pelvic symptoms.
- An episode of pelvic inflammatory disease threatens a woman's future fertility causing both ectopic pregnancy and tubal infertility.
- It is important that re-infection after treatment is prevented by pursuing partner notification vigorously.

Urinary tract infection

See Chapter 17.

New developments

DNA based tests such as polymerase chain reaction (PCR) or ligase chain reaction (LCR) offer the possibility of non-invasive sample collection to screen for infections such as *Chlamydia* and gonorrhoea. A national screening pro-gramme will reduce the incidence of *Chlamydia*, pelvic inflammatory disease, and subsequent ectopic pregnancy and infertility.

Screening for and treating genital infections such as bacterial vaginosis in pregnancy may significantly reduce the incidence of miscarriage, preterm birth and subse-quent neurological impairment.

The development of antiviral drugs continues. New agents are being developed which are likely to be effective against human papilloma viruses, herpes viruses and HIV. Novel immune stimulators which can be applied topically are also being evaluated.

Vaccines are being developed for the same chronic infections. If successful this approach should reduce the incidence of carcinoma of the cervix related to HPV infection.

References for further reading

Holmes KK, Mårdh PA, Sparks PF, Wiener PJ, eds. *Sexually Transmitted Diseases* 2nd ed. New York: McGraw Hill, 1990
Pastorek-II JG (ed). *Obstetric and Gynecological Infectious Disease*. New York: Raven Press, 1994.
Centers for Disease Control and Prevention. 1998 Guidelines for treatment of sexually transmitted diseases. *MMWR* 1998; **47**: 1–118. Also available at http: //www.cdc.gov/publications.htm.
Barton S, Hay P (eds). *The Handbook of Genitourinary Medicine.*, London: Arnold, 1999.
Website of the Medical Society for the Study of Venereal Disease. http: //www.mssvd.org.uk

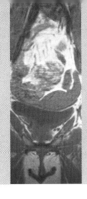

Chapter 17

Urogynaecology

OVERVIEW

Urogynaecological conditions include urinary incontinence, voiding difficulties, prolapse (see also Chapter 18), frequency and urgency, urinary tract infection and urinary fistulae. Increasingly it is recognized that the pelvic floor is one structure and this has led to an awareness of faecal incontinence and its treatment.

CLINICAL CONDITIONS

Introduction

Urinary incontinence is defined as the involuntary loss of urine that is objectively demonstrable and is a social or hygienic problem. It is an increasingly prevalent problem as the ageing population expands. It affects an individual's physical, psychological and social well-being and is associated with a significant reduction in quality of life. The prevalence increases with age, with approximately 5 per cent of women between 15 and 44 years of age being affected, rising to 10 per cent of those aged between 45 and 64 years and approximately 20 per cent of those greater than 65 years. It is even higher in women who are institutionalized and may affect up to 40 per cent of those in residential nursing homes.

Urinary incontinence is classified according to pathophysiological concepts rather than symptomatology, but the following definitions of symptoms are commonly used.

Common symptoms associated with incontinence

- Stress incontinence is a symptom and a sign and means loss of urine on physical effort. It is not a diagnosis.
- Urgency means a sudden desire to void.
- Urge incontinence is an involuntary loss of urine associated with a strong desire to void.
- Overflow incontinence occurs without any detrusor activity when the bladder is overdistended.
- Frequency is defined as the passing of urine seven or more times a day, or being awoken from sleep more than once a night to void.

Urethral causes

- Urethral sphincter incompetence (genuine stress incontinence)
- Detrusor instability or the unstable bladder – this is either neuropathic or non-neuropathic
- Retention with overflow.
- Congenital
- Miscellaneous

Extra urethral causes

- Congenital
- Fistula

Urethral causes of incontinence

Genuine stress incontinence

Genuine stress incontinence (GSI) occurs when the bladder pressure exceeds the maximum urethral pressure in the absence of any detrusor contraction.

Symptoms
Stress incontinence is the usual symptom but urgency, frequency and urge incontinence may be present. There may also be an awareness of prolapse.

On clinical examination stress incontinence may be demonstrated when the patient coughs. Vaginal examination should assess for prolapse and in particular assess the vaginal capacity and the woman's ability to elevate the bladder neck as this may alter management. It is quite usual to find a cystourethrocele in women with stress incontinence.

Urodynamic studies will define the cause of incontinence and are particularly important when there has been a previous, unsuccessful continence operation or if the symptomatology is complex (these are covered later in this chapter).

Detrusor instability

An unstable bladder is one that is shown objectively to contract, either spontaneously or on provocation, associated with symptoms during the filling phase of cystometry whilst the patient is attempting to inhibit

P   Understanding the pathophysiology

Likely causes of GSI are:
1. Abnormal descent of the bladder neck and approximal urethra, so there is failure of equal transmission of intra-abdominal pressure to the proximal urethra, leading to reversal of the normal pressure gradient between the bladder and urethra with a resultant negative urethral closure pressure.
2. An intraurethral pressure which at rest is lower than the intravesical pressure; this may be due to urethral scarring as a result of surgery or radiotherapy. It also occurs in the older woman.
3. Laxity of suburethral support normally provided by the vaginal wall, endopelvic fascia, arcus tendineus fascia and levator ani muscles acting as a single unit, results in ineffective compression during stress and consequent incontinence (Fig. 17.1).

The aetiology of GSI is thought to be related to a number of factors.
a) Damage to the nerve supply of the pelvic floor and urethral sphincter caused by childbirth leads to progressive changes in these structures resulting in altered function. In addition, mechanical trauma to the pelvic floor musculature and endopelvic fascia and ligaments occurs as a consequence of vaginal delivery. Prolonged second stage, large babies and instrumental deliveries cause the most damage.
b) Menopause and associated tissue atrophy may also cause problems to the pelvic floor.
c) A congenital cause may be inferred as some nulliparous women suffer from incontinence. This may be due to altered connective tissue, particularly collagen.
d) Chronic causes, such as obesity, chronic obstructive pulmonary disease, raise interabdominal pressure and constipation may also cause problems.

micturition. If there is evidence of neuropathy this condition is called detrusor hyper-reflexia.

Symptoms
The presenting symptoms include urgency, urge incontinence, frequency, nocturia, stress incontinence, enuresis and, sometimes, voiding difficulties.

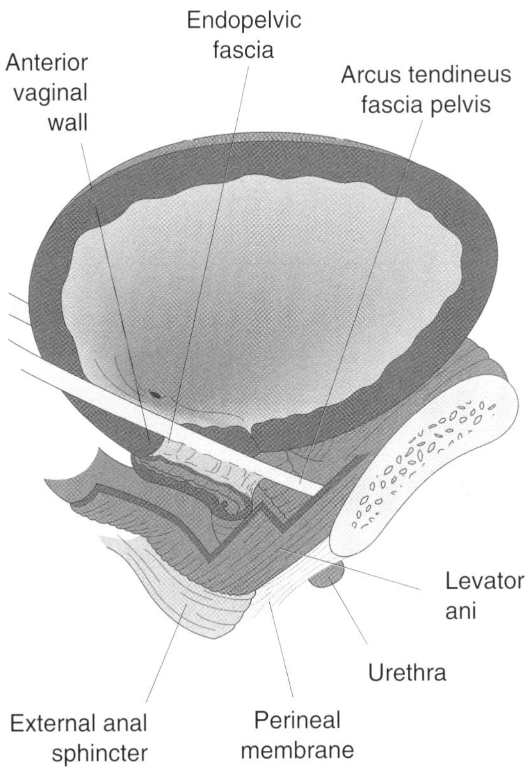

Figure 17.1 Diagram showing the suburethral support mechanism.

Examination

Any masses that cause compression of the bladder must be excluded and prolapse must be examined for as this may cause some of the symptoms. If there is vaginal atrophy this may also cause some urgency and frequency.

Investigations are considered later in the chapter.

Retention with overflow

Insidious failure of bladder emptying may lead to chronic retention and finally, when normal voiding is ineffective, to overflow incontinence. The causes may be:

- lower motor neurone or upper motor neurone lesions;
- urethral obstruction;
- pharmacological.

P | **Understanding the pathophysiology**

Detrusor instability

The pathophysiology of detrusor instability is poorly understood and the etiological factors require substantiation. Poor toilet habit training and psychological factors have been implicated.

The largest group of women with this condition have an idiopathic variety. Neuropathy appears to be the most substantiated factor. Incontinence surgery, outflow obstruction and smoking are also associated with detrusor overactivity.

The patient may be aware of and present with increasing difficulty in bladder emptying or she may present only with frequency. Ultimately normal emptying stops and a stage of chronic retention with overflow develops.

Symptoms

Symptoms include poor stream, incomplete bladder emptying and straining to void, together with overflow stress incontinence. Often there will be recurrent urinary tract infection.

Cystometry is usually required to make the diagnosis and bladder ultrasonography or intravenous urogram may be required to investigate the state of the upper urinary tract to exclude reflux.

Congenital

Epispadias, which is due to faulty midline fusion of mesoderm, results in a widened bladder neck, shortened urethra, separation of the symphysis pubis and imperfect sphincteric control.

The patient complains of stress incontinence which may not be apparent when lying down, but is noticeable when standing up. The physical appearance of epispadias is pathognomonic and a plain X-ray of the pelvis will show symphysial separation.

It is unlikely that a conventional suprapubic operation to elevate the bladder neck will be sufficient. It may be wiser to proceed straight to urethral reconstruction or an artificial urinary sphincter.

Miscellaneous

Acute urinary tract infection or faecal impaction in the elderly may lead to temporary urinary incontinence. A urethral diverticulum may lead to postmicturition dribble, as urine collects within the diverticulum and escapes as the patient stands up.

Extra urethral causes of incontinence

Congenital

Bladder exstrophy and ectopic ureter
In bladder exstrophy there is failure of mesodermal migration with breakdown of ectoderm and endoderm, resulting in absence of the anterior abdominal wall and anterior bladder wall. Extensive reconstructive surgery is necessary in the neonatal period.

An ectopic ureter may be single or bilateral and presents with incontinence only if the ectopic opening is outside the bladder, when it may open within the vagina or onto the perineum. The cure is excision of the ectopic ureter and the upper pole of the kidney that it drains.

Fistula

A urinary fistula is an abnormal opening between the urinary tract and the outside (Fig. 17.2). Urinary fistulae have obstetrical and gynaecological causes. The former includes obstructive labour with compression of the bladder between the presenting head and the bony wall of the pelvis. The gynaecological causes are associated with pelvic surgery or pelvic malignancy or radiotherapy.

Whatever the cause the fistula must be accurately localized. It can be treated by primary closure or by surgery and can be delayed until tissue inflammation and oedema have resolved at about four weeks. The surgical techniques involve isolation and removal of the fistula tract, careful debridement, suture and closure of each layer separately and without tension and, if necessary, the interposition of omentum which brings with it an additional blood supply.

Frequency and urgency

Frequency and urgency are two common urinary symptoms that present singularly or combined. Approximately 15–20 per cent of women have frequency and urgency. Clinical examination and investigation can be directed towards discriminating between the common causes. These include masses that cause compression and prolapse. Investigations should rule out infection, stones and malignancy. A simple urinary diary may show signs of increased fluid intake or evidence of ingestion of too much caffeine.

Voiding difficulties

Voiding difficulty, acute and chronic urinary retention represent a gradation of failure of bladder emptying. Of women attending a urodynamic clinic, 10–15 per cent may have voiding difficulties. The underlying mechanism is either failure of detrusor contraction or sphincteric relaxation, or urethral obstruction and this may be due to causes such as an impacted retroverted gravid uterus.

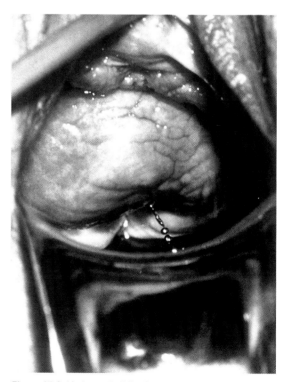

Figure 17.2 Vesicovaginal fistula.

Symptoms

The main symptoms are poor stream, incomplete emptying and straining to void. As the residual of urine increases in amount frequency occurs and urinary tract infection develops. Incontinence may follow and chronic retention and overflow may develop.

Examination

A full bladder may be palpated and there may be the primary signs of the cause of voiding difficulty. Investigations include uroflowmetry, cystometry and a lumbar sacral spine X-ray. Part of the assessment involves taking an accurate drug history as drugs such as anticholinergic agents may have been taken and the patient may be predisposed to retention.

Urinary tract infection

Acute and chronic urinary infection are important and avoidable sources of ill-health among women. The short urethra which is prone to entry of bacteria during intercourse, poor perineal hygiene and the occasional inefficient voiding ability of the patient and unnecessary catheterizations are all contributory factors.

A significant urinary infection is defined as the presence of a bacterial count $>10^5$ of the same organism per mL of freshly plated urine. On microscopy there are usually red blood cells and white blood cells. The common organisms are *E. coli*, *Proteus mirabilis*, *Klebsiella aerogenes*, *Pseudomonas* and *Streptococcus faecalis*. These gain entry to the urinary tract by a direct extension from the gut, lymphatic spread via the blood stream or transurethrally from the perineum. Symptoms include dysuria, frequency and occasionally haematuria. Loin pain and rigors and a temperature above 38°C usually indicate that acute pyelonephritis has developed.

A culture and sensitivity of mid-stream specimen of urine is required. Intravenous urography or venal ultrasonography may be required in patients with recurrent infection to define anatomical or functional abnormalities.

With acute urinary infection, once a mid-stream urine specimen has been sent for culture and sensitivity, antimicrobial therapy can begin. If the patient is ill the treatment should not be delayed and an antimicrobial drug regime can be started immediately. The regime can be changed later according to the results of the urine culture and sensitivity. Commonly used drugs include Trimethoprim 200 mg twice daily or Nitrofurantoin 100 mg four times daily or a Cephalosporin.

Recurrent urinary tract infection for which an identifiable source has not been found may be managed by long-term low-dose antimicrobial therapy, such as Trimethoprim. Recently Ciprofloxacin and Norfloxacin have been used with good efficacy.

It is important to treat urinary tract infections effectively, especially in the younger woman. The development of acute pyelonephritis during pregnancy can be a cause of faecal morbidity.

Investigations

An accurate and detailed history and examination provide a framework for the diagnosis but there is often a discrepancy between the patient's symptoms and the urodynamic findings. The aim of urodynamic investigations is to provide accurate diagnosis of disorders of micturition and involves investigation of the lower urinary tract and pelvic floor function.

Investigations range from simple procedures performed in the GP's surgery to sophisticated studies only available in tertiary referral centres. The clinician should pursue a streamlined yet meticulous evaluation, tailoring the investigations to the patient's clinical findings.

Mid-stream urine specimen

Urinary infection can produce a variety of urinary symptoms including incontinence. A nitrate stick test can suggest infection but a diagnosis is made from a clean, mid-stream specimen with a pure growth of more than 10^5 organisms per mL of urine. The presence of increased white blood cells alone suggests an infection and the test should be repeated. Invasive urodynamics can aggravate infection and test results are invalid when performed in the presence of infection.

Urinary diary

A urinary diary is a simple record of the patient's fluid intake and output (Fig. 17.3). Episodes of urgency and leakage and precipitating events are also recorded. There is no recommended period for diary keeping; a suggested practice is one week. These diaries are more accurate than patient recall and provide an assessment of functional bladder capacity. In addition to altering fluid intake, urinary diaries can be utilized to monitor conservative treatment, e.g. bladder re-education, electrical stimulation and drug therapy.

Pad test

Pad tests are used to verify and quantify urine loss. The International Continence Society pad test takes one hour. The patient wears a preweighed sanitary towel, drinks 500 mL of water and rests for 15 minutes. After a series of defined manoeuvres the pad is reweighed; a urine loss of more than 1 g is considered significant. If indicated, methylene blue solution can be instilled intravesically prior to the pad test to differentiate between urine and other loss, e.g.

insensible loss or vaginal discharge. The popularity of 24- and 48-hour pad tests is increasing because they are believed to be more representative. The woman performs normal daily activities and the pad is reweighed after the preferred period.

Uroflowmetry

Uroflowmetry is the measurement of urine flow rate and is a simple, non-invasive procedure that can be performed in the out-patient department (Fig. 17.4). It provides an objective measurement of voiding function and the patient can void in privacy.

Although uroflowmetry is performed as part of a general urodynamic assessment the main indications are complaints of hesitancy or difficulty in voiding in patients with neuropathy or a past history of urinary retention. It is also indicated prior to bladder neck or radical pelvic cancer surgery to exclude voiding problems that may deteriorate afterwards.

Time	Day 1			Day 2			Day 3	
	Input	Output		Input	Output		Input	Output
0700 hrs	250	150		200	160	W	250	170
0800 hrs		75	W		50			75
0900 hrs	200	140		200	55		150	60
1000 hrs		100			70			
1100 hrs	150			150		W	200	55
1200 hrs		60	W		100			60
1300 hrs	100	55		100	50			
1400 hrs		75						
1500 hrs			W	100				
1600 hrs	100							
1700 hrs								
1800 hrs								

Figure 17.3 Urinary diary.

The normal flow curve is bell-shaped. A flow rate below 15 mL on more than one occasion is considered abnormal in females. The voided volume should be above 150 mL as flow rates with smaller volumes are not reliable. A low peak flow rate and a prolonged voiding time suggest a voiding disorder. Straining can give abnormal flow patterns with interrupted flow. Uroflowmetry alone cannot diagnose the cause of impaired voiding: simultaneous measurement of voiding pressure allows a more detailed assessment.

Cystometry

Cystometry involves the measurement of the pressure–volume relationship of the bladder. It is still considered the most fundamental investigation. It involves simultaneous abdominal pressure recording in addition to intravesical pressure monitoring, during bladder filling and voiding. Electronic subtraction of abdominal from intravesical pressure enables determination of the detrusor pressure (Fig. 17.5).

Cystometry is indicated for the following.
1. Previous unsuccessful continence surgery.
2. Multiple symptoms, i.e. urge incontinence, stress incontinence and frequency.
3. Voiding disorder.
4. Neuropathic bladder.
5. Prior to primary continence surgery: this is still debatable if stress incontinence is the only symptom

Prior to cystometry, the patient voids on the flowmeter. A 12 French gauge catheter is inserted to fill the bladder and any residual urine is recorded. Intravesical pressure is measured using a 1 mm diameter fluid-filled catheter, inserted with the filling line, connected to an external pressure transducer. A fluid-filled 2 mm diameter catheter covered with a rubber finger cot to prevent faecal blockage, is inserted into the rectum, to measure intra-abdominal pressure. Microtip transducers can be used but are more expensive and fragile. The bladder is filled (in sitting and standing positions) with a continuous infusion of normal saline at room temperature. The standard filling rate is between 10 and 100 mL/min and is provocative for detrusor instability. During filling, the patient is asked to indicate her first and maximal desire to void and these volumes are noted. The presence of symptoms of urgency and pain and systolic detrusor contractions are noted. Any precipitating factors such as coughing or running water are recorded. Pressure rises during filling or standing are also noted. At maximum capacity, the filling line is removed and the patient stands. She is asked to cough and any leakage is documented. The patient then transfers to the uroflowmeter and voids with pressure lines in place. Once urinary flow is established she is asked to interrupt the flow if possible.

The following are parameters of normal bladder function.
1. Residual urine of less than 50 ml.

Figure 17.4 Normal uroflowmetry.

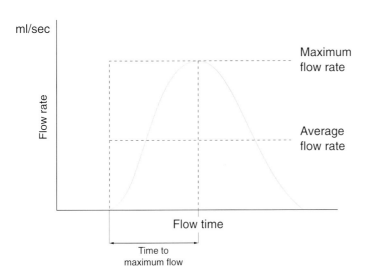

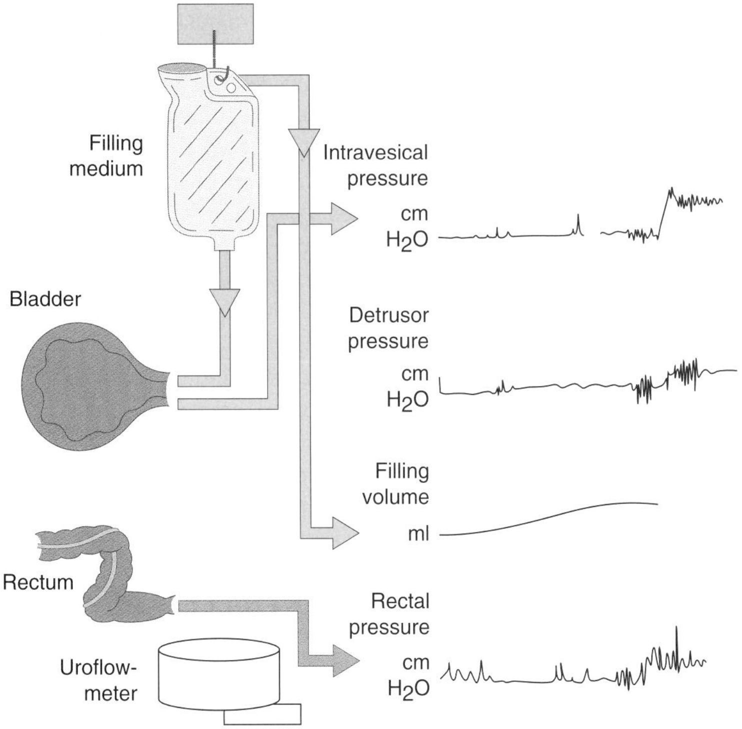

Figure 17.5 Schematic representation of subtracted cystometry.

2. First desire to void between 150 and 200 mL.
3. Capacity between 400 and 600 mL.
4. Detrusor pressure rise of less than 15 cm H_2O during filling and standing.
5. Absence of systolic detrusor contractions.
6. No leakage on coughing.
7. A voiding detrusor pressure rise of less than 70 cm H_2O with a peak flow rate of greater than 15 mL/s for a volume over 150 mL.

Detrusor instability is diagnosed when spontaneous or provoked detrusor contractions occur which the patient cannot suppress. Systolic detrusor instability is shown by phasic contractions, whilst low compliance detrusor instability is diagnosed when the pressure rise during filling is greater than 15 cm H_2O and does not settle when filling ceases. Genuine stress incontinence is diagnosed if leakage occurs as a result of coughing, in the absence of a rise in detrusor pressure.

Videocystourethrography (VCU)

If a radio-opaque filling medium is used during cystometry, then the lower urinary tract can be visualized by X-ray screening with an image intensifier. There are only a few situations in which VCU provides more information than cystometry. During bladder filling, vesico-ureteric reflux can be seen. As the screening table is moving to the erect position, any detrusor contraction and leakage can be noted. In the erect position the patient is asked to cough; bladder neck and base descent and leakage of contrast can be evaluated. During voiding, vesico-ureteric reflux, trabeculation and bladder and urethral diverticulae can be noted (Fig. 17.6).

Intravenous urography

This investigation provides little information about the lower urinary tract but is indicated in cases of haematuria, neuropathic bladder and suspected ureterovaginal fistula.

Ultrasound

Ultrasound is becoming more widely used in urogynaecology. Postmicturition urine residual estimation can be performed without the need for urethral catheterization and the associated risk of infection. This is useful in the investigation of patients with voiding difficulties, either idiopathic or following postoperative catheter removal. Urethral cysts and diverticula can also be examined using this technique.

Magnetic resonance imaging

Magnetic resonance imaging (MRI) produces accurate anatomical pictures of the pelvic floor and lower urinary tract and has been used to demarcate compartmental prolapse. Although still mostly experimental, the use of endopelvic coils allows fine detail imaging which may be useful in visualizing damage to the urethral sphincter mechanism.

Cystourethroscopy

Cystourethroscopy establishes the presence of disease in the urethra or bladder. There are few indications in women with incontinence.
1. Reduced bladder capacity.
2. Short history (<2 years) of urgency and frequency.
3. Suspected urethrovaginal or vesicovaginal fistula.
4. Haematuria or abnormal cytology.
5. Persistent urinary tract infection.

Urethral pressure profilometry

To maintain continence, the urethral pressure must remain higher than the intravesical pressure and various methods have been devised to measure urethral

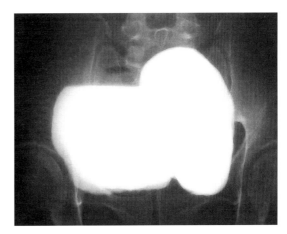

Figure 17.6 Videocystourethrography showing bladder diverticulum.

pressure. Urethral pressure profiles can be obtained using a catheter tip dual sensor microtransducer. Measurement of intraluminal pressure along the urethra at rest or stress (e.g. coughing) appears to be of little clinical value because of a large overlap between controls and women with GSI.

Ambulatory monitoring

During ambulatory monitoring, fine microtip transducers are inserted into the bladder and rectum and data is recorded and stored in a portable device carried by the patient. The pressures are recorded for 4–6 hours with physiological bladder filling and emptying. The data is subsequently downloaded on to computer software and a chart recording produced. It has become apparent that differences exist between values obtained for artificial and natural filling urodynamic systems in relation to pressure rise during filling and voiding pressure. Ambulatory monitoring appears to be more sensitive in the detection of detrusor instability than cystometry.

TREATMENT

Simple measures such as exclusion of urinary tract infection, restriction of fluid intake, modifying medication, e.g. diuretics, and treating chronic cough and constipation play an important role in the management of most types of urinary incontinence.

Genuine stress incontinence

Prevention

Shortening the second stage of delivery and reducing traumatic delivery may result in fewer women developing stress incontinence. The benefits of hormone replacement therapy have not been substantiated. Pelvic floor exercises either before or during pregnancy need to be evaluated.

Conservative management

Physiotherapy is the mainstay of the conservative treatment of stress incontinence. The rationale behind pelvic floor education is the reinforcement of cortical awareness of the levator ani muscle group, hypertrophy of existing muscle fibres and a general increase in muscle tone and strength.

With appropriate instruction and regular use between 40–60 per cent of women can derive benefit from pelvic floor exercises to the point where they decline any further intervention.

Premenopausal women appear to respond better than their postmenopausal counterparts. Motivation and good compliance are the key factors associated with success. Use of biofeedback techniques, e.g. perineometry and weighted cones can improve success rates. Maximal electrical stimulation is gaining popularity. A variety of devices have been used but have not been very successful.

Surgery

For women seeking cure the mainstay of treatment is surgery. The aims of surgery are:
1. restoration of the proximal urethra and bladder neck to the zone of intra-abdominal pressure transmission;
2. to increase urethral resistance;
3. a combination of both.

There is no general agreement on the best surgical procedure for women with GSI. The choice of operation depends on the clinical and urodynamic features of each patient, and the route of approach. The colposuspension operation (Fig. 17.7) is associated with the highest success rates in the hands of most surgeons. The success rate is over 95 per cent at one year, falling to 78 per cent at 15-year follow-up. However, for the elderly or frail patient with a scarred, narrowed vagina, an endoscopic bladder neck suspension, e.g. Pereyra, or Stamey, may be more appropriate because it is less invasive and allows quicker postoperative recovery. Laparoscopic colposuspension is gaining popularity but is associated with lower success rates than the traditional procedure.

When the bladder neck is adequately elevated and aligned with the symphysis pubis it is presumed that the incontinence is due to a defect in the sphincteric mechanism producing a low resistance, poorly functioning, drainpipe urethra. The procedures in these circumstances to increase outflow resistance are the artificial urinary sphincter and periurethral injections.

The artificial sphincter has been used since 1972. It is used where conventional surgery has failed and the patient is mentally alert and manually dexterous. It is a major procedure performed only in tertiary referral centres because of the level of expertise required. Most of the procedures have been performed on patients with neuropathic bladders but results for persistent female stress incontinence range from 66 to 85 per cent.

Periurethral bulking has attracted considerable interest because of the inherent simplicity of the technique, its applicability in cases where other surgery has failed and its use in the frail patient. With increasing consumer demand it is being used as a first-line surgical therapy for stress incontinence. Contigen collagen, subcutaneous fat, and microparticulate silicon (Macroplastique) have all been evaluated in the last decade. Subcutaneous fat, although cheap, has poor efficacy and therefore has lost popularity.

Contigen collagen is usually injected paraurethrally and Macroplastique transurethrally. Most authors inject collagen under local anaesthetic and Macroplastique under general anaesthetic. The principle is to inject the agents into the periurethral tissues at the level of the bladder neck aiming for bladder neck coaptation (Fig. 17.8).

Early success at three-month follow-up ranges from 80–90 per cent, but there is a time-dependent decline to approximately 50 per cent at 3–4 years. Complications are uncommon and minor. Dysuria, urinary tract infection and retention requiring overnight catheterization are occasionally encountered. When

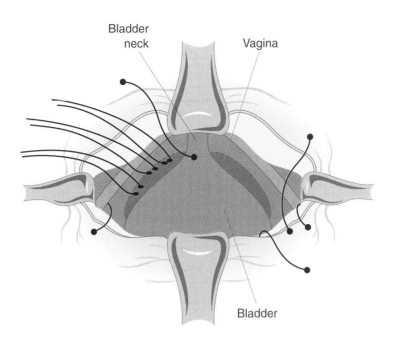

Bladder neck

Vagina

Bladder

Figure 17.7 Diagram showing colposuspension.

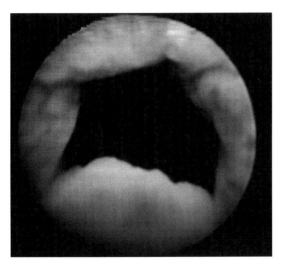

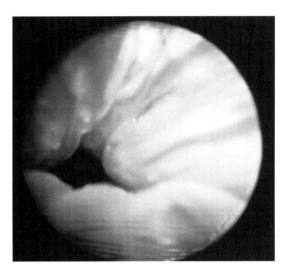

Figure 17.8 The bladder neck before (a) and after (b) collagen injection.

injectables fail, other bladder neck surgery can be performed without additional problems.

Detrusor instability and voiding difficulty

Detrusor instability can be treated by bladder retraining, biofeedback or hypnosis, all of which tend to increase the interval between voids and inhibit the symptoms of urgency. This is effective in between 60–70 per cent of individuals. Anticholinergic agents such as Oxybutynin 2.5 mg twice daily or Tolterodine 2 mg twice daily can be effective in 60–70 per cent of individuals. The latter has fewer side effects, such as dry mouth and constipation. Imipramine is often used for enuresis and Desmopressin (an antidiuretic hormone analogue) is useful for nocturia.

Neuropathic and non-neuropathic detrusor instability can be treated with anticholinergic drugs and when symptoms are resistant then intravesical therapy can be used.

At the end stage, bladder augmentation can be performed or even a ureterostomy. Bladder emptying can be achieved either by use of clean intermittent self-catheterization or by an indwelling suprapubic or urethral catheter. Drug therapy to encourage and aid detrusor contraction or relax the urethral sphincter is relatively ineffective.

New developments

The move towards evidence-based medicine has shown colposuspension to be the most widely practised and most effective operation for stress incontinence. The anterior repair and end stage bladder neck suspensions are not good operations in the medium- or long-term for this condition. The most important point is that the primary operation is the best chance of achieving success as the success rate falls with subsequent attempts.

A new operation called a tension-free vaginal tape, which is based on the theory of suburethral support, has been developed. This involves insertion of a Prolene tape underneath the midurethra and this is inserted through a very small vaginal incision with two tiny abdominal incisions. The novel part of the tape is that it is self-retaining and does not require fixation. Early and medium-term results are very encouraging. There is a short operative time and the procedure can be performed under local anaesthetic and may be one of the major advances in surgery for stress incontinence of recent times.

Key Points

- Urinary incontinence has a high prevalence affecting approximately 20–30% of the adult female population
- The most common causes are GSI and DI
- The mainstays of treatment for GSI are physiotherapy and surgery
- The most appropriate treatment for detrusor instability includes bladder retraining and anticholinergic medication
- Urinary tract infection must always be excluded as it can cause most urinary symptoms
- A woman with voiding difficulty may present with similar symptoms to women with GSI or DI
- Subtracted cystometry is the most useful investigation for the management of the incontinent patient
- Surgery for incontinence should be the patient's decision and must be tailored to clinical and urodynamic findings

CASE HISTORY

Mrs U Loss
54-year-old married caucasian, 95 kg.
Non-smoker, works as a library administrator.

Presents with a long history of stress incontinence, since the birth of her first child, which has worsened recently. There is also urgency and urge incontinence but this is not as severe as the stress incontinence. There is daytime frequency and nocturia but no history of voiding difficulty. She has had a previous total abdominal hysterectomy for menorrhagia.

She has four children, the first was a forceps delivery. The heaviest birth weight was 4 kg.

She is very fit and well but drinks a lot of coffee. She is sexually active.

Examination reveals a normal vaginal capacity and

mobility, the bladder neck can be elevated and there is no sign of any major prolapse.

Discussion

What is the most likely diagnosis?

This patient has mixed symptoms but probably has genuine stress incontinence. Urodynamics will help to elucidate the cause.

What treatments can she be offered?

Conservative measures would include weight loss and also reduction in caffeine intake.

It would be beneficial to offer her pelvic floor exercises first before considering surgery. If surgery was to be considered, as the bladder neck can be elevated, the operation of choice might be a colposuspension. Anterior repair carries much lower success rates and therefore should not be considered.

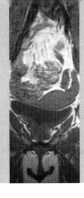

Uterovaginal prolapse

OVERVIEW

Uterovaginal prolapse is extremely common with an estimated 11% of women undergoing at least one operation for this condition. Conservative management involves the use of pessaries but surgery is the most appropriate management for the physically fit woman.

Definition

A prolapse is a protrusion of an organ or structure beyond its normal confines (Fig. 18.1). This is classified according to its location and the organ contained within it.

Prevalence

It is estimated that prolapse affects 12–30 per cent of multiparous and 2 per cent of nulliparous women. In the UK approximately 30 000 prolapse operations are performed each year and in the USA the number is 400 000. A woman has an 11 per cent lifetime risk of having an operation for prolapse.

Grading

Three degrees of prolapse are described and the lowest or most dependent portion of the prolapse is assessed whilst the patient is straining.

1st   descent within the vagina.
2nd   descent to the introitus.
3rd   descent outside the introitus.

In the case of uterovaginal prolapse the most dependent portion of the prolapse is the cervix and careful examination can differentiate uterovaginal descent from a long cervix. Third-degree uterine prolapse is termed procidentia and is usually accompanied by cystourethrocele and rectocele.

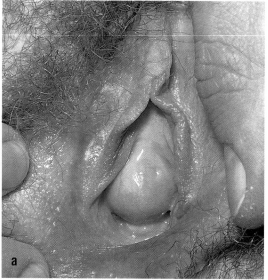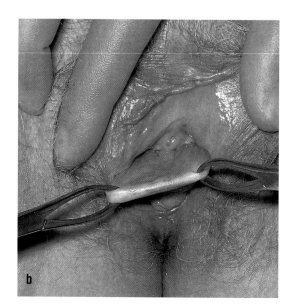

Figure 18.1 (a) A cystourethocele. (b) A vaginal vault prolapse.

Classification

Anterior vaginal wall prolapse		**Apical vaginal prolapse**	
Urethrocele	- urethral descent	Uterovaginal	- uterine descent with inversion of vaginal apex
Cystocele	- bladder descent		
Cystourethrocele	- descent of bladder and urethra	Vault	- post-hysterectomy inversion of vaginal apex
Posterior vaginal wall prolapse			
Rectocele	- rectal descent		
Enterocele	- small bowel descent		

Aetiology

The connective tissue, levator ani and intact nerve supply are vital for the maintenance of position of the pelvic structures, and are influenced by pregnancy, childbirth and ageing. Whether congenital or acquired, connective tissue defects appear to be important in the aetiology of prolapse and urinary stress incontinence.

Congenital

Two per cent of symptomatic prolapse occurs in nulliparous women implying that there may be a congenital weakness of connective tissue. In addition

genital prolapse is rare in Afro-Caribbean women suggesting genetic differences exist.

Childbirth and raised intra-abdominal pressure

The single major factor leading to the development of genital prolapse appears to be vaginal delivery. Studies of the levator ani and fascia have shown evidence of nerve and mechanical damage in women with prolapse, compared to those without, occurring as a result of vaginal delivery.

Parity is associated with increasing prolapse. The WHO Population Report (1984) suggested that prolapse was up to seven times more common in women who had more than seven children com-

P Understanding the pathophysiology

There are three components that are responsible for supporting the position of the uterus and vagina:

- ligaments and fascia by suspension from the pelvic side walls;
- levator ani muscles by constricting and thereby maintaining organ position;
- posterior angulation of the vagina which is enhanced by rises in abdominal pressure causing closure of the 'flap valve'.

Damage to any of these mechanisms will contribute to prolapse.

Endopelvic fascia is derived from the paramesonephric ducts and is histologically distinct from the fascia investing the pelvic musculature although attachments exist between the two. It is a continuous sheet that attaches laterally to the arcus tendineus fascia pelvis and levator ani muscles and extends from the symphysis pubis to the ischial spines. This network of tissue lies immediately beneath the peritoneum, surrounds the viscera and fills the space between the peritoneum above and the levators below and in parts it thickens to form ligaments, e.g. the uterosacral–cardinal complex. This complex is probably the most important component of the support. The segment of fascia that supports the bladder and lies between the bladder and vagina is known as pubocervical fascia and that which prevents anterior rectal protrusion and lies between rectum and posterior vagina is termed rectovaginal fascia.

(The levator muscles are described in Chapter 1)

pared to those who had one. Prolapse occurring during pregnancy is rare but is thought to be mediated by the effects of progesterone and relaxin. In addition the increase in intra-abdominal pressure will put an added strain on the pelvic floor and a raised intra-abdominal pressure outside of pregnancy (e.g. chronic cough or constipation) is also a risk factor.

Ageing

The process of ageing can result in loss of collagen and weakness of fascia and connective tissue. This effect is noted particularly during the post-menopause as a consequence of oestrogen deficiency.

Postoperative

Poor attention to vaginal vault support at the time of hysterectomy leads to vault prolapse in approximately 1 per cent of cases. Mechanical displacement as a result of gynaecological surgery such as colposuspension may lead to the development of a rectocele or enterocele.

Clinical features

History

Women usually present with non-specific symptoms. Specific symptoms may help to determine the type of prolapse. Aetiological factors should be enquired about.

Abdominal examination should be performed to exclude organomegaly or abdominopelvic mass.

Vaginal examination

Prolapse may be obvious when examining the patient in the dorsal position if it protrudes beyond the introitus; ulceration and/or atrophy may be apparent.

Vaginal pelvic examination should be performed and pelvic mass excluded.

The anterior and posterior vaginal walls and cervical descent should be assessed with the patient straining in the left lateral position, using a Sims

S Symptoms

Non-specific: Lump, local discomfort, backache, bleeding/infection if ulcerated, dyspareunia or apareunia. Rarely in extremely severe cystourethrocele, uterovaginal or vault prolapse renal failure may occur as a result of ureteric kinking.

Specific: Cystourethrocele - urinary frequency and urgency, voiding difficulty, urinary tract infection, stress incontinence.

Rectocele: Incomplete bowel emptying, digitation, splinting.

speculum. Combined rectal and vaginal digital examination can be an aid to differentiate rectocele from enterocele (Fig. 18.2).

Differential diagnosis

* Anterior wall prolapse - congenital or inclusion dermoid vaginal cyst, urethral diverticulum.
* Uterovaginal prolapse - large uterine polyp.

Investigations

There are no essential investigations. If urinary symptoms are present then urine microscopy, cystometry and cystoscopy should be considered. The relationship between urinary symptoms and prolapse is complex. Some women with cystourethrocele have concurrent incontinence, as the prolapse increases in severity, urethral kinking may restore continence but lead to voiding difficulty (see Chapter 17). Should renal failure be suspected then serum urea and creatinine should be evaluated and renal ultrasound performed.

Treatment

The choice of treatment depends on the patient's wishes, frailty and wish to preserve coital function.

Prior to specific treatment, attempts should be made to correct obesity, chronic cough or constipation. If the prolapse is ulcerated then a seven-day course of local oestrogen should be administered.

Prevention

Shortening the second stage of delivery and reducing traumatic delivery may result in fewer women developing a prolapse. The benefits of episiotomy and hormone replacement therapy at the menopause have not been substantiated.

Medical

Silicon rubber-based ring pessaries are the most popular form of conservative therapy. They are inserted into the vagina in a similar fashion to the

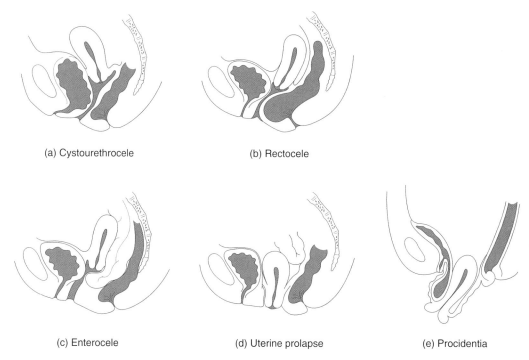

(a) Cystourethrocele   (b) Rectocele

(c) Enterocele   (d) Uterine prolapse   (e) Procidentia

Figure 18.2 Varieties of prolapse: (a) cystourethrocele; (b) rectocele; (c) enterocele; (d) uterine prolapse; (e) procidentia.

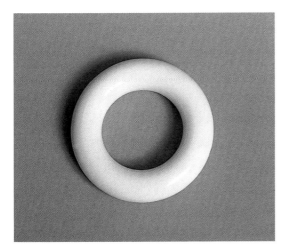

Figure 18.3 Ring pessary.

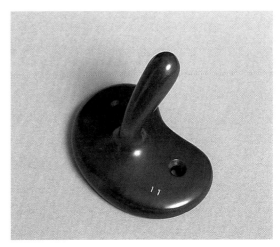

Figure 18.4 Shelf pessary.

contraceptive diaphragm and need replacement at annual intervals (Fig. 18.3). Shelf pessaries are rarely used but may be useful in women who cannot retain a ring pessary (Fig. 18.4). The use of pessaries can be complicated by vaginal ulceration and infection. The vagina should therefore be carefully inspected at the time of replacement.

Indications for pessary treatment

- Patient's wish.
- As a therapeutic test.
- Childbearing not complete.
- Medically unfit.
- During and after pregnancy (awaiting involution).
- While awaiting surgery.

Surgery

The aim of surgical repair is to restore anatomy and function. There are vaginal and abdominal operations designed to correct prolapse and choice often depends on a woman's desire to preserve coital function.

Cystourethrocele
Anterior repair or colporrhaphy is the commonest performed surgical procedure but should be avoided if there is concurrent stress incontinence. An anterior vaginal wall incision is made and the fascial defect allowing the bladder to herniate through is

identified and closed. With the bladder position restored any redundant vaginal epithelium is excised and the incision closed.

Rectocele
Posterior repair or colporrhaphy is the commonest procedure performed. A posterior vaginal wall incision is made and the fascial defect allowing the rectum to herniate through is identified and closed. With the rectal position restored any redundant vaginal epithelium is excised and the incision closed.

Enterocele
The surgical principles are similar to anterior and posterior repair but the peritoneal sac containing the small bowel should be excised. In addition, the pouch of Douglas is closed by approximating the peritoneum and/or the uterosacral ligaments.

Uterovaginal prolapse
If the woman does not wish to conserve her uterus for fertility or other reasons then a vaginal hysterectomy with adequate support of the vault to the uterosacrals is sufficient. If uterine conservation is required then the Manchester operation or sacrohysteropexy are alternatives.

The Manchester operation involves partial amputation of the cervix and approximation of the cardinal ligaments below the retained cervix remnant (it is usually combined with anterior and posterior repair. Sacrohysteropexy is an abdominal procedure and involves attachment of a synthetic

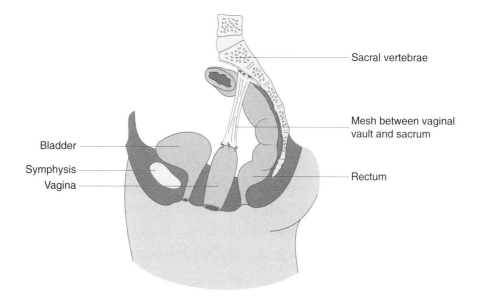

Figure 18.5 Sacrocolpopexy.

mesh from the uterocervical junction to the anterior longitudinal ligament of the sacrum. The pouch of Douglas is closed.

Vault prolapse

Sacrocolpopexy (Fig. 18.5) is similar to sacrohysteropexy but the inverted vaginal vault is attached to the sacrum using a mesh and the pouch of Douglas

is closed. Sacrospinous ligament fixation is a vaginal procedure where the vault is sutured to one or other sacrospinous ligament.

New developments

Collagen metabolism in vaginal skin from pre-menopausal women with uterovaginal prolapse and controls has been compared. There is a significant reduction in total collagen and an increase in immature cross-linking. Activity of matrix metalloproteinases (enzymes that break down collagen) was elevated. This suggests that the primary problem in genitourinary prolapse is increased collagen degradation causing a decrease in the mechanical strength of supporting fascia.

Fascial defect repairs - A variety of operations are described for the correction of prolapse most of them use either fascial or muscle plication or attachment to ligaments to support the vagina in its presumed original position. The recognition of specific fascial defects at three different levels of vaginal support resulting in different combinations of incontinence and prolapse, has prompted the development of surgical techniques aiming to repair these site-specific defects.

Key Points

- A prolapse is a protrusion of an organ or structure beyond its normal confines and is extremely common in multiparous women
- Damage to the major supports of the vagina, i.e. ligaments, fascia and levator ani muscles leads to prolapse
- Childbirth injury is the major aetiological factor
- Most women with prolapse present with non-specific symptoms such as a lump and backache
- Women with cystourethrocele often have urinary symptoms
- Women with rectocele often have bowel symptoms
- Diagnosis is made by clinical examination
- Surgery is the mainstay of treatment

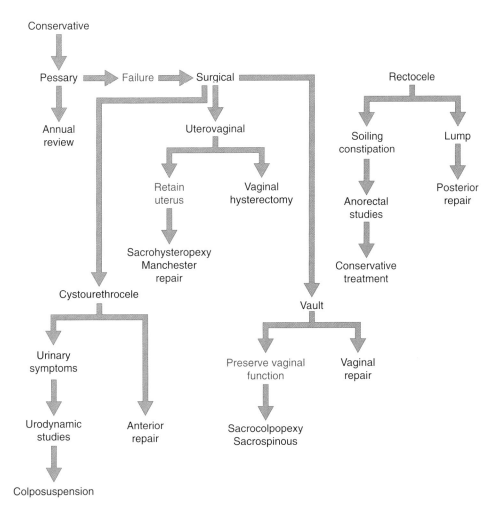

Figure 18.6 Treatment of prolapse.

Mrs PS

48 years old, married, Caucasian, 89 kg.
non-smoker, works as a nursing assistant in a nursing home.

Presents with an eight-month history of 'feeling a lump down below' and backache. The lump is bigger when she has been on her feet all day. She also complains of poor urinary stream and a feeling of incomplete emptying of her bladder. She admits to no urinary incontinence or bowel symptoms. She had a total abdominal hysterectomy three years previously for menorrhagia.

She has two children aged 24 and 22 years. Both were delivered vaginally, the heaviest at birth was 3.8 kg.

She suffers from asthma and uses Salbutamol and Becloforte inhalers. She is married and is sexually active.

Discussion

What is the most likely diagnosis?

Anterior vaginal wall prolapse is the most likely in view of her urinary symptoms, however vault prolapse and rectocele can also cause obstructive urinary symptoms.

What risk factors does she have for the development of prolapse?

- Vaginal delivery of a large infant can cause damage to pelvic nerves, endopelvic fascia and levator ani which can result in prolapse.
- She is overweight and this will increase the effect of abdominal pressure on the pelvic floor.
- She has a chronic cough and her job involves heavy lifting. Both these factors increase abdominal pressure.

References for further reading

Mallett VT, Bump RC. The epidemiology of female pelvic floor dysfunction. *Current Opinion in Obstetrics and Gynaecology* 1994; **6**:308–12.

Jackson SR, Avery NC, Tariton JF, Eckford SD, Abrams P, Bailey A. Changes in metabolism of collagen in genitourinary prolapse. *Lancet* 1995; **347**:1658–61.

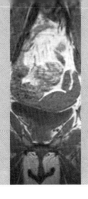

Chapter 19

Menopause

OVERVIEW

The term menopause is often misapplied and it is therefore worthwhile to define its origin and precise meaning. A derivation of the ancient Greek words *menos* (month) and *pausos* (ending), the term means the end of the monthly or menstrual cycle, the central external marker of human female fertility. A natural menopause, therefore, is deemed to have occurred after six months of secondary amenorrhoea in a woman aged 45 years or over.

Introduction

The menopause takes place at a modal age of 51 years in first-world countries – and therein lies the central demographic problem, for life expectancy in the UK is now at a modal age of 81 years for women. Thus, a woman at menopause today can expect to live for some 30 years, or 40 per cent of her life, in a state of relatively profound oestrogen deficiency (Fig. 19.1).

The considerable concentration of births in the late 1940s and early 1950s – popularly known as the baby boom – has resulted in some 40 per cent of the female population of the UK now being peri- or post-menopausal. Hence, any symptomatic or metabolic disturbance consequent of menopause that requires medical investigation will impose a significant effect upon the public health and a significant call upon the public purse in the form of NHS resources.

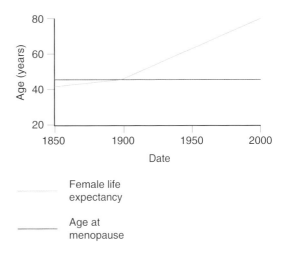

Figure 19.1 Age of menopause and age of mean life expectancy in females in the UK since 1850.

The menopause, as defined above, is simply one event in the whole range of anatomical, physiological and psychological events which contribute to the climacteric, a term also worthy of definition. Derived from the Greek *klimakter* (rung of a ladder), the climacteric was so termed to describe a major movement on life's ladder. It is the global expression for what the general public succinctly calls 'the change'. It is the transition from fertility to infertility, and occupies that decade, from 45–55 years, when a woman passes from her reproductive into her postreproductive years. It is attended by a wide variety of symptoms, signs and metabolic adjustments, the ultimate cause of which is a major reduction in the level of circulating oestrogen.

Pathophysiology

Premature ovarian failure

Secondary amenorrhoea due to ovarian failure to generate oestrogen may occur at any age and if below age 45 years may be reasonably accounted as premature. These patients exhibit low plasma E_2, usually below 150 pmol/L, high levels of follicle stimulating hormone (FSH), luteinizing hormone (LH) and a symptom pattern suggestive of oestrogen deficiency. The term resistant ovary syndrome describes a group of such women in whom the biological appearances of the ovary are normal, with abundant primordial follicles. In premature ovarian failure (POF), by contrast, the appearances are those of a postmenopausal ovary. POF is associated with other autoimmune endocrinopathies and in about half of patients other antibodies are present. However, the precise site of action of an antibody attack on the hypothalamic-pituitary ovarian axis is unknown.

Surgical menopause

Obviously, if for any reason both ovaries require to be surgically removed an obligatory menopause is immediate. At hysterectomy in premenopausal patients, even if both ovaries are conserved, a premature ovarian failure may supervene. Studies have indicated that the median age of menopause in

P | **Understanding the pathophysiology**

The human ovary basically consists of an outer cortex containing follicles at various stages of development, and a central medulla which is heavily vascularized. Both cortex and medulla contain stroma of mesenchymal origin which, in addition to their supportive function, are actively involved in steroid synthesis, principally of androgens. Stromal cells are recruited to form the thecal cells which surround the follicles. The primordial follicles number some 1.5 million at birth, the number having sharply declined from a peak of 7 million midway through gestation (Fig. 19.2). The vast majority of these primordial follicles become atretic and, in the reproductive lifetime of a healthy woman, only some 400 of the 400,000 follicles present at puberty will progress to ovulation. It is important to realize that it is the developing follicle that produces the bulk of the oestradiol circulating in the plasma of a premenopausal woman, the median level of which is usually between 400–500 υmol/L. Synthesis is principally from androstenedione and testosterone to oestradiol in the granulosa cells, which form the internal lining cells of the follicle. The androgen to oestrogen conversion is catalyzed by the aromatase enzyme cascade and is promoted by FSH. Theca cells also produce oestradiol from androgens whose elaboration from cholesterol is stimulated by LH.

The first signs of approaching menopause is a decline in fertility, where a downturn is apparent after the commencement of the fourth decade in most studies. The first endocrine change is a fall in inhibin production by the ovary. This glycoprotein inhibits the production of FSH by the anterior pituitary and hence, with this loss restraint, the plasma FSH concentration begins to rise above the premenopausal upper limit of <5 IU/L. The rise in LH values above the premenopausal limit of 12 IU/L is of later onset. Plasma values of both gonadotrophins remain elevated into old age. It is important to state that a significant amount of the postmenopausal androgen production is stimulated by FSH and LH, the principal site of oestrogen production being androstenedione conversion to oestrone in adipose tissue.

The cessation of cyclic bleeding takes many forms. The menstrual cycle may stop abruptly or may cease after a prolonged stage of oligomenorrhoea. Even after a substantial period of amenorrhoea a further cycle may occur which, if six months from the last, will be correctly classed as postmenopausal bleeding and will hence require investigation.

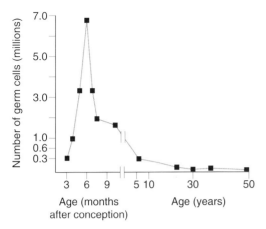

Figure 19.2 Total number of oocytes in the human ovary at different ages.

hysterectomized patients may be advanced by some 2–3 years but no prediction can be given at the time of operation as to which patients may or may not be affected. Such a menopause is, of course, occult due to the postoperative amenorrhoea and hence must be diagnosed on symptomatic and endocrine grounds.

A considerable debate still continues as to whether in women over the age of 45 oophorectomy should accompany hysterectomy. The principle argument for oophorectomy is the absolute prevention of subsequent ovarian cancer, and the principle argument for conservation is the retention of the steroid output from developing follicles until natural menopause, and from the ovarian stroma thereafter.

Other causes of menopause

Suppression of ovarian steroid output is physiological during lactation when the recurrent cycles of prolactin release on suckling inhibit both gonadotrophin drive to the ovaries and, possibly, intra-ovarian steroidogenesis. Therapeutically, the use of gonadotrophin-releasing hormone agonists in the treatment of endometriosis or in the preoperative containment of leiomyomata fibroids results in virtually complete suppression of ovarian steroid output. Such treatment, if given for over six months continuously, may result in major metabolic consequences such as significant loss of skeletal tissue.

The management of malignant disease in young women may provoke menopause in two ways. In premenopausal women with breast cancer radiation,

menopause may still be used to suppress oestrogen output, although this management may be superceded by pure oestrogen antagonists in future. The use of chemotherapeutic agents in such cases as breast cancer or the lymphomas may suppress and indeed arrest ovarian cyclic activity. Patients entering the management of such conditions should have the implications for their fertility and ovarian hormonal output fully discussed.

Symptoms of menopause

It is important to realize that the symptoms of oestrogen deficiency, loosely termed menopausal symptoms, may begin long before the cessation of menstruation which, as noted above, defines the menopause itself. These symptoms are often triggered by a relative fall in circulating oestradiol and hence may afflict the patient before the absolute level of circulating oestradiol reaches the levels of the fully developed postmenopause at <100 pmol/L. The physical symptoms of menopause include the classical vasomotor symptoms of hot flushing and night sweats. These are common and occur in at least 70 per cent of perimenopausal women. Their frequency varies widely from a few to several dozen per day and the duration may be from a few weeks to many years. Hot flushes are not contemporaneous with LH pulses and are essentially a vascular response to a central

S Symptoms

Physical
- Tiredness
- Hot flushes
- Night sweats
- Insomnia
- Vaginal dryness
- Urinary frequency

Psychological
- Mood swings
- Anxiety
- Loss of short-term memory
- Lack of concentration
- Loss of self-confidence
- Depression

disturbance of the thermoregulatory centre in the hypothalamus. There is a downshift of the set point of the centre in such that there is a frequent central misapprehension of excess body temperature. This in turn leads to activation of the physiological mechanisms such as cutaneous flushing and perspiration, which result in heat loss by radiation and by the loss of the latent heat of vaporization. If the episode occurs at night the patient, in addition to the vasomotor discomfort, may experience repeated awakening from sleep with consequent loss of sleep quantity and quality. In turn, this chronic incursion into the deep sleep–REM sleep–deep sleep rhythm may promote certain pyschological symptoms of which menopausal women frequently complain.

Vaginal dryness is a vitally important symptom of menopause, not least because it is frequently missed. Some patients find it difficult to give a sexual history and thus a gentle, courteous but full enquiry should be made regarding the presence of dryness and associated dyspareunia. This, in turn, can lead to significant disharmony between partners in a relationship. The vaginal skin is dependent on oestrogen for the depth and lubrication of its squamous epithelium and with loss of plasma oestrogen the skin becomes thin and poorly moisturized.

The physical symptoms of menopause are partnered by a set of psychological symptoms that can be equally distressing and disabling. The degree to which these symptoms are due to a lack of oestrogen *per se* or to chronic sleep deprivation is not settled. In addition, the perimenopausal years are frequently marked by life events such as divorce, departure of children, death of partner or parents and other stressful occurrences that may contribute to the overall psychological picture. Intrinsic personality type may also exert influence with the symptoms being more marked among those with a tendency to anxiety, neurosis and low self-esteem. There does not, however, appear to be a true increase in formal psychiatric disorders at this time.

Overall, it should be stressed that the severity, duration and nature of menopausal symptoms are highly variable. Symptoms may be absent, fleeting and mild or they may be severe and continue for years. The duty of the clinician is to assess the global effect of the symptom complex presented and to decide whether or not an exogenous replacement of the lost oestrogen is likely to result in a significant reduction in the symptom load.

Urinary symptoms

Menopausal women frequently complain of frequency, dysuria and urgency symptoms which suggest urinary tract infection (UTI) but which are not associated with a positive urine culture. The presence of oestrogen receptors in the trigone and proximal urethra may explain certain symptoms which should only be assigned to menopause if other causes have been excluded. Similarly, stress incontinence is also a frequent symptom at this time and in the absence of interovaginal prolapse may be attributed to oestrogen deficiency. However, direct experimental evidence of a true relationship is absent.

The skeletal system

The skeleton consists of 203 bones but of only two types of bone. Some 80 per cent of the skeleton is compact bone and is found, for example, in the shafts of the long bones. It is relatively insensitive to oestrogen. The remaining 20 per cent of bone is, in contrast, highly oestrogen-sensitive and is named after its trabecular structure. It is found at such sites as the vertebrae, the distal radius, the femoral neck and the calcaneus.

The relationship beween oestrogens and trabecular bone is complex and intimate. In summary, oestrogen acts as a physiological restraint on bone turnover and acts to hold the balance between bone resorption and bone formation. Over a four month period, each of the half million or so bone turnover sites in the skeleton moves through the unvarying sequence of bone removal and then bone replacement (Fig. 19.3). It is obvious that these processes should be balanced or be coupled to preserve bone mass.

However, with the loss of circulating oestrogen after menopause, a decoupling takes place that is characterized by a greater bone resorption than formation in the context of a general increase in the activation of new bone turnover sites on bone surfaces. Trabecular bone with its high surface area is thus particularly at risk. Trabecular bone is shock-absorbing bone. Its function is to absorb, dissipate and dispense incident kinetic-energy. This it accomplishes by means of the vast network of interconnecting trabeculae or struts that comprise its internal architecture. Hence when this network is degraded by the progres-

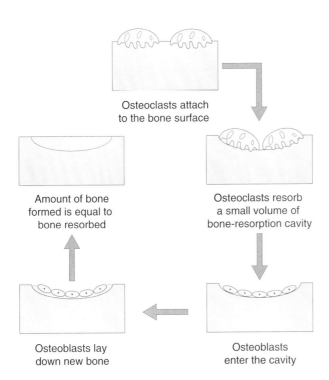

Osteoclasts attach
to the bone surface

Osteoclasts resorb
a small volume of
bone-resorption cavity

Amount of bone
formed is equal to
bone resorbed

Osteoblasts lay
down new bone

Osteoblasts
enter the cavity

Figure 19.3 The bone remodelling cycle shown clockwise from top. Some 0.5 million sites are operational simultaneously and each cycle takes approximately five months to complete.

sive loss of trabecular number, thickness and interconnection (Fig. 19.4), the bone becomes more liable to fracture after minimal or moderate trauma. The net result is that after menopause there is a progressive rise in the incidence of fracture of the trabecular sites. Traumatic fracture affects distal radius and femoral neck while non-traumatic fracture affects the vertebrae (Fig. 19.5).

Cardiovascular system

The function of the heart and great vessels is now known to be affected by the presence and by the relative absence of oestradiol. It has been known for many years that the incidence of such clinical events as myocardial infarction is much lower in premenopausal women than in men of the same age but a precise elucidation of the protective role of oestrogen has been slow to emerge. The decline in plasma oestrogen is attended by changes in the lipid profile that is conducive to atherogenesis.

- Total cholesterol   ↑
- HDL cholesterol   ↓
- LDL cholesterol   ↑
- Triglycerides   ↔

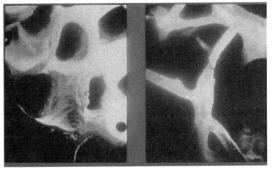

Figure 19.4 Normal bone is shown on the left. Osteoporotic bone is shown on the right. Note the reduction in trabecular number, breadth and connectivity.

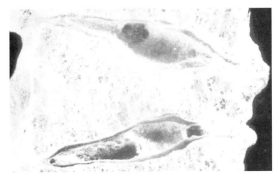

Figure 19.5 Sagittal section of human osteoporotic thoracic vertebrae. Note the wedging effect due to collapse of the trabecular structure anteriorly.

In addition to the lipid effects, oestrogen is now known to exert direct effects on the vessel wall. Oestradiol is known to stimulate the enzyme nitrogen synthase whose product, nitric oxide, is both a vasodilator and an oxidant for lipoprotein accumulating in the subintima. Loss of oestrogen can thus result in a promotion of both atherogenesis and vasoconstriction.

Hormone replacement therapy

Strong and opposing views on hormone replacement therapy (HRT) are held by professional and lay groups, extending from the view that the menopause is natural and physiological, and thus requires no intervention, to the view that it is a true hormonal deficiency state and thus should be treated with replacement therapy for life. Between these views is the compromise position that each patient should be examined and counselled on the individual nature of her problems, with HRT being offered when the presence of such symptoms or effects of oestrogen deficiency are such as to interfere with her personal, marital or occupational welfare. What is vital is that the woman herself has the final say in whether or not she will initiate and continue with such therapy.

Consultation

A full history is taken with concentration on those symptoms that are, or are likely to be, due to oestrogen deficiency – as listed above. Not only the presence of these symptoms but also the impact of them upon the patient's personal, domestic and occupational efficiency and fulfilment should be ascertained. It should be emphasized that gentle and courteous enquiry into sexual difficulties including loss of libido and dyspareunia should be made. In view of the longer term effects of oestrogen deficiency, the family history should include history of cardiovascular disease, particularly angina pectoris, myocardial infarction and stroke, and of skeletal disease in particular a history of osteoporosis manifested in relatives through height loss and low-trauma fracture to wrist, hip and other sites. The presence of Alzheimer's disease or other neurogenerative disease in the family is of relevance. The history of any gastrointestinal or liver disease that might interfere with the normal pharmacodynamics of oestrogen therapy must be sought.

The gynaecological history should include a record of all previous medical and surgical interventions, and in particular the presence of any conditions influenced by ambient plasma oestrogen, such as leiomyomata or endometriosis. A history of benign or malignant breast disease must be sought. Histological reports on any breast biopsy material should be scrutinized to determine whether or not cellular atypia was present as this may affect future management. The patient's mammographic record should be ascertained and she should be encouraged to accept all triennial recalls from age 50–64 in the national breast screening campaign. Any heavy, or persistently irregular, bleeding should be further investigated by pelvic ultrasonic examination proceeding, if required, to hysteroscopy and endometrial biopsy.

Examination

Any patient who is being considered for HRT must have a physical examination by a qualified practitioner. This is principally to identify the presence of potentially oestrogen-sensitive turnover in breast or pelvis. Thus, the patient should have a breast examination when she should also be advised, if necessary, on the techniques of breast awareness and examination. A pelvic examination should be performed and record made of any abnormality particularly uterine enlargement, the presence of fibroids and any signs suggestive of past or present endometriosis. Adnexal palpation to seek any ovarian turnover completes the examination. The blood pressure should be checked in the semi-recumbent position.

Modes of treatment

Oestrogen and the progestogens may be delivered by many routes. Most common in the UK is the oral route where the oestrogen is absorbed from the stomach and duodenum and is therefore passed up the portal system and through the liver *en route* to its other target sites. Oestradiol is largely converted in the liver parenchyma into oestrone, which is then released via the hepatic veins. This results in an oestradiol:oestrone ratio of 1:2, which is the reverse of the normal premenopausal position. Oral oestrogen can be taken at any time of the day. It is cheap and convenient and is usually well-tolerated.

The oral route does, however, result in the activation by oestrogen of certain hepatic enzymes resulting in the synthesis and release of such problems as cortical-binding globulin, resin substrate and sex hormone-binding globulin. No pronounced effects upon hepatic release of the proteins of the coagulation cascade have been observed. Nevertheless, some effect on this system is likely since there has been a recently reported increase in the risk of venous thromboembolism (VTE), from approximately 1.5 to approximately 3.5 per 10,000 per year.

Formerly oral oestrogen was given for three weeks out of four as in the combined oral contraceptive pill but the modern practice is to give oestrogen daily thus mimicking the perimenopausal daily release of hormone by the ovary. The oral oestrogens in common use are:

- oestradiol valerate 1 mg or 2 mg;
- conjugated equine oestrogen 0.625 mg or 1.25 mg;
- oestrone 1.25 mg.

Transdermal oestrogen

The advent of transdermal oestrogen, first by reservoir and now by matrix patches is a further attempt to mimic the physiology of the premenopause. The oestrogen which, being lipid soluble may transit across the epidermis, passes directly into the systemic circulation thus avoiding the hepatic first pass which is obligatory with the oral route. This maintains the oestradiol:oestrone ratio of 2:1 and is thus highly physiological. The reservoir patch in which the oestrogen is linked to an alcohol carrier may cause skin irritation and is being superseded by the matrix patch in which the oestradiol is incorporated into an adhesive matrix lined by a backing membrane. Skin reactions are few and absorption is steady with therapeutic plasma levels of oestradiol being achieved within four hours. Patches are available in varying strengths usually delivering 28 μg, 50, 75 or 100 μg of oestradiol per day and can be tailored to the individual patient's needs. Seven-day patches are now also available.

Transdermal HRT is of particular use in the older patient with, for example, osteoporosis in whom a very gradual build-up of oestrogen is required in order to avoid adverse start-up effects. Thus, the patient can be given a 25 μg patch for three months before advancing to the 50 μg therapeutic level. In general terms, the 50 μg patch has been found to have equivalent effects to 0.625 mg of conjugated equine oestrogen and 2 mg of oral oestradiol.

A variant of the transdermal patch is the percutaneous gel. In this mode of HRT delivery oestradiol is spread onto a convenient surface such as an upper arm, the metered dose from the container being some 2.5 g. Absorption produces therapeutic plasma levels within four days of commencement and the treatment is well-tolerated.

Subcutaneous implantation

This mode of delivery is restricted in the UK to patients who have undergone hysterectomy with or without oophorectomy. The procedure involves the positioning of a pellet of oestradiol in the subcutaneous tissue, usually of the lower abdomen, under sterile conditions and local anaesthetic. Implants are available at 25, 50 and 100 mg strengths and are usually reviewed at intervals of six months. They are very well tolerated and, of course, they obviate the need for daily or weekly action by the patient. Reports of tachyphylaxis have appeared in which patients are described as requesting re-implantation at progressively shorter intervals. In practice, however, this is rare but nevertheless re-implantation should be preceded by an annual check on plasma oestradiol which in most centres is not allowed to rise above 1000 pmol/L.

This mode of treatment successfully treats menopausal symptoms and also protects against bone loss. Indeed, there is now evidence that long-term E_2 implantation may be associated with a significant gain in bone mass at hip and spine.

Progestogens

In the premenopausal state, progesterone from the corpus luteum transforms the oestrogen-primed endometrium, which then sheds when progesterone production fails. In the 1970s early attempts to give oestrogen alone resulted in a significant degree of endometrial hyperplasia and neoplasia, and it was realized that, again, the physiology of the premenopause would have to be mimicked. To this end, studies showed that the administration of a progestogen for 12 days per month resulted in the secretory transformation of the endometrium and in satisfactory shedding (Table 9.1).

Unfortunately, the use of progestogens, particularly those of the 19-*nor* group which are derived

Table 19.1 – Progestogens used in conjunction with oestrogen (minimum treatment – 12 days/month)

Progestogen	Daily dose
C-21 Group	
Micronized progesterone	200 mg
Medroxytogesterone	10 mg
Dydrogesterone	10 mg
C-19-*nor* Group	
Norethisterone	1 mg
Norgesterel	0.15 mg

from testosterone, may cause adverse effects which may be of sufficient severity for the patient to give up treatment. These adverse effects include bloating, mastalgia and a PMS-like syndrome involving irritability and mood swings. When one considers that these are the very symptoms for which HRT is often prescribed in the first place, the necessary use of progestogen is seen to be a major potential problem.

In one method of avoiding cyclic progestational effects, the progestogen is given daily combined with the oestrogen in oral or transdermal therapy. This continuous combined approach has the effect of suppressing oestrogen receptor production in the endometrium thus preventing proliferation and rendering the patient free of the cyclic bleeding which many find unacceptable. Fears that the use of concomitant progestogen would annul the cardioprotective regime of oestrogen have proved unfounded in practice. Some 80 per cent of UK women at age 50 retain the uterus and should receive continuous or cyclic progestogen if being treated with HRT. Progestogen is not necessary in hysterectomized patients.

The progestogens commonly used for 12 days per month include, a C-21 group derived from native progesterone and a C-19-*nor* group derived from testosterone.

Gonadomimetic therapy

The only licensed product in this group is Tibolone, which is a synthetic steroid which exhibits oestrogenic, progestogenic and androgenic activity. Given in a dose of 2.5 mg per day to women at least one year

after menopause, it results in suppression of symptoms and the prevention of bone loss. Mild androgenic side effects may occur but in general the preparation is well-tolerated and the amenorrhoea, which is present in 80 per cent of patients by six months, is usually warmly welcomed.

Contraindications to HRT

- Absolute
  - Present or suspected pregnancy
  - Suspicion of breast cancer
  - Suspicion of endometrial cancer
  - Acute active liver disease
  - Uncontrolled hypertension
  - Confirmed venous thromboembolism
- Relative
  - Presence of uterine fibromyomata
  - Past history of benign breast disease
  - Unconfirmed venous thromboembolism
  - Chronic stable liver disease
  - Migraine

The presence of any of the above conditions in a patient being considered for HRT should result in a specialist referral so that further investigations can refine the balance between indication and contraindication. For example, the presence of benign breast fibrocystic disease but without atypia may allow treatment to proceed. Similarly, the finding of a normal thrombophilic screen in a patient with a history of unconfirmed DVT may allow oestrogen to be given.

Management of the patient receiving HRT

The first essential in management is the preparation of the patient for those symptoms that mark the reintroduction of oestrogen and progestogen into the circulation. The longer the elapsed time since menopause, the more likely these symptoms are to arise. Forewarned is forearmed and, equipped with the knowledge that the start-up symptoms are likely to be temporary and to remit by three months the patient is more likely to persevere over the first twelve critical weeks.

The similarity with certain symptoms of early pregnancy is striking and useful. Parous women will remember these symptoms and the fact that they

S Symptoms

The start-up symptoms of HRT include:
- breast tenderness
- nipple sensitivity
- appetite rise
- weight gain
- calf cramps

tend to remit at bout 12–14 weeks' gestation. If a patient is not so forewarned then the occurrence of, say, breast tenderness will distress and alarm her and she will be minded to stop treatment.

The time for the first critical review is at three months. At this stage enquiry should be made about the resolution of menopausal symptoms and of start-up effects. At three months the incidence of vasomotor symptoms reaches baseline and hence a critical review prior to this time may falsely indicate that treatment is failing. If no untoward effects are encountered the patient may be reviewed six months later and thereafter annually.

Annual review
There is no general agreement as to the constitution of an annual review.

Breast
The patient's participation in the national campaign should be verified. If the patient is breast aware, performing self-examination regularly, and in the mammographic programme, a full clinical breast examination is probably not necessary. If, however, there is any doubt over her breast awareness then an examination should be performed.

Blood pressure
This should be checked.

Pelvic examination
If the patient is amenorrhoeic on a continuous combined oestrogen/progestogen or gonadomimetic treatment or if she is bleeding on time and with normal flow on a cyclic regime, then routine pelvic examination is unlikely to disclose an abnormality. However, unscheduled bleeding, especially if it is heavy, prolonged or recurrent should always trigger a specialist consultation with a view to hysteroscopy

and biopsy if indicated. Further information may be obtained from ultrasonic evaluation of the pelvis either abdominally or, preferably transvaginally when leiomyomata or endometrial polyps may be identified.

Central nervous system

The favourable impact of HRT upon psychological symptoms of oestrogen deficiency has prompted enquiry into its possible role in the prevention and treatment of Alzheimer's disease and other related neurodegenerative disorders. The physiological basis for such studies rests upon the known ability of oestrogen to enhance central blood flow, its action as a monoamine oxidase inhibitor and the presence of oestrogen receptors in key areas of the CNS, such as the hippocampus, which is the point of interface between the short- and long-term memory.

To date, cognitive function has been shown to improve in symptomatic but not in asymptomatic perimenopausal women. A recent meta-analysis of ten observational studies addressing the incidence of dementia concluded that the prior use of oestrogen was associated with a decrease in incidence of about one-third. These observations held firm after adjustment for potentially confounding variables such as ethnic group, education and APO-E genotype.

The true relationship between HRT exposure and subsequent Alzheimer's disease and related dementia now urgently require testing by an interventional study, such as a randomized placebo-controlled trial. Treatment of established Alzheimer's disease with oestrogen has been reported in several small uncontrolled studies. No clear picture has emerged and hence the use of HRT in the established condition is not indicated. At present, HRT products are not licensed for the prevention of neurodegenerative disease.

Local oestrogens

The treatment of symptoms originating in the lower genital tract and in the bladder and urethra may be approached through the use of locally-applied oestrogen. In the form of a cream, pessary or vaginal tablet oestrogen may be inserted into the upper vagina where it will disperse and engage the local receptors. This route of delivery is suitable for those women whose symptoms are of genitourinary origin and in whom systemic delivery of oestrogen is unacceptable or hazardous. For example, in patients with a past history of breast cancer it may be beneficial to relieve local symptoms without elevating the plasma oestradiol. Presently licensed preparations for local use include: dinoestrol, oxestin, etc.

Other sites of action

The oestrogen receptor is now known to be of extremely wide distribution and it is likely that its presence in a specific tissue implies, but does not mandate, a role for the hormone in the optimal function of the tissue concerned.

The clinical importance of postmenopausal oestrogen deficiency and the usefulness of HRT have yet to be established in the majority of these tissues but several promising clinical leads are now to hand. It has recently been reported that the incidence of colonic cancer in HRT-treated women is lower than would have been expected in a control population.

New developments

Selective oestrogen receptor modulators (SERMs)

Recently clinical trial data has begun to appear concerning the SERMs. These agents are special or, in other words, specific. They do not engage the oestrogen receptor in all tissues but do so selectively with the central object of avoiding the two key disincentives to HRT continuation – bleeding and fear of breast cancer.

The first SERM, Raloxifene, is now licensed in the US and the EU for the prevention and treatment of bone loss. In summary, Raloxifene is a benzothiophene, and is related to Tamoxifen. It engages the oestrogen receptor and locks into the ligand-binding cavity at its core (Fig. 19.6a and b). However, in doing so the side chain of Raloxifene disables one of the activation function domains of the receptor (the AF-2 domain) necessary for oestrogen action at certain tissues, such as breast and uterus. The other activation domain function (AF-1) is unaffected and at sites, such as the skeleton, where its action is required Raloxifene behaves like an oestrogen.

Raloxifene does not modify the vasomotor symptoms of menopause and its use will initially be restricted to patients at risk of developing osteoporosis, such as those with premature menopause, steroid therapy and positive family history.

CASE HISTORY

Mrs CJ

54 year old; Caucasian, staff nurse

Presents with a history of early menopause at 44 years accompanied by vasomotor symptoms which have now ceased. Vaginal dryness and dyspareunia persist. She is overweight but not obese, BMI 29 and smokes occasionally. A breast biopsy three years ago led to local resection of a fibromyoma with atypia. Her mother died following a femoral neck fracture aged 83 and had previously lost height. Her father died of a myocardial infarction. She lives with a partner and is sexually active.

Discussion

The patient presents several risk factors for osteoporosis including premature menopause, positive family history and cigarette smoking. A bone mineral density scan, to include hip and spine is indicated.

Treatment

The absence of vasomotor or psychological symptoms of oestrogen deficiency together with the prior breast histology mitigate against the use of systemic oestrogen. However, for relief of the lower genital tract dryness, a local oestradiol by tablet or cream may be used.

If the densitometry scan confirms osteopenia (bone density was 1–2.5 Standard Deviations below the mean for young adults) then treatment with a selective oestrogen receptor modulator may be considered. Alternatively, bone loss may be prevented by means of a bisphosphonate. Dietary intake of calcium should be established and, if ≤1000g/day, should be supplemented. A weight bearing physical exercise programme of 20 minutes, three times per week, should be encouraged.

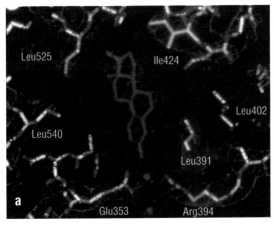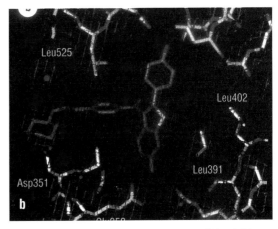

Figure 19.6 Electron crystallographic image of the ligand-binding domain of the oestrogen receptor with (a) oestradiol and (b) Raloxifene occupying the central cavity.

Key Points

- Median age of menopause is 51 years in the UK
- The central change is a tenfold reduction in plasma E_2
- Oestrogen's activities range far beyond the reproductive system
- Premenopausal amenorrhoea of >6 months should be investigated
- Physical and/or psychological symptoms should be treated if causing distress to the patient
- Bone loss after menopause may be arrested by exogenous oestrogen
- Progestogen is required for endometrial protection
- Selective oestrogen receptor modulators avoid withdrawal bleeding and breast cancer risk
- A careful breast and pelvic examination should precede HRT treatment
- Withdrawal bleeding and fear of breast cancer impede acceptance and continuance with HRT

References for further reading

Panney J, *et al.* Management of the Menopause. In: Grossman A. (ed.) *Clinical Endocrinology*. Oxford: Blackwell, 1998, 769–86.

Carr BR. Disorders of the Ovary. In: Wilson JD, Foster DW (eds). *Williams' Textbook of Endocrinology*. Philadelphia: W B Saunders Co. 1992, 733–98.

The British Menopause Society Handbook (available from BMS Offices, Marlow, Bucks SL7 2NB).

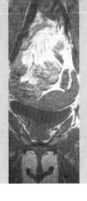

Psychological aspects of gynaecology

OVERVIEW

A woman is likely to experience a variety of changes to her body throughout her life: puberty, the menstrual cycle, pregnancy and the menopause are all states defined by physical change. The ability to adapt to these and other life events is important and if there are difficulties the woman's sense of wellbeing may be adversely affected, which, in turn, may have an effect on her ability to function in other areas of her life. Understanding the psychosocial aspects of gynaecology is therefore important and will help ensure a holistic approach is adopted, integrating physical, psychological and cultural dimensions.

Introduction

Puberty

With puberty there are enormous physical changes and the young woman must come to terms with her changing body shape, menstruation and awareness of her own femininity and sexuality. Through the phase of adolescence that follows, the main tasks are separation from the family, formation of identity and coming to terms with sexuality and its attendant demands for decisions about sexual orientation, behaviour and relationships. Risk-taking behaviour is a natural part of this growing up process. Not all adolescents complete the above tasks and therefore some remain dependent and insecure.

Transition to parenthood

With parenthood comes loss of freedom. Depression and sexual difficulties are common following childbirth. A woman's withdrawal from her partner, both emotionally and sexually, may be an expression of her perceived inadequacy in the face of extra responsibility.

Menopause

At the time of the menopause emotional upset comes from several sources. Loss of oestrogen causes physical discomfort and symbolizes the loss of youth and potential. As elderly parents die the sense of personal mortality grows and as children leave home a new purpose in life needs to be found.

Menstrual problems

Emotional problems can affect the menstrual cycle. Most women experience this at some time, such as missing a period when anxious about exams. The emotional disturbance can be more protracted and can lead to amenorrhoea, e.g. in anorexia nervosa.

Menorrhagia and psychosomatic factors may interact in one of the following ways.

- Heavy periods and consequent anaemia may lead to considerable distress and lethargy.
- Anxious or depressed women may be less tolerant of their periods and therefore report menorrhagia or dysmenorrhoea more frequently as an acceptable symptom to obtain medical help.
- Chronically anxious or depressed women may unconsciously use the complaint of menorrhagia to avoid sexual intimacy or pregnancy.

Psychosocial factors from the history should alert the gynaecologist to the possibility of an emotional disturbance underlying the presentation of menorrhagia and other gynaecological problems. These are:

- multiple social problems;
- relationship problems;
- recent life stress, e.g. divorce, bereavement;
- dysfunctional family background;
- history of self abuse, e.g. alcohol, drugs, self harm, eating disorders;
- symptoms suggestive of chronic anxiety or depression.

If several of these factors are present in the history, together with normal findings on examination and investigation, it is important to refer to a counsellor or psychologist and not to resort to surgery in the first instance. Some women will not accept that there could be a psychological component to their problem and as part of this denial will insist that surgery is the answer. It is easy for the gynaecologist to collude and perform a hysterectomy only to find that the underlying depression gets worse. The woman is often dissatisfied after surgery and will look for other surgical solutions to cut out her unacceptable psychic pain.

Referral for psychological help can be very threatening for women who have a heavy investment in denial. They may feel they are being accused of malingering and that the problem is 'all in the mind'. It is important that the gynaecologist does not give the impression that they think the woman is malingering but instead is able to accept and believe the woman's story and empathize with the importance and reality of her symptoms. At the same time a non-judgemental link between psychological distress and physical illness can be made.

Premenstrual syndrome

Research has shown that women who keep diaries about premenstrual symptoms and who are aware of the purpose of the diary over-report psychological symptoms compared to women who are ignorant of the purpose of the diary. Under these conditions a correlation between the premenstrual phase and negative mood has not been made so readily. The only symptoms consistently linked to the premenstrual phase are pain and water retention and not the psychological ones.

Psychological symptoms are more likely to present in women with pre-existing psychological or social problems. Evidence suggests that in a society where women are expected to be emotionally out of control premenstrually, negative emotions expressed premenstrually will be attributed to being governed by female hormones. The danger in attributing negative feelings to internal uncontrollable forces is that women may avoid solving situational and relationship problems. Gynaecologists should be wary of colluding in this avoidance. It is too easy to prescribe hormones or other drug therapies without attending to the woman's background or current environment.

Transactional analysis (TA), originated by the American psychiatrist Eric Berne in the 1960s, is a model for understanding human personalities, relationships and communication. Using TA concepts, Stephen Karpman devised a model for looking at dysfunctional relationships. He proposed that people who play games may be in one of three roles, Persecutor, Rescuer or Victim. A Persecutor is someone who discounts other people by putting them down. A Rescuer is someone who discounts other people by helping them because they assume they are incapable of helping themselves. A Victim discounts themselves and will agree with the put down or the concept that they are helpless. These three roles together form the Drama Triangle (Fig. 20.1).

Women with premenstrual mood disturbance tend to adopt the role of Rescuer during the first half

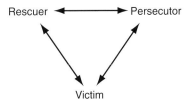

Figure 20.1 The Drama Triangle.

of their cycle when they feel full of energy. They often perceive a change of energy levels as they approach their next period and change to being a Victim, put upon by others. They become resentful of doing everything for their friends and family and turn into the irritable Persecutor. A psychological approach to working with women with PMS can therefore help the sufferer to gain insights into these shifts and to learn assertiveness skills and relaxation techniques. These will reduce the tendency to rescue others in the first half of the cycle and be aggressive in the second.

Menopause

Attitudes to the menopause range from relief to acute dread. It is reasonable to assume that no-one wishes to get older and lose their physical and mental abilities. Since the menopause is often seen as the beginning of these changes, it is likely that the woman who affects indifference will be denying her anxiety. If the denial worked it would be a satisfactory way of dealing with the anxiety, but it often fails and anxiety emerges in other ways such as physical symptoms or as excessive emotional reaction to ordinary situations.

For many women the menopause coincides with a variety of stressful life events that can affect how they perceive and cope with the physical changes.

- Empty nest syndrome.
- Retirement.
- Divorce.
- Bereavement.
- Elderly parents.
- Teenage children.
- Moving home.

Hormone replacement therapy (HRT) can be used for the short- and long-term alleviation of unpleasant symptoms and health risks associated with oestrogen loss. Some women also see it as a means of retaining youth or of denying the stress of co-existing life events. Inability to adjust to the reality of aging can lead to depression, especially when long-term HRT is withdrawn.

Infertility

Infertility is very stressful, with cycles of continual hope and disappointment (loss). Life for these women centres around having a baby. Nothing else seems important and partners blame each other and become frustrated and guilty.

The more advanced technology becomes, the more difficult it is to accept infertility, and it is partly the gynaecologist's role to help a patient judge when to withdraw from what may become an obsession. By the very nature of her problems the infertile woman becomes increasingly divorced from any normal doubts about having a child. The more it seems she may be denied her natural inheritance, the more desperate she becomes in her efforts to obtain it. Paradoxically, it is the woman who always wanted children who is best able to accept disappointment and to adopt, or to seek fulfilment by working with children. The woman who originally did not want children may become desperate, depressed and unable to face life without a child. There are many unconscious reasons why some women do not want a child.

- Their mother's life was a drudgery therefore motherhood is to be avoided.
- Hatred of younger siblings displacing them leading to a fear that they hate babies.
- A successful career is valued more highly than motherhood.
- Avoidance of having a child of a gender that is hated or feared.
- Desire to have been born be a boy. Motherhood is the ultimate proof they are 'only a woman'.

The question of adoption can give insight into these problems, and much can be learned from the women's response to the idea of adoption. The woman who realistically wants a baby will consider adoption. Those who will not consider adoption may be unconsciously wanting a baby to prove some point about themselves, or may be ambivalent to motherhood.

Fertility choice and control

The responsibility of controlling conception and choosing when to conceive ideally rests with the couple, although frequently the woman takes it on as her sole responsibility.

Women need a sense of positive self worth and the ability to make decisions in order to exercise this responsibility. It is not uncommon for personal issues relating to low self-esteem and impulse control to present as contraceptive problems or unwanted pregnancy. It is important to be aware of the possibility of such problems in women who present with multiple symptoms that prevent them settling with one contraceptive method. When method failure has been excluded, an unwanted pregnancy is likely to be the end result of some inner conflict over an unconscious need.

- To love or be loved.
- To right the wrongs of their own childhood experiences.
- To establish control by rebelling.
- To be successful at something.

Chronic pelvic pain without pathology

Chronic pelvic pain is a common symptom presenting in gynaecology outpatients.

Following laparoscopy about two-thirds of women will be found to have no pathology, but even the presence of pathology does not mean that the cause of the pain has been found. It may be a somatic expression of psychic pain. The unconscious pay-off being avoidance of conflict relating to issues such as sex, intimacy or pregnancy.

Self-monitoring and a heightened awareness of pain is particularly apparent in women who have a past history of pelvic pathology or who have a family history of pelvic disease. This increased awareness leads to distress and the discomfort is relabelled pain, which heightens the distress and sets up a vicious circle. The distress can be reinforced by family members.

Sexual problems

Sexual intimacy is a fundamental aspect of humanity, which is of much deeper significance than the reproductive element. Sexual problems in women can be primary, secondary, situational or total and may occur in any of the phases of the sexual response cycle. Sexual dysfunctions are difficult to classify and several dysfunctions may overlap. Common precipitating and predisposing factors for sexual problems are summarized in the box.

Sexual expression is complex. There is interaction between:
- the instinctive reproductive drive;
- emotional responses;
- thought processes;
- physical actions;
- physiological changes.

The possibility of conflict surrounding sexual expression may be due to:
- lack of information;
- belief in sexual myths;
- poor communication skills;
- expectations from past generations leading to guilt;
- expectations from current generation leading to performance pressure.

Difficulty in any of these areas can interfere with the final integration of responses necessary for the sexual fulfilment of two people. Failure in any aspect of the sexual response is likely to feed into a fear of failure on future occasions thus perpetuating a vicious cycle.

Female sexual behaviour

The 1994 Sexual Attitudes and Lifestyles Survey has extended understanding of female sexual behaviour in Great Britain.
- Women are experiencing first intercourse at a younger age.
- Vaginal intercourse is the most common activity.
- Non-penetrative sex including fellatio and cunnilingus contribute to the sexual experiences of the majority of the female population.
- Anal sex is a minority activity.
- Younger women tend to have more partners than the older cohort.
- Serial monogamy remains the main pattern.
- Homosexual activity is reported by a minority of women; 4.5 per cent sexual attraction, 3.5 per cent sexual contact and 1.5 per cent genital contact.

P Understanding the pathophysiology

Physiological/organic or iatrogenic factors:

- Child birth, menopause and aging
- Directly affecting the sexual response, e.g. diabetic autonomic neuropathy
- Alteration of genital anatomy, e.g. postsurgery or radiotherapy for gynaecological cancers
- Mobility for sexual activity affected, e.g. spinal cord injury, cerebrovascular accident
- Musculoskeletal pain limiting sexual activity, e.g. rheumatoid arthritis
- Genital pain limiting sexual activity, e.g. vestibulitis, episiotomy scar
- General ill health leading to fatigue, e.g. anaemia, renal failure
- Secondary to medication side effects, e.g. antidepressants, antihypertensives

It is important to remember that although organic or iatrogenic factors can affect sexual function, a psychological component usually coexists. Loss of previous sexual function can lead to a grief reaction and loss of confidence because of a poor self/body image.

Psychosocial factors:

Lack of, or incorrect, information about sex: Many adults still lack knowledge about sexual anatomy, physiology and behaviour. They may have received inadequate information due to a restrictive upbringing, incorrect information from peers or a false impression of sexual behaviour from the media.

Sexual myths and taboos: Our values systems, beliefs and attitudes develop within our family, social, cultural and religious experiences. Myths and taboos about sexual behaviour evolve within different cultural frameworks and perpetuate guilt and shame about sexual activity.

Examples of sexual myths:

- Performance is everything
- The man is responsible for the woman's orgasm
- The woman is responsible for the man's erection
- Good sex is spontaneous sex
- Only loose women initiate sexual activity
- Sex equals intercourse.
- Mind-reading – when in love one doesn't need to tell one's partner what is wanted because they already know.

Communication problems: Talking about sex can be embarrassing. One partner may think they can mind-read the other partner's needs and the other partner may fear upsetting them if they are honest and tell them that their sexual technique is not enjoyable. Also fear, anger, resentment or guilt can build up in a relationship because of general communication problems and these can be acted out as sexual avoidance.

Predisposing, precipitating and perpetuating factors: Past experiences, life events and behaviour patterns for dealing with problems can all contribute to the onset and maintenance of sexual problems.

Differing and unrealistic expectations: Problems can arise when partners have a different need for sexual expression, particularly if they have different levels of sex drive. Problems can also arise due to unrealistic expectations which lead to performance pressure and fear of failure.

Examples of unrealistic expectations:

- No change in sexual interest when ill, tired or bereaved
- To always achieve orgasm during intercourse
- Mutual orgasm on every occasion
- To return to the same interest in sex after childbirth
- Performance to remain unchanged by age

Other studies indicate that:
- eighty-five per cent of women have masturbated;
- most women find it easier to reach orgasm through clitoral stimulation rather than coitus.

The sexual response cycle

Sex drive underlies the sexual response cycle, which consists of four phases.

1 Desire.
2 Arousal (subdivided into excitement and plateau).
3 Orgasm.
4 Resolution.

Compared to men, on average women take longer than men to reach the plateau phase of arousal.

Effects of aging – the time to reach plateau phase increases further and intensity of orgasm declines.

The physiological changes occurring in the female genitalia during the sexual response cycle are summarized in Figure 20.2 and Table 20.1.

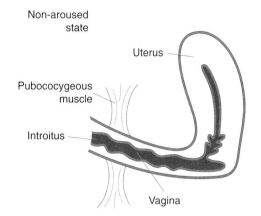

Non-aroused state

Uterus

Pubococygeous muscle

Introitus

Vagina

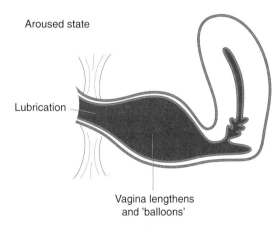

Aroused state

Lubrication

Vagina lengthens and 'balloons'

Figure 20.2 Physiological changes occuring in the female genitalia during the sexual response cycle.

Classification of sexual disorders

The DSMiV classification is:

Sexual desire disorders	Hypoactive sexual desire
	Sexual aversion disorder
	Excessive sexual desire

Arousal disorder

Orgasmic disorder

| Sexual pain disorder | Dyspareunia |
| | Vaginismus |

Prevalence

The prevalence of female sexual problems in the population is unknown. A variety of scientific and unscientific studies, on general or clinic populations, have attempted to quantify the frequency of sexual problems and it appears that about 60 per cent of women will have a sexual problem at some time.

The most commonly presenting problems are:

- decreased frequency either due to low desire or avoidance;
- problems with penetration;
- problems with orgasm.

Assessment

Taking a sexual history
The first concern of the doctor in history taking must be to accurately identify the area of difficulty, i.e. emotional or physical, since it is easy for trouble

Table 20.1 – Physiological changes occurring in the female genitalia during the sexual response cycle

	Excitement	Plateau	Orgasm	Resolution
Labia	—	Vaso-congestion red >> burgundy	—	10–15 secs
Clitoris	Vaso-congestion	Retracts flat under hood	—	5–10 secs
Vagina	Lubrication Vaso-congestion Ballooning of inner two-thirds	The same plus orgasmic platform of outer third	Contracts 0.8 secs × 3–15	10–15 secs
Uterus	Engorged Rises from pelvic floor	Completes ascent	Cervix opens and contracts	20–30 mins

Sexual history

Childhood and adolescent experiences

- Family background and relationships
- Cultural and religious background
- Family attitudes to sexuality, intimacy and expression of emotion
- Traumatic sexual or other life experiences
- Sex education
- Experience of puberty
- Sexual opportunities, masturbation, non-coital and coital experiences

Adult experiences

- Past relationships
- Traumatic life events

Current experiences

- History of the presenting problem
- Details of the current sexual dysfunction
- Present sexual practices and preferences including masturbation
- Present relationship(s)
- Sexual orientation
- Use of fantasy, erotic material or sex aids

Medical history

- Past medical and surgical history
- Past gynaecological and obstetric history
- Drug history both social and therapeutic
- Contraception/infertility

in one area to be mistaken for trouble in the other. Experience shows that when symptoms seem to be physical there is a risk that the more elusive and difficult emotional cause may be ignored. Taking a sexual history therefore requires sensitivity, careful attention to detail and good communication skills.

Whenever there is a sexual problem the patient is likely to be embarrassed when talking about the problem. It is therefore important that health professionals develop an open, non-judgemental style that encourages talking about such sensitive matters as sexual orientation, masturbation, fantasies and affairs. It is important to be confident about the use of language and sexually explicit words and to check a patient's understanding of these words. The patient's verbal and body language can be a window into their belief systems, their fears and their shame.

Examination

When examining a patient with a sexual problem it is important to progress at a pace the patient can cope with. This is particularly important in patients who have been sexually abused. The patient needs to feel in control of the situation. The way in which a patient responds to the genital examination can give insight into how they feel about their sexuality. This insight can be used diagnostically and therapeutically.

Investigations

Investigations (Table 20.3) should be performed selectively depending on the possible underlying causes for a sexual problem (Table 20.2).

Table 20.2 – Common precipitating and predisposing factors underlying causes for sexual problems

Precipitating factors	Predisposing factors
Parenthood	Physical, emotional or
Illness	sexual abuse in childhood
Random failure	Restrictive upbringing
Life stresses	Lack of information
Performance pressure	Poor self-esteem
Traumatic sexual	Poor body image
experience	Communication identity
	Psychiatric illness

Sexual therapy/psychosexual counselling

All health professionals should be trained to offer first line education, advice and guidance especially if they work in a specialty that deals specifically with aspects of sexuality, such as gynaecology.

Outcome research in the field of sex therapy is notoriously difficult. Many couples and individuals present with more than one dysfunction and with mixed organic and psychogenic factors. The variables involved are complex and confuse outcome results. Further confusion has arisen because of failure to define dysfunctions by internationally agreed classifications. Finally, a successful outcome defined by the

Table 20.3 Investigations to consider for a sexual problem

Sexual problem	Disorder	Investigation
Loss of desire	Anaemia	FBC
	Renal disease	U&Es
	Liver disease	LFTs
	Hyperprolactinaemia	Prolactin
	Hypothyroidism	TFTs
Superficial dyspareunia	Genital infections	STD screen
	Dermatological problem	Skin biopsy
Deep dyspareunia	Urinary tract infection	MSU/IVU
	Pelvic inflammatory disease	Ultrasound/laparoscopy

patient may not be a resolution of the dysfunction. Sometimes the individual or couple find ways of adapting to the dysfunction and therefore satisfaction with the outcome maybe more relevant than 'success'.

Management of sexual problems due to physiological or pathological change

Most NHS services that work with sexual problems offer general management such as:
• education, advice and guidance – including recommendation of self help-books;
• physical treatments as appropriate;
• brief counselling/therapy – this may be with individuals or couples.

If long-term counselling or psychotherapy is required then patients will need referral to a counsellor or psychotherapist who can undertake this work either within the NHS or privately.

In the following sections sexual problems are considered with specific management options that are additional to the general management outlined above.

Postchildbirth

Many women experience reduced interest in sex in the first six months after childbirth and do not return to previous sexual activity until one year later. Exhaustion and sleep-deprivation play a part, as may the raised prolactin and low oestrogen levels in women who are breastfeeding. Following a vaginal delivery physical changes to the labia minora and introitus may affect the woman's ability to grip the penis and achieve the same sensations during penetration as before. This reduces the indirect stimulation to the clitoral head from the tugging effect on the clitoral hood produced by the thrusting penis, thus the woman's ability to achieve orgasm with penetration may be reduced. Other adverse factors after childbirth can be painful scars or temporary incontinence of urine, flatus or even faeces. Fear of pain or embarrassment may lead to sexual avoidance.

Specific management will include the following:
• the female superior position and the simultaneous manual stimulation of the clitoris may overcome a difficulty with achieving coital orgasm;
• added lubrication and the female superior position may help overcome fear of pain (see dyspareunia);
• pelvic floor muscle tone can be improved with pelvic floor exercises.

Postmenopause

The loss of oestrogen and testosterone has been linked psychologically with loss of sexual interest. Physical factors such as night sweats and atrophic changes to the urogenital tissues can lead to sexual avoidance because of exhaustion or fear of pain. Women may present problems with arousal or orgasm because with ageing it takes longer to become aroused and orgasm becomes less intense. Some women have described either hyper- or hyposensitivity to touch with the menopause that leads to sexual avoidance. Stress incontinence can also present at this time and this also leads to sexual avoidance.

Specific management will include:
• HRT for night sweats, atrophic urogenital changes and touch impairment;
• testosterone implant for loss of interest;
• weighted cones for stress incontinence;
• surgery for persistent stress incontinence.

- Growing up with negative or over-romanticized messages about sex leading to fear of intimacy or loss of control
- Women of small stature who believe that their vagina is too small
- Fear of pain, either primary or secondary after childbirth
- Traumatic past sexual experiences

Organic/iatrogenic factors

Organic disease can lead to sexual problems because of physical and psychological factors (see the box on aetiology above).

Specific management comprises:

- treatment of the specific pathological condition;
- information about the disease and/or treatment effect on the sexual response;
- practical advice to adapt sexual activity to the limitations of the disease process;
- couple therapy can be helpful to open up communication about the sexual relationship that may otherwise be avoided for fear of hurting or being hurt.

Management of specific sexual problems

Desire phase

Lack or loss of desire

The problem may have always existed or may develop after a period of normal sexual interest. It is possible for low desire to exist in isolation, but commonly it is secondary to some other sexual problem so that repeated unsatisfactory experiences lead to a loss of desire. Deep seated personal problems, sexual orientation dilemmas or relationship difficulties often present in this way. Chronic physical illness frequently leads to low desire because of fatigue, loss of self-esteem, altered body image or as a side effect of medication.

Specific management will involve the following.

- Exclude physical factors, or if they exist, recognize their significance to the maintenance of the sexual problem and manage appropriately.
- Self-pleasuring or sensate focus exercises to improve understanding and communication of sexual needs (see p 247).

- Bromocryptine for hypoprolactinaemia.
- Testosterone implants for postmenopausal women (especially if the menopause occurs prematurely through a natural or iatrogenic loss of ovarian function).
- Antidepressants if clinically depressed.

Sexual aversions and phobias

Problems may stem from receiving negative messages about sex so that sex is feared as it leads to feelings of guilt or shame. They can also follow on from some traumatic sexual experience. Sexual aversion may be confused with low desire because both present with reduced frequency of sexual activity. There is a difference between sexual interest being present but the activity avoided rather than no interest and therefore no activity. Sexual aversion and phobias can be total, in which case all sexual activity is avoided, or situational when specific sexual activities trigger the aversion or phobic response, e.g: masturbation, penetration, breast stimulation or oral sex. The sense of impending loss of control with mounting arousal can also trigger a panic response.

Specific management includes the following.

- Individual therapy is usually required to help to discover the predisposing or precipitating factors.
- Abuse resolution therapy when there is a history of past sexual abuse.
- Gradual desensitization to sexual activities that lead to the aversive response.
- Serotonin re-uptake inhibitors can reduce the physical phobic response.

Excessive sexual desire

This sexual problem is also referred to as sexual addiction. Sexual behaviour in this condition is self-destructive and compulsive and like other addictions can lead to loss of family, money, job and even life. Most sexual addicts come from dysfunctional families and were abused as children, sexually, physically or emotionally. Many exhibit other addictions such as alcohol, drugs or gambling. Sexual addicts are powerless to control their compulsion to be sexual despite the negative consequences.

Specific management covers the following.

- Long-term individual therapy.
- Group therapy. Most groups function along similar lines to Alcoholics Anonymous with a 12-step recovery programme.

Arousal phase

Failure of genital response

The physiological arousal response in the female is invisible, unlike the male erection. Most men and women know that vaginal lubrication indicates arousal but have no knowledge of the pelvic congestion and ballooning of the inner two-thirds of the vagina that occurs with high arousal (see Fig. 20.2). Sometimes problems arise because the woman allows her partner to penetrate her too soon because she is too shy to communicate her need for longer foreplay. Arousal problems can present as painful sex, which can trigger avoidance. Lack of lubrication leads to superficial dyspareunia and lack of vaginal ballooning can lead to deep dyspareunia.

Arousal requires:
- that what you see, hear, smell, taste and touch;
- a time and place that will enhance and not sabotage positive sexual feelings;
- positive tactile stimuli to genital and other sensual areas;
- switching off distracting thoughts.

Specific management encompasses:
- self-pleasuring exercises (see p 247);
- sensate focus (see p 248);
- exploring the use of fantasy, erotic material or vibrators;
- HRT if oestrogen deficiency is a factor in failure of lubrication;
- lubricants, e.g. KY jelly, Senselle or Replens.

Orgasmic phase

Orgasmic dysfunction

There is controversy about whether all women are potentially orgasmic or whether some women are unable to reach an orgasm. Studies suggest that 5–10 per cent of women never experience an orgasm. The female orgasm is not essential for fertility, and anorgasmia is linked with late onset menarche and chronic constipation, which suggests possible physiological explanations. Psychologically, anorgasmia is related either to inadequate stimulation or to difficulty in losing control. It is often situational so that orgasm may occur with masturbation but not with a partner. Half of the women who are orgasmic find it easier to orgasm with manual stimulation rather than during coitus.

Specific management is:
- same as for arousal problems;
- nipple stimulation during sexual arousal may help enhance the orgasmic response due to oxytocin release.

Vaginismus

Vaginismus is caused by an involuntary spasm of the pubocoxygeous muscle. The muscle tightens in anticipation of pain and if penetration is forced through the tight muscle then pain is experienced re-enforcing the problem. Women with vaginismus frequently enjoy full non-penetrative sex to orgasm. Specific management involves the following.

- Gradual desensitization using such items as cotton buds, tampon covers, fingers, etc. (plenty of lubrication helps). Alternatively there are specifically designed vaginal trainers in different sizes, e.g. Amielle trainers (Fig. 20.3).
- Desensitization using visualization techniques.
- Transition to penile penetration – best achieved in gradual steps with the woman maintaining control. She is likely to feel most relaxed in the female superior or side-to-side position.
- Serotonin re-uptake inhibitors may be useful to overcome a phobic response if this is blocking progress.

Dyspareunia

Dyspareunia can be either superficial or deep. There can be an organic component and therefore a full medical history, examination and appropriate investigations are necessary. About 70 per cent of women will have no obvious disease process. Emotional pain related to penetrative sex can also be expressed as genuine physical pain.

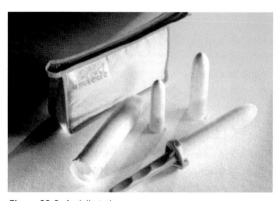

Figure 20.3 Amielle trainers.

Non-organic dyspareunia can be divided into type I (intrapersonal) and type II (interpersonal). In type I the presentation involves guilt, misinformation, previous traumatic experiences or previous physical factors such as episiotomy. Type I responds well to permission giving and systemic desensitization as outlined in the section on vaginismus.

Type II is where relationship problems exist and dyspareunia is an expression of unconscious fear or anger in the relationship providing an excuse to avoid sex. Type II requires therapy.

Specific management is as follows.

- Management is similar to vaginismus.
- Adaptation of sexual positions to minimize pain.
- Adequate lubrication is essential and use of artificial lubricant is beneficial.
- Low-dose amitriptyline may be beneficial.
- Topical steroids may help if dermatological problems exist.
- Topical oestrogens may improve atrophic changes.
- Local anaesthetic gel applied to the painful area.

Specific sex therapy concepts and strategies

The sexual response staircase

The sexual response staircase can be used educationally, diagnostically and therapeutically. Information about the human sexual response is given as an analogy to going up stairs (Fig. 20.4).

- Ground level is non-sexual.
- Step 1 is desire without any physical change.

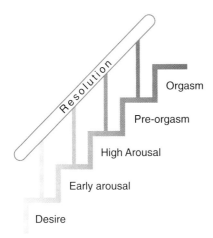

Figure 20.4 The sexual response staircase.

- Step 2 arousal begins. The woman begins to lubricate and for the man the penis begins to get firm, but not firm enough for penetration.
- Step 3 arousal progresses and for the woman there is more lubrication and vaginal ballooning. For the man there is a firm erection that could achieve penetration.
- Step 4 orgasm is recognized as being imminent.
- Step 5 orgasm itself.
- Sliding down the bannisters is the process of resolution and is accompanied by all the thoughts and feelings from that particular sexual encounter. It is possible to choose to climb on to the bannister from any step on the staircase.

It is normal for both men and women to spend time going up and down the steps and not go directly to step 5 in one dash up the stairs. Men and women often progress up the stairs at different rates. Physiologically a man on step 3 can penetrate a woman who can still be on step 1 or even on the ground level. The reverse is impossible. A common problem occurs when the man is ahead of his partner and reaches step 5 to slide down the bannisters leaving her to feel frustrated still on step 1 or 2.

The important concept for both partners to understand is that each is responsible for their own progression up the stairs. The woman is responsible for her orgasm and the man for his. Communication is therefore essential. There is no need to aim for synchronicity. What is important is that each individual feels comfortable with their own progress and if they do not wish to reach orgasm on that occasion this is also acceptable. For sex to be seen as a positive experience the thoughts and feelings that are around when returning down the bannisters need to be those of fulfilment and contentment not anger, resentment or a sense of failure.

Self-discovery and self-pleasuring

Information about the physiology of the sexual response cycle is given. With this knowledge women can embark on learning about their own body and sexual needs through a process of self-discovery and self-pleasuring. They can experiment at home in private through a series of exercises which will give them insights into their sexual likes and dislikes. The information gained can then be communicated to their partner.

Sensate focus
This is an extension of the self-discovery programme into couple work. It is a strategy for overcoming sexual problems by addressing all the possible blocks to arousal. 'Homework' assignments are set for the couple and can be tailor-made to meet specific needs.

Step 1
Sexual intercourse is banned, thus removing performance pressure. The couple set aside two or three one-hour sessions during the week to be together. Difficulty in finding the time may highlight other issues such as privacy or a busy schedule indicating that time for intimacy has a low priority or is being avoided. Setting the scene is important. Attention is paid to ensuring privacy and selecting an environment will enhance the experience. The couple takes turns to touch and be touched in all areas of the body excluding the breasts and genitals. Focusing on the sensation of touch and being touched helps overcome distracting thoughts. Each individual focuses on getting pleasure from the experience for themselves but not at the expense of the partner. In this way each person takes responsibility for their own enjoyment but also cares about the other person's enjoyment. If talking is difficult then feedback can be given by the receiver moving the hands of the giver to achieve the desired effect.

Step 2
Once the couple are comfortable with step 1 they can move on to introduce genital touching. Arousal is still not the goal and it is important for the couple to discuss what they will do should the exercise lead to arousal in one or other of the partners. The ban on sexual penetration is continued so that the couple experiences the pleasure of arousal for its own sake and trust is maintained.

Step 3
The final step is to remove the ban on intercourse and bring back the concept of pleasure leading to arousal. When there has been a problem with penetration a further sequence of gradual steps may be required before full penetrative sex can be achieved.

Key Points

- Treat the whole person and consider psychological causes and consequences of gynaecological and sexual problems
- Good communication skills: Talk openly, be non-judgemental and avoid jargon. Observe non-verbal messages. Listen carefully and avoid assumptions
- Know your professional limitations and resources and for referral

CASE HISTORY

Mrs A V
33-year-old married teacher, presents with superficial dyspareunia leading to loss of interest in sex since the difficult assisted delivery of her first child two years previously. She has been married for four years to a busy lawyer. Sex prior to the pregnancy was satisfactory. Six months after the birth of her son she returned to work as a part-time supply teacher. Her husband's legal practice seems to have got busier and he spends long hours at work. Their relationship is under stress and separation is possible if the sexual problem is not resolved.

Discussion
What is the most likely diagnosis? Is it dyspareunia leading to sexual avoidance, or sexual avoidance leading to dyspareunia? There may have been organic factors such as initial high prolactin and low oestrogen levels if she was breastfeeding, or a painful episiotomy scar. Alternatively it could be psychosocial with her symptoms secondary to fear of a further pregnancy and delivery, coming to terms with her new role as mother or a relationship problem if she is resenting the time her husband spends at work or is suspicious he is having an affair.

Management options
Include brief individual or couple therapy to give information and improve general and sexual communication. Attention should also be paid to exclude organic factors and if found to manage them appropriately.

New developments

Sildenafil Citrate (Viagra) has recently been introduced for the treatment of male impotence. There is much speculation that it may also increase female sexual arousal and libido and research trials are in progress to substantiate this claim. Early results have been encouraging.

References for further reading

Hunter M. *Counselling in obstetrics and gynaecology.* Leicester: The British Psychological Society, 1994.

Reader F. Female sexual problems. In: Studd J. (ed.), *The Year Book of the Royal College of Obstetricians and Gynaecologists 1996.* London: RCOG, 1996.

Skrine R. *Blocks and freedoms in sexual life – a handbook of psychosexual medicine.* Oxford: Radcliffe Medical Press, 1997.

Webster L, Riley A, Mostyn P, Clark A, Griffin M. Mini symposium – Psychosexual disorders. *The Diplomate* 1997; **4**: 264–84.

Wellings K, Field J, Johnson M, Wadsworth J. *Sexual behaviour in Britain – the national survey of sexual attitudes and lifestyles.* London: Penguin, 1994.

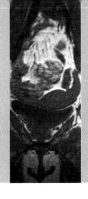
Medico-legal aspects of gynaecology

OVERVIEW

Litigation has become a major feature of medical practice over the last two decades. Not only has the frequency of claims escalated but also the basis for these claims has changed. Complications that were once viewed as acceptable hazards of common surgical procedures are now commonly the source of litigation. In other words, the Bolam Principle that has provided the guidelines for judgements about negligence in the past is no longer being applied. The fact that actions taken by a doctor may be considered to be reasonable by a significant number of medical colleagues is no longer always a defence and in reality a complication is increasingly taken as evidence that there has been substandard practice. It is therefore important, both as a basis for good practice and to avoid litigation, to minimize the risk of complications.

The case records

Case records are medico-legal documents and whilst they are of great importance in the general care of the patient, they also provide the basis for the defence of a case in medico-legal claims. Case records should be kept for a minimum of seven years in gynaecology and 25 years in obstetrics. It is essential to remember that case records may be scrutinized in a Court case line by line, so they should contain nothing that is not accurate, factual and contemporaneous (see box opposite).

All entries in case notes must be dated and signed in a legible fashion. Too often it is impossible to decipher the signature after a case note entry and as

Rules for case records

- The information should be:
  contemporaneous
  accurate
  factual
- All entries signed and dated
- No alterations should be made unless they are signed and dated
- Stored for a minimum of seven years

medical staff in the training grades commonly move on to other jobs, it can be subsequently very difficult to trace the persona in an individual case. The same principle applies to entries that are made into computer records although it may be easier to trace the authors through their access codes.

If it is necessary to alter or modify an entry in the case notes, it is important to countersign and date any modifications so that the alteration is seen to be a deliberate act. Attempts to alter case records are nearly always apparent and arouse suspicion where an attempt is made to simply delete an entry.

Nursing records also provide valuable information on the progress of a patient and the measurement of vital signs: the same rules of entry apply as for the medical entries.

Important reports, such as histopathology reports, should be signed and dated at the time of receipt and when they are placed in the records to demonstrate that the report has been noted and the appropriate action taken.

Consent

The following is the legal definition of consent as laid down by the Medical Defence Union.

'The competent adult patient has a fundamental right to give, or withhold, consent to examination, investigation or treatment. This right is founded on the moral principle of respect for autonomy. An autonomous person has the right to decide what may or may not be done to him (or her). Any treatment or investigation or, indeed, even deliberate touching, carried out without consent may amount to battery. This could result in an action for damages, or even criminal proceedings, and in a finding of serious professional misconduct by the healthcare professional's registration body.'

Consent must be informed or it becomes invalid. In obtaining consent, it is important that the patient understands the nature of any procedure that is to be performed and the attendant risks of that procedure.

In most instances, consent is obtained in writing but consent may be implied by the patient's actions or by oral consent. Material risks must be made clear to the patient and the consent form must be signed before premedication is given. However, there is no longer any certainty about what constitutes a 'material risk'.

The consent form should be signed by the patient and, ideally, by the surgeon who will perform the procedure. It must, however, be emphasized that consent forms are only of value if it is evident that the consent is informed.

CASE HISTORY

A 19-year-old physical education instructor was admitted to hospital with lower abdominal pain. On examination, she was found to have a cystic mass arising from the pelvis. The diagnosis of an ovarian cyst was confirmed by ultrasound and, in view of the pain, the possibility of torsion was considered. The woman had no previous abnormal medical history and no history of any pregnancies.

A decision was made to perform a laparotomy and to remove the ovarian cyst. The Senior Registrar performed the operation in the Emergency Theatre on the day of admission. Consent was obtained for an ovarian cystectomy and if necessary for the removal of the affected ovary.

At laparotomy, although there was only a small quantity of free fluid, it was clearly apparent that the cystic mass was malignant with numerous small serosal and omental deposits. The Senior Registrar rang the Consultant on call from the theatre to ask how he should proceed. The Consultant decided that there was no option but to proceed to total hysterectomy, bilateral oophorectomy, and omentectomy.

Despite surgery and extensive chemotherapy, the patient was dead within three months.

The issue of consent was fully discussed at the time but in view of the fact that the only hope of survival was to perform a pelvic clearance, the action was authorized by the Consultant. The issues were fully discussed subsequently with the patient and with her parents and they agreed that the appropriate action had been taken.

This case exemplifies the difficulties that arise from issues of consent. It could be argued that the surgeon exceeded the authority of the consent form. No one under these circumstances would have obtained a consent form for such an extensive procedure because the possibility of malignant disease in a woman of this age was extremely remote.

Under these circumstances, the decision to proceed was based on the premise that the operation was necessary for the preservation of the patient's life.

Patients should be informed of material risks that may result from the procedure. However, in the British and Irish courts, it is generally agreed that a medical practitioner is not negligent if they follow a practice generally approved by their peers of similar specializations and skills.

Consent forms should not be altered after they have been signed and the doctor should not exceed the authority given. However, there are always exceptions where the surgeon, on the grounds of common humanity, has an obligation to act in the patient's interests without complete consent.

Consent for minors

The legal age for consent for medical and surgical treatment is 16 years or over. Under the age of 16 years, the situation is more complex. When an under-age child consents to treatment, the doctor may proceed with that treatment. If the child refuses treatment, that refusal can be over-ridden by someone with parental authority.

The situation is particularly complicated in issues of contraception.

Having sexual intercourse under the age of 16 years is unlawful and therefore providing contraceptive advice to a minor could be regarded as aiding and abetting a crime. This matter was tested in the courts in the case of Gillick versus West Norfolk and Wisbech Area Health Authority in 1985 where Mrs Gillick took action against a doctor for providing contraceptive advice to her under-age daughter. The matter was finally reviewed by the Law Lords and the summary of their judgement is shown in Table 21.1.

In general terms, in all cases of consent in minors, it is sensible to obtain the consent of the parents as well as that of the child.

Limitation

Under normal circumstances, the Limitation Act 1980 states that action must be taken within three years from:
(a) the date on which the cause of action accrued; or
(b) the date of knowledge (if later) of the person injured.

However, there are exceptions to this rule, particularly in obstetric claims. The extension to the Limitation period may be made to the following provision: 'if on the date when any right of action accrued for which a period of limitation is prescribed by the Limitation Act, the person was under a disability, the action may be brought at any time before the expiration of six years from the date when the disability ceased or death occurred'.

Surgery and foreign bodies

In all surgical procedures, it is essential to ensure that all swabs and instruments are accounted for at the completion of the operation. This is done firstly, by knowing at the commencement of a procedure the number and disposition of all the instruments, packs and swabs, and secondly, by checking at the completion of the procedure with the Theatre Sister that the count is complete before wound closure is achieved.

If any instrument, pack or swab is missing, it is essential to search manually and if it cannot be located, an X-ray should be performed to locate the missing object. Failure to take these precautions may result in an instrument being lost in the abdominal cavity with the consequent complications of a retained foreign body and all such complications are inevitably indefensible.

Table 21.1 – Summary of the Gillick judgement

1. The doctor may give contraceptive advice to a minor without parental consent provided she understands the advice
2. The doctor may do so even if he cannot persuade her to tell her parents that she is seeking contraceptive advice
3. The advice may be provided if she is likely to begin or continue to have sexual intercourse with or without contraceptive treatment
4. That without contraceptive advice her physical and mental health are likely to suffer
5. Her best interests require him to give her the advice, with or without parental consent

COMMON CAUSES OF LITIGATION IN GYNAECOLOGY

Failed sterilization

The purpose of sterilization in either the male or the female is to render the individual permanently infertile and incapable of bearing further, or any, children. There is a failure rate for nearly all sterilization procedures and litigation commonly arises from the failure of the procedure and the conception of an unwanted pregnancy and the failure to inform the patient of the risk of failure.

It is now standard practice to inform the patient of the risk of failure and to include reference to this risk in the case notes and in the consent form. In the past, it has been a common event for legal action to be taken in a case of failed sterilization. The basis of these claims is that had the patient known that there was a risk of failure they would not have had the procedure or they would have continued to take contraceptive precautions.

Sterilization of the female is generally performed by occluding or removing the fallopian tubes. This is achieved by ligation, diathermy or clipping. In the UK, the most commonly used procedure is the application of Filshie clips, which are made of titanium lined by silastic rubber. The advantages of this method of female sterilization lie in its safety and simplicity and the fact that there is a high success rate when the procedure is reversed.

Whilst it is advisable to warn the patient that the operation should be considered as permanent, it is incorrect to say that it is irreversible although no guarantees can be given about the success of reversal in any one procedure.

Failure of sterilization with subsequent conception carries a significant risk that the pregnancy will be ectopic. One of the advantages of warning the patient that there is a risk of pregnancy is that early notification of a possible pregnancy can be achieved with the offer of termination at an early stage if this is the wish of the woman.

Failure of the procedure arises from two sources. The failure may occur because of incomplete occlusion of the tubal lumen. This may occur because the wrong structure is ligated or because occlusion of the tube is incomplete at the time of the initial procedure. Secondly, the tube may be successfully occluded at the time of the original procedure but subsequently the tube recanalizes and the tubal lumen becomes patent.

In general terms, failure within six months is related to method failure but after six months, failure is more commonly associated with recanalization. If the tubes are not completely occluded at the original procedure, then although the clips may appear to be correctly applied across the tubes, occlusion of the tubal lumen may not be complete. In the case of the Filshie clip, the manufacturers recommend that the applicators should be regularly serviced to ensure that the clips are completely closed.

Recanalization is a recognized risk of the procedure and can only be avoided by removal of the tubes and ovaries but that is a difficult procedure to justify as the risk of recanalization is small and the side effects of bilateral oophorectomy may be profound.

The application of clips to the wrong structure is impossible to defend in court whereas recanalization can be successfully defended.

Induced abortion

Induced or therapeutic abortion is regulated by statute in the UK and in most countries where therapeutic abortion is permissible.

The fundamental regulations controlling abortion under the Abortion Act 1967 and as amended in 1990 are shown below.

1. That gestation is not in excess of 24 weeks and that continuation of the pregnancy involves greater risk to the physical and mental health of the woman or her family, than termination.
2. Termination is necessary to prevent grave permanent injury to the physical or mental health of the woman.
3. That there is substantial risk that if the child were born, it would suffer such physical or mental abnormalities as to be seriously handicapped.

The decision should be made by two registered medical practitioners acting in good faith, i.e. they have considered, independently, the effects that continuation of the pregnancy would have on the woman and formed a judgement that termination is in her best interests.

The Law as it operates in England and Wales specifies that the abortion must be performed in an NHS hospital or a place approved for this purpose by the Secretary of State for Health and that the appropriate Certification and Notification is completed and returned to the Chief Medical Officer.

It must be remembered that the original Abortion Act 1967 includes a clause that states that 'no person shall be under any duty to participate in any treatment authorized by the Act to which he has conscientious objection.'

Complications of abortion

Abortion may be induced by medical or surgical means. The commonest complications that lead to litigation are those resulting from surgical procedures. The complications are shown in the box below.

With the exception of the continuing pregnancy, all of these complications may occur in the management of spontaneous abortion and all may lead to medico-legal claims. However, the three complications that most commonly lead to litigation are perforation, failed termination and retained products of conception.

Perforation
The uterus is particularly vulnerable to perforation at the time when the uterine wall is soft. Perforation may arise from the cervical dilator, from the suction curette or from the use of forceps during the removal of products of conception.

Perforation usually occurs through the uterine fundus and is recognized by the instrument visibly penetrating too far into the uterine cavity or by fatty tissue from the mesentery or omentum seen in the forceps when the instrument is withdrawn.

Complications of abortion

- Haemorrhage
- Infection
- Perforation of the uterus
- Continuing pregnancy
- Retained products of conception
- Cervical damage

Perforation is a particular risk when the uterus is retroverted and, on occasions, it may result in injury to the bowel.

Having ascertained that the uterus is empty, if there is clear evidence that perforation has occurred, laparoscopy should be performed and the perforation site identified.

It is also important to look for bowel damage. If the bowel is intact, the perforation should be cauterized and haemostasis secured.

If it is not possible to close the perforation site or there is a suspicion that the bowel has been perforated, then a laparotomy should be performed. Inexperienced medical staff should not undertake any of these procedures unless they are properly supervised.

Failed termination
Continuation of a pregnancy after attempted termination has been shown to occur in up to 2.6 per cent of evacuations before 6 weeks' gestation. The likelihood of failure diminishes to 0.38 per cent by 9 weeks' gestation. Thus, the pregnancy may be missed because it is small or because the implantation is cornual or because the uterus may be bicornuate.

If this complication is not to be missed it is advisable, in the author's view, to follow up all women who have had a termination of pregnancy with a six-week pelvic examination. If this is not done, there is always a possibility that the pregnancy may be too advanced for termination by the time the woman returns. Despite the fact that it is common practice to offer a repeat termination, women often decline this offer and then take legal action for the failure of the initial procedure on the basis of the need for financial support to raise the child.

Retained products of conception
This is a common complication of either induced or spontaneous abortion and in many cases, cannot be avoided. Occasionally following termination, a significant quantity of fetal material may be retained and this may cause distress when the products are passed at a later date. Provided that the appropriate steps are taken to remove the placental or fetal material, to correct the blood loss and where necessary, to give antibiotics for any infection, claims made concerning retained products of conception should be defensible.

However, procedures to remove retained products should be undertaken by experienced staff, or,

Mrs X was admitted to hospital with a history that she had been bleeding continuously since her discharge from hospital after the delivery of her second child seven weeks earlier. She was seen by Dr Y who arranged for an ultrasound scan of the pelvis: this showed the presence of retained products of conception. Dr Y who was an experienced Senior House Officer took the patient to theatre on the evening of admission for uterine evacuation.

During the procedure, he thought he had perforated the uterine fundus. The uterus was bulky and soft and the ovum forceps penetrated well beyond the measured length of the cavity, and furthermore, there was some fatty material in the forceps that did not look like placental tissue.

He called for the Duty Registrar and she decided to perform a laparoscopy. At this procedure, she could see the perforation in the anterior wall of the uterus but could not be certain about the condition of the bowel. She therefore performed a laparotomy and found that there was a small tear in the mesentery of the pelvic colon, but no damage to the wall of the bowel. The uterine perforation and the mesenteric tear were oversewn and the abdomen was closed. The patient made an uneventful recovery and was discharged home five days later. The woman subsequently lodged a claim for pain and suffering and for the anxiety induced by the knowledge that she was now more prone to uterine rupture in any subsequent pregnancy. In fact, she had a further four pregnancies, two of which went on to full term normal deliveries and two were terminated.

The judge found in the Plaintiff's favour on the basis that the uterus was probably retroverted and that this should have been recognized by the surgeon and the risk of perforation minimized. The woman was paid a modest settlement, which was the same as the sum paid into Court before the commencement of the five-day hearing.

if inexperienced, staff who are supervised by senior staff. This particularly applies where an initial procedure has failed to remove all the placental tissue and this has resulted in continuous bleeding. A further curettage under these circumstances should always be performed by an experienced gynaecologist.

Ectopic pregnancy

The diagnosis of a tubal pregnancy is often missed at the first contact because the symptoms and signs may be confusing and atypical. As a result, the woman is sent away with a diagnosis of threatened or incomplete abortion and she presents later with a sudden collapse and acute abdominal pain. Legal action is often subsequently taken by the patient on the grounds that the diagnosis should have been made at the earlier visit and that the failure to make the diagnosis has resulted in additional pain and suffering and has potentially reduced the subsequent fertility of the woman.

Whilst it is often difficult to establish the diagnosis at an early stage, in many cases the diagnosis of ectopic pregnancy is overlooked. Under these circumstances, it may be difficult to defend the doctor's actions. It is therefore essential that the diagnosis of tubal pregnancy should be automatically considered in any woman presenting with a short period of amenorrhoea followed by vaginal bleeding and abdominal pain. The diagnosis should be assumed until proven otherwise by using a sensitive pregnancy test, pelvic ultrasound and, where necessary, by diagnostic laparoscopy.

Assisted reproduction

The regulation of procedures involved in assisted reproduction is provided by the Code of Practice of the Human Fertilization and Embryology Authority in the UK under the rules of the Human Fertilisation and Embryology Act. Breach of this Code of Practice and the Terms of the Act may lead to criminal prosecution.

Litigation is relatively uncommon and often arises from financial disagreements as much of this work is done in the private sector. However, whilst there are many potential hazards, the common complications are those of high multiple gestations and ovarian hyperstimulation. However, provided adequate counselling is given, these complications rarely lead to litigation.

Contraception

Despite the widespread nature of contraceptive practice, only 10 per cent of gynaecological claims are associated with problems that arise from contraceptive problems. Most of the problems arise from the use and insertion of intrauterine contraceptive devices, particularly where perforation occurs and the device is not in the uterine cavity. Oral contraception may lead to a variety of complications which, if they occur in a woman where there is a specific contraindication to the use of the pill, will often lead to litigation.

If the guidelines for all forms of contraception are carefully observed and the patient is kept fully informed it should be possible to both avoid and successfully defend complications arising from any particular form of contraceptive practice.

Surgical complications

Complications of surgical procedures are a common source of litigation. It is therefore important to recognize the areas of potential risk. A summary of the common complications leading to litigation are shown in Table 21.2.

Laparoscopic procedures

With the safeguards now built in to modern insufflators, it is uncommon to experience massive gas embolism and if the correct line of insertion is followed and the gas pressure does not exceed 15mmHg at a flow rate of 1 L per minute, then insufflation should be uneventful. The only common problem occurs when insufflation is extraperitoneal so that subsequently, the risk of damage to viscera is exaggerated at the time of insertion of the trochar as there is no pneumoperitoneum.

The most common complication is to the bowel, particularly where there are already adhesions, and that damage may be caused by the Veress needle or by the trochar.

Provided the damage is recognized at the time and steps are taken to close the perforation or to institute expectant management where the puncture site is small and inflicted by the needle, such injuries

Table 21.2 – Common surgical complications leading to litigation

Laparoscopic procedures
Insufflation	gas embolism
	penetrating injuries from the Veress needle
Trochar injuries	perforation of the bowel
	perforation of blood vessels
Diathermy	damage to bowel and bladder

Hysteroscopic procedures
Haemorrhage
Uterine perforation
Bowel or bladder damage (diathermy injuries)

Abdominal and vaginal procedures
Damage to bowel
Damage to bladder
Damage to ureters
Damage to major blood vessels

should be viewed as the inevitable consequence of a blind procedure such as laporoscopy.

The difficulty with diathermy injuries to the bowel is that leakage tends to occur some days after the procedure leading to faecal peritonitis. These difficulties have largely been minimized by the use of bipolar diathermy. Litigation usually arises out of delays in recognizing the injuries. Pain that persists or worsens over the first few days after a laparoscopic procedure should be viewed with great suspicion and particular notice taken of the vital signs.

Hysteroscopic procedures

Despite the fact that hysteroscopy as a diagnostic procedure is now very common, it is rarely a source of litigation as injuries tend to be limited to perforation of the uterus and fluid overload, particularly where the infusion fluid contains glycine and the procedure is prolonged. Fluid overload may result in abnormal volume expansion and hyponatraemia with intravascular haemolysis and hepatorenal failure. It is essential to keep a continuous record of the amount of fluid infused and the amount returned.

Transcervical endometrial resection

This procedure involves the diathermy excision of the endometrium. If the cut is too deep, then perforation of the uterine wall can occur with possible diathermy injury to the bowel. This risk can be reduced by the use of the rollerball or by laser diathermy. If the uterus is displaced laterally, the perforation at the uterotubal junction may lead to damage of the major vessels or the ureter.

Most serious injuries occur with inexperienced operators and as with all procedures, and particularly with endoscopic surgery, it is essential that the surgeon has been properly trained.

Abdominal and vaginal procedures

The most commonly performed major gynaecological operation is hysterectomy and this may be achieved through the abdominal or vaginal route.

The uterus lies between the bladder and the pouch of Douglas and the rectum. Both ureters are adjacent to the uterine cervix and are particularly prone to injury at this site or at the pelvic brim where the ureters enter the true pelvis. Pelvic masses wedged in the pouch of Douglas and adherent to the rectum and pelvic colon may cause problems with bowel damage and ureteric injury.

Injuries to the urinary tract

These injuries may be directly to the bladder or to one or both ureters.

Bladder injuries

The bladder may be opened when the abdominal incision is made or, commonly as the bladder is separated from the cervix, particularly following a previous Caesarean Section.

If the injury is recognized at the time, it is a simple matter to close the hole and drain the bladder and it usually gives rise to no further problems. However, if the injury is not recognized, it may give rise to leakage of urine into the peritoneal cavity or into the retropubic space. More commonly, with vaginal surgery, a suture is placed through the bladder wall during the closure of the vaginal vault and this may result in the development of a vesicovaginal fistula. Unless there are particular reasons for the difficulties experienced during surgery, such patients are commonly compensated out of court.

CASE HISTORY

Miss B presented to a gynaecological clinic with a history of severe dysmenorrhoea and a sensation of pressure in her pelvis. She was 25 years old and had not had any pregnancies. On pelvic examination, there was a fixed ovarian mass in the pelvis approximately 8 cm in diameter. The following week, she was admitted to hospital for ovarian cystectomy. The operation was performed on a Friday afternoon by an experienced gynaecological surgeon. At operation, the ovarian cyst was found to be densely adherent in the pouch of Douglas. During attempts to remove the cyst it ruptured, releasing thick, brown fluid typical of an endometrioma. It was difficult to remove the capsule which was adherent to the rectum deep in the pelvic cavity. Removal was eventually achieved with considerable venous bleeding which was controlled by packing. The surgeon was on leave after completing his operating list so the patient was left in the care of the resident medical staff.

The following day, the patient complained of persistent abdominal pain and the abdomen became distended. The staff suspected that there might be bowel damage and she was taken back to theatre within 24 hours of the original procedure and a tear was identified in the rectum deep in the pouch of Douglas. There was intraperitoneal leakage of faecal material. A defunctioning colostomy was performed and the tear was closed.

Despite the prompt action taken by the resident staff in detecting and correcting the injury, she developed a pelvic abscess and subsequently a deep vein thrombosis and a sympathetic arterial thrombosis. Thrombectomy was performed but the femoral artery thrombosed again leading to the necessity for a mid-thigh amputation of her left leg.

Despite the appalling sequelae of her surgery, it was not felt that the staff had been negligent. However, it was considered highly unlikely that any judge would fail to award her compensation and on this basis, an out of court settlement was made.

Ureteric injuries

Ureters may be cut, crushed, partially sutured or completely ligated on one or both sides. This may result in the loss of kidney function on one side or the development of a hydronephrosis if occlusion is not complete. It may also result in an ureterovaginal fistula. Injury to one ureter can sometimes be defended in court, particularly where difficulties, such as in malignant cervical disease, may lead to difficult surgery. However, increasingly, these cases are settled out of court, as there is a significant risk that they will be lost if they do go to court.

Ligation or damage to both ureters is generally indefensible.

Pelvic malignant disease

Most claims arising in relation to malignant disease arise from either wrongful diagnosis or delay in diagnosis.

Cervical cytology

In recent years, there have been a number of cases where wrong reports have been issued on cervical smears leading to over- or underdiagnosis of the staging of cervical smears. Errors also arise because of the failure to take action on an abnormal smear test or by the incorrect filing or labelling of an abnormal smear test.

In the NHS, guidelines have been laid down for the responsibilities of the originator of the smear and the laboratory and these are outlined in Table 21.3.

The efficacy of any screening programme depends on the fact that the smear is taken properly and that it is interpreted correctly. Failures at any given point in this sequence may result in litigation. It is uncommon for legal action to be taken over the failure to cure an individual of malignant disease outside of the delay in making the diagnosis. Such cases stand or fall on the judgement of the gynaecologist's peers as to the adequacy of the management and the knowledge of what is 'best treatment' at any given point in time.

Risk management

With the rapid escalation in litigation against gynaecologists, the profession has to some degree been protected in the UK by the introduction of Crown

Table 21.3 – Responsibilities in cervical screening

The originator
Check that all smear reports are received
Reports should be initialled before filing
Inform the woman of the result
Undertake further investigations
Keep the GP informed

The cytology laboratory
Send the report to the originator and/or GP
Maintain a register of women whose smears require
  further investigation
Add histology reports to the register
Add repeat smears to the register
Contact the originator if repeat smears are not
  received
Inform the local cervical screening programme
  manager of women for whom all attempts at
  follow-up have failed

Indemnity. However, 'Insurers' in one form or another now tend to insist that risk management procedures become an integral part of day-to-day practice. In any case, risk management constitutes good practice for by definition, 'risk management is the process of reducing or eliminating losses due to accident or misadventure'. Each Directorate should be responsible for providing a risk management group (RMG) and a suggested composition of this group is shown in Table 21.4.

To work effectively, a full-time coordinator should be appointed. They may be from the nursing/midwifery or medical staff. The role of this person is to ensure that all incidents that may have medico-legal implications are reported to the group and to take statements from all the staff involved in the management of the particular incident.

Table 21.4 – Risk management group

Lawyer (with experience in medical litigation)
Clinical director
Senior resident
Hospital claims manager
Senior nursing/midwifery officer
Coordinator

These reports can not be considered privileged but should be a truthful description of the events leading to the particular complication or to a near miss. Staff should never be asked to appear before the committee unless they wish to attend. There should be a list available to all staff of the complications that need to be notified.

The reports are considered by the RMG and a decision made as to whether the incident is likely to lead to litigation or whether the complication is acceptable and unavoidable.

Information is fed back to the Clinical Directorate via the Clinical Director and management policies are changed where this is appropriate.

Staff are encouraged to keep their patients fully informed about the nature of their problems, their causes and likely outcome.

The establishment of a system that allows for monitoring of clinical standards and the development of appropriate protocols is important. Furthermore, a good record of events often enables a good defence to be mounted in a case where it is considered that the standard of care has been acceptable even where there is an adverse outcome.

Most Directorates are both obstetrical and gynaecological and under these circumstances, the group where possible should include a neonatologist, an obstetric anaesthetist and a fetomaternal specialist.

Key Points

- Litigation in gynaecology is common and increasing in frequency
- The keeping of detailed clinical case records is an essential part of modern gynaecological practice
- Due attention must be paid to all issues of consent
- Many procedures in gynaecology are regulated by legal statutes and by the Criminal Law such as the Abortion Act and the Human Fertilization and Embryology Act
- Complications that often lead to litigation are failed sterilizations, complications of abortions, operative injuries from laparoscopic procedures and damage to bowel and bladder during vaginal and abdominal surgery
- Risk management is essential for the maintenance of high standards of practice

References for further reading

Clements RV. *Safe Practice in Obstetrics and Gynaecology.* Churchill Livingstone, 1994.

Consent to Treatment. The Medical Defence Union Ltd. 1997.

James, C. Family Planning. *Journal of the Medical Defence Union* 1991; **7**: 96.

Senior OE, Symonds EM. Risk Management. A 'do-it-yourself' package. *Clinical Risk.* 1996; **2**: 107–13.

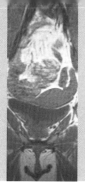

Appendix

Common gynaecological procedures

Hysteroscopy

Hysteroscopy involves passing a small diameter tele-scope, either flexible or rigid, through the cervix to directly inspect the uterine cavity. Excellent images can be obtained. A flexible hysteroscope is used as an out-patient procedure and uses carbon dioxide as a filling medium. Rigid instruments use fluids and therefore can be used even if there is bleeding present.

Indications
Any abnormal bleeding from the uterus can be inves-tigated by hysteroscopy including:

- postmenopausal bleeding;
- irregular menstruation, intermenstrual bleeding and postcoital bleeding;
- persistent menorrhagia;
- persistent discharge;
- suspected uterine malformations;
- suspected Asherman's syndrome.

Complications
- Perforation of the uterus.
- Cervical damage – if cervical dilatation is neces-sary.
- If there is infection present hysteroscopy can cause ascent.

An operating hysteroscope can also be used to resect endometrial pathology such as fibroids and polyps.

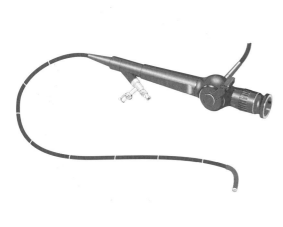

Figure 1 Flexible fibreoptic hysteroscope

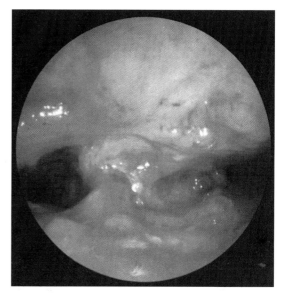

Figure 2 Hysteroscopic view of endometrial cavity

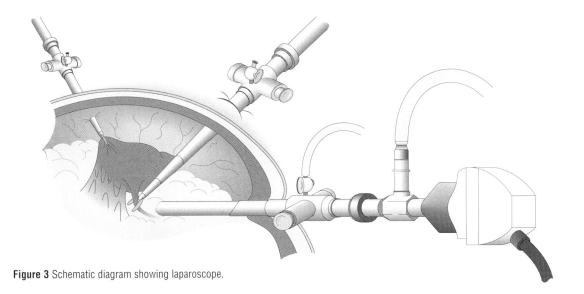

Figure 3 Schematic diagram showing laparoscope.

Laparoscopy

Laparoscopy allows visualization of the peritoneal cavity. This involves insertion of a needle called a veress needle into a suitable puncture point in the umbilicus. This allows insufflation of the peritoneal cavity with carbon dioxide so that a larger instrument can be inserted. The majority of instruments used for diagnostic laparoscopy are 5 mm in diameter and 10 mm instruments are used for operative laparoscopy. More recently there is a 2 mm laparoscope available.

Indications
- Suspected ectopic pregnancy.
- Undiagnosed pelvic pain.
- Tubal patency testing.
- Sterilization.

Operative laparoscopy can be used to perform ovarian cystectomy or oophorectomy and treat endometriosis with cautery or laser. Reversal of sterilization is also possible using laparoscopy.

Complications
Complications are uncommon but include damage to any of the intra-abdominal structures including bowel and major blood vessels. The bladder is always emptied prior to the procedure to avoid bladder injury. Incisional hernia has been reported.

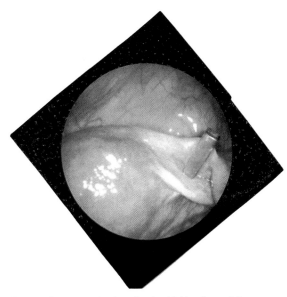

Figure 5 Laparoscopic view showing Fishie clip on right fallopian tube.

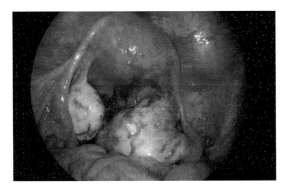

Figure 4 Laparoscopic view of bilateral endometriomas.

Abdominal and vaginal hysterectomy

Vaginal hysterectomy is associated with a much quicker recovery than abdominal hysterectomy and therefore is preferred for that reason. However, vaginal hysterectomy is not indicated when there is malignancy as the ovaries often need to be removed and lymph nodes examined and sampled. If the uterus is larger than that of a 12-week pregnancy and has outgrown the pelvis then usually again an abdominal hysterectomy is preferred and is thought to be safer. The main reason a vaginal hysterectomy is associated with faster recovery is the lack of abdominal incision.

Most abdominal hysterectomies are performed through a Pfannenstiel incision, which is a low (bikini line) suprapubic transverse incision. Patients recover more quickly from this incision than from than a midline incision and the cosmetic result is more acceptable. For larger masses and malignancies a midline incision is utilized.

Although a complete description of abdominal hysterectomy is outside the scope of this chapter, the procedure involves taking three pedicles:
- the infundibulo-pelvic ligament which contains the ovarian vessels;
- the uterine artery;
- the angles of the vault of the vagina which contain vessels ascending from the vagina. The ligaments to support the uterus can be taken with this pedicle or separately.

In the vaginal hysterectomy the same steps are taken but in the reverse order.

Indications for abdominal hysterectomy
- Uterine, ovarian, cervical and fallopian tube carcinoma.

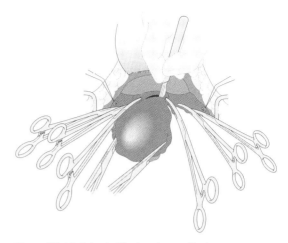

Figure 6 Total abdominal hysterectomy with clamps on

- Pelvic pain from chronic endometriosis or chronic pelvic inflammatory disease where the pelvis is frozen and vaginal hysterectomy is impossible.
- Symptomatic fibroid uterus greater than 12-week size.

Indications for vaginal hysterectomy
- Menstrual disorders with a uterus less than 12 weeks in size.
- Microinvasive cervical carcinoma.
- Uterovaginal prolapse.

Complications
Specific complications of hysterectomy include:
- haemorrhage;
- ureteric injury;
- bladder and bowel injury.

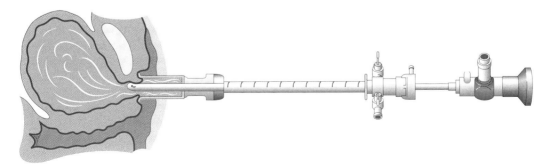

Figure 7 Schematic representation of cystoscopy

Cystoscopy

Cystoscopy involves passing a small diameter telescope, either flexible or rigid, through the urethra into the bladder. Excellent images of both these structures can be obtained.

Indications
- haematuria
- recurrent urinary tract infection
- sterile pyuria
- short history of irritative symptoms
- suspected bladder abnormality (e.g. diverticulum, stones, fistula)
- assessment of bladder neck

Complications
- urinary tract infection
- rarely bladder perforation

A cystoscope with an operative channel can be used to biopsy any abnormality, perform bladder neck injection, retrieve stones and resect bladder tumours.

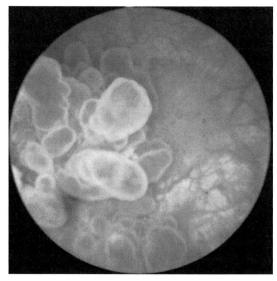

Figure 8 Cystoscopic view of bladder papilloma

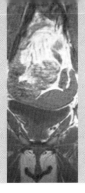

Index